Management of Diabetic Complications

Georgi Abraham • Jothydev Kesavadev
Priyanka Govindan • Nanditha Arun
Suneeta Teckchandani
Editors

Management of Diabetic Complications

Calling for a Team Approach

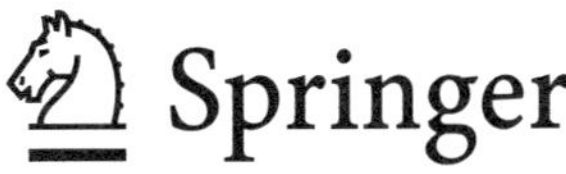

Editors
Georgi Abraham
Department of Nephrology
MGM healthcare
Chennai, Tamil Nadu, India

Priyanka Govindan
Department of Nephrology
The nephrology clinic
Fort Collins, CO, USA

Suneeta Teckchandani
Department of Acute Medicine
Chesterfield Royal Hospital
Calow, Derbyshire, UK

Jothydev Kesavadev
Jothydev's Diabetes Research Centre
Trivandrum, Kerala, India

Nanditha Arun
Dr. A. Ramachandran's Diabetes Hospitals
& India Diabetes Research Foundation
Chennai, Tamil Nadu, India

ISBN 978-981-97-6408-2 ISBN 978-981-97-6406-8 (eBook)
https://doi.org/10.1007/978-981-97-6406-8

This Springer imprint is published by the registered company Springer Nature Singapore Pte Ltd.
The registered company address is: 152 Beach Road, #21-01/04 Gateway East, Singapore 189721, Singapore

Foreword

It is my great privilege and pleasure to write this foreword to this unique book on diabetic complications. It has been rightly said that "diabetes is a sweet disease but with sour complications". Complications of DM are the most important and challenging issues, accounting for the majority of morbidity and mortality in T2DM. This book is a good combination of basic and clinical science on the topic. This book focuses on epidemiology, early diagnosis and monitoring and addresses various challenges related to diabetic complications, including screening, monitoring, management and prevention.

For every chapter discussed, there is a brief overview of the clinical perspective on managing diabetes, including specific complications and relevant comorbidities. This book mainly focuses on arguably the most devastating complication of diabetes, that is, long-term vascular complications. The cardiovascular complications include heart failure and coronary artery disease, which account for about 75% of all vascular complications. These have been extensively covered. Similarly, the kidney complications in diabetes which are on the rise have been covered very well with chapters on acute kidney injury, conservative management of chronic kidney disease, and the renal replacement therapy in diabetic kidney disease. This book provides contemporary information about each important complication in diabetes.

The screening, morbidity and mortality and their early detection have been very well emphasised. The stress of current guidelines to "catch them young and catch them early" has been well projected.

Therefore, this book assumes paramount importance and should be in the hands of undergraduate and post-graduate students, teachers, clinicians and researchers in this field.

All the important chapters have been very well covered.

Many unique areas, less discussed but of great importance like management of obese diabetic, musculoskeletal system in DM, oral complications, and hearing loss in T2DM are this book's exclusive feature.

I must say that this book appears to be an integral resource on diabetic complications, providing practical clinical guidelines. All important and commonly encountered problems, whether it is hypoglycaemia or sexual dysfunction, diabetic ketoacidosis or infections, psychiatry disorders or diabetic foot disease, have been given prominence.

The chapters on technologies for preventing diabetes and its complication are a special new theme. Neurological and Psychiatric manifestations are well covered, as is imaging in T2DM.

The language used in the book is very simple and appealing, with the inclusion of flow charts and figures that are visually appealing.

This book is also a ready reckoner of all that we need for practical, clinical management. These are rich sources of information on diabetic complications, usable by all who care for such patients.

The ravages of diabetic complications are relentless, but the advances in monitoring and managing them are also equally relentless.

All the contributors are eminent experts in their respective field, and their chapters have been highly informative, advanced and clinically enriching.

I would like to extend my congratulations to all the editors on this outstanding endeavour, and I am confident that this book will be an exceptional addition to the world's literature on diabetes and its complications.

Department of Medicine and Endocrinology
MGMCRI, Dean Academic, SBV
Puducherry, India

Ashok Kumar Das

Preface

As the global prevalence of diabetes mellitus continues to rise, we face significant challenges in managing the associated complications, largely due to non-adherence to therapy. Uncertainties encountered in patients with T1DM and T2DM pose a real threat, standing as a significant barrier to achieving euglycaemia.

Knowledge of the complications and ways to prevent them is often overlooked. As microvascular and macrovascular involvement is a hallmark of diabetes mellitus, organ systems should be a regularly evaluated during each visit to the treating facility. Many patients with diabetes mellitus present with complex, multi-organ complications that can range from mild to life-threatening, necessitating prompt attention and effective management. Confronting and solving these challenges requires paradigms and state-of-the-art facilities to reduce morbidity and mortality. Visits and consultation at primary and secondary care facilities for early detection of complications can either slow down or arrest the progression.

This book "Complications of Diabetes Mellitus Multidisciplinary Approach" is a comprehensive compilation of the pathophysiology, clinical manifestations, investigation and timely intervention. The contributors are renowned specialist in their fields of specialisation. The chapters have been selected after detailed discussion and are written in a clear and lucid manner. The book is targeted towards medical students, interns, post-graduates, physicians, nurses and other specialists.

The editors extend their gratitude to the thousands of patients with diabetes mellitus who have contributed to our learning and improvement in diabetic care. The publication of this book would not have been possible without the dedicated support of our spouses Rene, Sunitha, Arjun, Arun and Rishi.

Chennai, Tamil Nadu, India — Georgi Abraham
Trivandrum, Kerala, India — Jothydev Kesavadev
Fort Collins, CO, USA — Priyanka Govindan
Chennai, Tamil Nadu, India — Nanditha Arun
Calow, Derbyshire, UK — Suneeta Teckchandani

Contents

A Clinical Perspective on the Economic Burden of Diabetes Mellitus in India Book: Diabetic Complications—A Multidisciplinary Approach

1

Tarun K. George and Saiprasath Janarthanan

1.1 Introduction

Diabetes Mellitus is a chronic metabolic disorder characterised by an imbalance in insulin secretion, insulin action, or both. This leads to hyperglycaemia, or elevated blood sugar levels, which can cause insidious and gradual damage to organs.

The American Diabetic Association has an etiological classification shown in (Table 1.1). This has cost implications in the diagnostic tests to confirm subtypes of the disease and the medications used. The costs are higher in varieties where insulin is an absolute requirement [1].

It is an insidious disease that may present with a sudden complication or identified by screening. It can cause macrovascular complications involving the heart, brain, and peripheral vessels, and microvascular affectations of retinopathy, nephropathy, and neuropathy. These have significant economic implications as diabetes, which is identified early and controlled, has fewer complications, lower costs, and better quality of life.

T. K. George (✉)
Christian Medical College, Vellore, Tamil Nadu, India

S. Janarthanan
Mahatma Gandhi Institute of Medical Sciences, Wardha, Maharashtra, India

G. Abraham et al. (eds.), *Management of Diabetic Complications*, https://doi.org/10.1007/978-981-97-6406-8_1

Table 1.1 Etiologic classification of diabetes mellitus

1. Type 1 diabetes	A. Immune-mediated
	B. Idiopathic
2. Type 2 diabetes	
3. Other specific types of diabetes	A. Genetic defects of beta cell function
	B. Genetic defects in insulin action
	C. Diseases of the exocrine pancreas
	D. Endocrinopathies
	E. Drug- or chemical-induced
	F. Infections
	G. Uncommon forms of immune-mediated diabetes
	H. Other genetic syndromes associated with diabetes
4. Gestational diabetes mellitus	

1.2 Epidemiological Burden

The international diabetes federation estimated in 2021 that more than 53 crore people have diabetes worldwide and that by 2045, this number will rise to at least 78 crores (10.5% in 2021 to 12.2%) [2, 3]. Type 2 diabetes contributes about 90% to 95% of cases, and the remaining is contributed by type 1 diabetes. It is estimated that almost 80% of diabetes cases come from middle-income countries, and that many of these patients may not be able to afford diabetic medications. According to WHO, between 2000 and 2015, there was a 3% increase in premature mortality from diabetes [4, 5].

The highest growth is expected in middle-income countries, where the prevalence may rise 10.8% to 13.1% [6]. This is also reflected in past changes, as seen in Fig. 1.1. The age-standardised prevalence of diabetes by each country rises with age and is noted to be higher in men [7].

India's disease patterns have switched due to an epidemiological transition; thus, mortality from communicable, maternal, neonatal, and nutritional diseases (CMNNDs) has decreased significantly, while NCDs and injuries have markedly increased their contribution to overall disease burden and mortality. In India in 1990, total disability-adjusted life years (DALYs) were distributed as follows: 61% from CMNNDs, 30% from NCDs, and 9% from injuries. However, due to major epidemiological transitions in India over the years, total DALYs from CMNNDs have decreased to 33%, while those from NCDs and injuries have increased to 55% and 12%, respectively, in 2016. Across India, the disease burden or DALY rate in 2016 was fourfold for diabetes. When looking at the leading individual causes of DALYs in India, most NCDs have risen in rank since 1990, with diabetes showing a dramatic increase, from 35th place in 1990 to 13th place in 2016 [9].

The India State-Level Disease Burden Initiative Diabetes study collaborators reported that the prevalence and number of people with diabetes in India increased from 5.5% and 26 million in 1990 to 7.7% and 65 million in 2016. According to this report, Tamil Nadu had the highest prevalence in 2016, followed by Kerala, Delhi,

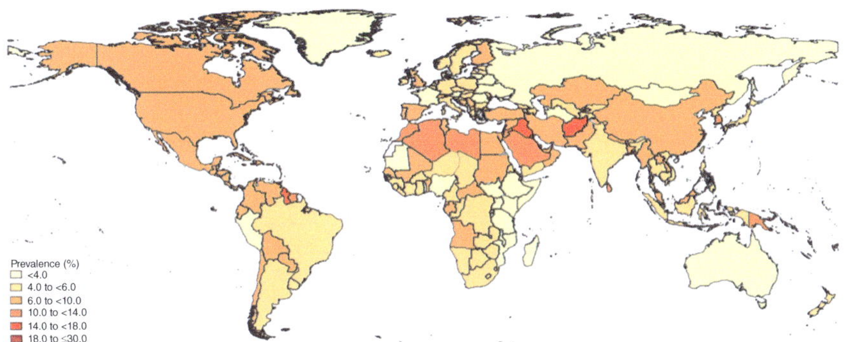

Fig. 1.1 Age-standardized prevalence rates of diabetes by country [8]. (Figure from publication—Global, regional, and national burden of diabetes from 1990 to 2021, with projections of prevalence to 2050: A systematic analysis for the Global Burden of Disease Study 2021—The Lancet, licensed under CC-BY 4.0)

Punjab, Goa, and Karnataka [10, 11]. The prevalence of diabetes was higher among states with higher per capita GDP and among individuals belonging to the higher SES. Studies demonstrate clear evidence of an epidemiological transition, with a higher prevalence of diabetes in the high socioeconomic status of urban areas in more economically developed states [12].

1.3 Health Care and Economic Scenario in India

In India, the health expenditure as a proportion of GDP was 2.96 (2020), and over the years, the government's proportion has increased from 1.6% in (FY2021 to 2.1% of GDP in FY2023 [13, 14]. About 60% of healthcare treatment is accessed in the private sector, and this is similar in several other developing countries [15]. India's GDP per capita for 2023 was ₹2,17,704.5 ($2612.45) and the average national income in India in 2023 was ₹14,356 ($172) monthly [16, 17]. The proportion of the population below the poverty rate of $2.15 a day (2017 PPP) was 11.90% in 2021 [17, 18]. A catastrophic health expenditure occurs when healthcare expenditure exceeds 10% of household consumption, and in 2018, this varied from 1.8% to 33.7% of the population in different Indian states [19]. There are positive trends with increased government health spending and reduction in CHE [19, 20].

This economic burden stems from two primary sources: direct medical costs associated with diagnosis, treatment, and management of diabetes and its complications and indirect costs arising from lost productivity, disability, and premature mortality [21]. Direct costs involve the cost of care, which is medication, professional fees, investigations during hospitalization, specialized care, and advanced treatments for complications like retinopathy, neuropathy, and nephropathy. Indirect costs, often underestimated, include absenteeism, reduced work efficiency, and early retirement due to diabetes-related complications [22]. The consequences of diabetes on the global and Indian economy are far-reaching and multifaceted. On a microlevel, individuals and families face financial hardship due to the high cost of treatment, which can lead to poverty and a diminished quality of life. On a macrolevel, the economic burden of diabetes can hinder economic growth and development, impacting national budgets, progress, and the healthcare systems' sustainability. Many families with diabetic patients tend to spend a sizable part of their income on treating the disease and its complications, as high as ₹17,000 ($203) a year [23].

A simple cost comparison of selected regimens for the treatment of diabetes in India is shown in Table 1.2. It is evident that with newer oral therapy and insulin regimens, the out-of-pocket costs can be very demanding on many households. One should also bear in mind that this may be associated with costs for treatment of comorbidities and complications.

Diabetes care, including treatment of its associated complications, often requires expensive healthcare resources such as hospitalization charges, laboratory tests, and drugs. An average person might require blood tests atleast four times and more frequently while on insulin. This has an equity dimension since people with higher affordability can obtain better diabetic care with proper follow-up, and potentially better control and outcomes than those who do not follow up. This cost can be highly variable where it can be free in the public sector and extremely high where professional fees, investigations, and drugs are exponentially greater in different private sector hospitals. The associated complications can also be prohibitive and catastrophic to most families, as seen in Table 1.3.

A study demonstrated with the high costs there can be distress mechanisms to payments especially at tertiary hospitals for diabetes related hospitalization Table 1.4 [24]. This demonstrates that over a third of people had to resort to adverse measures while paying for care.

Table 1.2 Monthly costs for diabetic medications in India

Category	Drug (oral/SC)	Representative daily dose	Average monthly cost for dose ₹ ($)[a]
Biguanide	Metformin (o)	1000 mg	52 (0.62)
Sulphonylureas	Glimeperide	2 mg	162 (1.94)
	Gliclazide	40 mg	110 (1.32)
Thiazolidenediones	Pioglitazone	15 mg	170 (2.04)
	Acarbose	25 mg	200 (2.4)
DPP-4 inhibitors	Sitagliptin	50 mg	300 (3.6)
	Linagliptin	5 mg	400 (4.8)
SGLT2 inhibitors	Dapagliflozin	10 mg	350 (4.2)
	Canagliflozin	100 mg	1500 (18)
GLP-1 agonists	Exenatide (s/c)	250 mg	13,800 (165.6)
	Semaglutide (o)	3 mg	9000 (108)

[a]Costs compiled from online pharmacies

Table 1.3 Cost of selected complications of diabetes mellitus

Condition	Cost ₹
Foot ulcer (2013) [24, 25]	Hospitalized direct cost due to foot ulcer was ₹19,020 and those who had two complications ₹17,633
Myocardial infarction (2019) [26]	The median (IQR) expenditure was ₹34,258 (8022 to 1,23,582) per acute myocardial infarction encounter across public and private sector
Stroke (2018) [27]	The mean cost for hospitalized stroke was ₹40,360 from National Sample Survey, across public and private sector
Hemodialysis (2018) [28, 29]	Per session health system cost was ₹4148 and out of pocket expense ₹2838. Under the public sector dialysis scheme the costs were ₹1595 and OOPEs were ₹1173
Peritoneal dialysis (PD) (2022) [29]	The annual health system cost and OOPEs incurred on PD were estimated as ₹6550 and ₹4,78,303, respectively, in the public sector dialysis scheme
Renal transplant (2013) [30]	The mean direct medical cost of transplant in a public hospital ranged from ₹64,243 to ₹1,81,033

OOPE out of pocket expenditure

Table 1.4 Mechanisms of out-of-pocket payment for diabetes in India [24]

Mode of payment	Percentage
Personal savings	48
Borrowing loan	14
Mortgage	8
Company reimbursement	12
Selling property	11
Medical insurance	7

The absence of insurance mechanisms leads to a dependence on personal savings and loans. Thus, an untimely hospitalization can derail the future social security of any family.

An analysis from 35 low- and middle-income countries, included in the World Health Survey, reported that diabetic individuals had a higher out-of-pocket expenditure and health insurance did not reduce the chance of catastrophic health expenditure when compared to nondiabetics. Furthermore, this was more pronounced in low- and middle-income countries [31].

Studies from India reported treatment costs for diabetics increase with duration of diabetes, presence of complications, surgery, hospitalization, insulin therapy, and urban setting. The study found that low-income groups spent the highest proportion of household income to diabetic care and medical reimbursement increased by tenfold over 7 years in the urban high-income group [32]. This has changed due to recent state and national health insurance schemes which cover lower SES families.

The direct diabetes costs revealed that the expense toward medications was considered a significant component (17%) of outpatient care and hospitalization contributed up to 35% [33].

1.4 Covid-19 and Diabetes

Diabetes was associated with more incidence of severe Covid infections, acute respiratory distress syndrome, critical care admissions, intubation, and mortality [34, 35]. In India, the high prevalence of uncontrolled diabetes led to higher admissions, complications, and poorer outcomes [36, 37]. In some studies, up to 28% of patients had diseases like diabetes or hypertension and the mortality rate increased with more comorbidities. During the second wave, there was a triple burden of mucormycosis in diabetic patients and Covid-19 [38]. This had multifactorial causes that resulted from poor control, unregulated immune response, and rampant steroid use. The need for steroids during Covid management, lack of access to medicine, and follow-up among other factors led to worsening of diabetic control. All these factors imposed a significant catastrophic impact [39].

1.5 Potential Solutions

Addressing the economic burden of diabetes requires a multipronged approach. The obvious goal is to reduce the incidence, prevalence, and hence the disease burden, but it is also important to be more efficient in managing prevalent cases. These are amenable to mitigation through early detection and prevention of diabetes-related complications. Given that diabetes mellitus is a lifestyle syndrome, alterations in dietary practices, physical activity, and behavioural modifications have the potential to mitigate financial adversity [40]. This requires prevention strategies aimed at promoting healthy lifestyles and eating habits, addressing modifiable risk factors like obesity and physical inactivity, strengthening healthcare systems to ensure access to affordable and quality diabetes care, and investing in research and development to optimise management protocols. The need to adopt a cost-effective approach while creating guidelines focusing on the Indian context will guide rational interventions and drug choices [41]. At the public sector level, this will provide clear guidance on when to escalate to more expensive drugs. At the private sector, it will require individualization of care based on affordability. A fair rule of thumb would be to provide information regarding therapeutic options, assess the financial capacity of the family, signpost to safe financing options, support the decision process, and strive to limit their annual health expenses to less than 10% of income. Thus, diabetes management, though guided by a protocol, must be contextualized based on affordability and preferences.

In conclusion, India will continue to face tremendous economic repercussions with both the medical costs and productivity loss of diabetes, associated lifestyle diseases, and their complications unless aggressive public health measures are adopted. At a clinical level, awareness of the cost implications at every stage, from diagnosis to complications, should guide rational and appropriate patient-centric management. There is an urgent need for context-relevant guidelines, monitoring adherence, economic evaluation of management protocols, public financial protection schemes, and aggressive public health measures to curb the rising burden of diabetes in India.

References

1. ElSayed NA, Aleppo G, Aroda VR, Bannuru RR, Brown FM, Bruemmer D, et al. 2. Classification and diagnosis of diabetes: standards of care in diabetes—2023. Diabetes Care. 2023;46(Suppl 1):S19–40.
2. Global, regional, and national burden and trend of diabetes in 195 countries and territories: an analysis from 1990 to 2025. https://pubmed.ncbi.nlm.nih.gov/32901098/. Accessed 11 Dec 2023.
3. National Diabetes Statistics Report | Diabetes | CDC [Internet]. 2023. https://www.cdc.gov/diabetes/data/statistics-report/index.html. Accessed 11 Dec 2023.
4. Emerging Risk Factors Collaboration, Sarwar N, Gao P, Seshasai SRK, Gobin R, Kaptoge S, et al. Diabetes mellitus, fasting blood glucose concentration, and risk of vascular disease: a collaborative meta-analysis of 102 prospective studies. Lancet. 2010;375(9733):2215–22.
5. Institute for Health Metrics and Evaluation [Internet]. GBD Results. https://vizhub.healthdata.org/gbd-results. Accessed 11 Dec 2023.
6. Magliano DJ, Boyko EJ, Committee IDA 10th Edition Scientific. Table 3.2, number of adults (20–79 years) with diabetes per World Bank income classification in 2021 and 2045 [internet]. Brussels: International Diabetes Federation; 2021. https://www.ncbi.nlm.nih.gov/books/NBK581940/table/ch3.t2/. Accessed 11 Dec 2023.
7. Magliano DJ, Boyko EJ, Committee IDA 10th Edition Scientific. Global picture. In: IDF DIABETES ATLAS [Internet] 10th. Brussels: International Diabetes Federation; 2021. https://www.ncbi.nlm.nih.gov/books/NBK581940/. Accessed 11 Dec 2023.
8. Global, regional, and national burden of diabetes from 1990 to 2021, with projections of prevalence to 2050: a systematic analysis for the Global Burden of Disease Study 2021—The Lancet [Internet]. 2023. https://www.thelancet.com/journals/lancet/article/PIIS0140-6736(23)01301-6/fulltext. Accessed 11 Dec 2023.
9. The increasing burden of diabetes and variations among the states of India: the Global Burden of Disease Study 1990–2016—The Lancet Global Health [Internet]. 2023. https://www.thelancet.com/journals/langlo/article/PIIS2214-109X(18)30387-5/fulltext. Accessed 11 Dec 2023.
10. Tandon N, Anjana RM, Mohan V, Kaur T, Afshin A, Ong K, et al. The increasing burden of diabetes and variations among the states of India: the global burden of disease study 1990–2016. Lancet Glob Health. 2018;6(12):e1352–62.
11. GDP per capita of Indian states—StatisticsTimes.com [Internet]. 2023. https://statisticstimes.com/economy/india/indian-states-gdp-per-capita.php. Accessed 6 Dec 2023.
12. Socioeconomic Gradients and Distribution of Diabetes, Hypertension, and Obesity in India—PubMed [Internet]. 2023. https://pubmed.ncbi.nlm.nih.gov/30951154/. Accessed 11 Dec 2023.
13. World Bank Open Data [Internet]. World Bank open data. 2023. https://data.worldbank.org. Accessed 6 Dec 2023.
14. Share of Government Health Expenditure in total health expenditure increases from 28.6 percent in FY14 to 40.6 percent in FY19 [Internet]. 2023. https://pib.gov.in/pib.gov.in/Pressreleaseshare.aspx?PRID=1894902. Accessed 6 Dec 2023.
15. Executive Summary on Report—Health in India, NSS 75th round | Ministry of Statistics and Program Implementation | Government of India [Internet]. 2023. http://164.100.161.63/announcements/executive-summary-report-health-india-nss-75th-round. Accessed 6 Jan 2023.
16. Press note on Provisional Estimates of National Income 2022–23 and quarterly estimates of gross domestic product for the fourth quarter (January-March) of 2022–23 [Internet]. 2023. https://pib.gov.in/pib.gov.in/Pressreleaseshare.aspx?PRID=1928682. Accessed 6 Dec 2023.
17. IMF [Internet]. Report for selected countries and subjects. 2023. https://www.imf.org/en/Publications/WEO/weo-database/2023/October/weo-report. Accessed 13 Dec 2023.
18. pip.worldbank.org/country-profiles/IND [Internet]. 2023. https://pip.worldbank.org/country-profiles/IND. Accessed 6 Dec 2023.
19. Sriram S, Albadrani M. A study of catastrophic health expenditures in India—evidence from nationally representative survey data: 2014-2018. F1000Res. 2022;11:141.

20. Share of Government Health Expenditure in total health expenditure increases from 28.6 percent in FY14 to 40.6 percent in FY19 [internet]. 2023. https://pib.gov.in/pib.gov.in/Pressreleaseshare.aspx?PRID=1894902. Accessed 6 Dec 2023.
21. Yesudian CA, Grepstad M, Visintin E, Ferrario A. The economic burden of diabetes in India: a review of the literature. Glob Health. 2014;10(1):80.
22. Bansode B, Jungari DS. Economic burden of diabetic patients in India: a review. Diabetes Metab Syndr. 2019;13(4):2469–72.
23. Nagarathna R, Madhava M, Patil SS, Singh A, Perumal K, Ningombam G, et al. Cost of management of diabetes mellitus: a pan India study. Ann Neurosci. 2020;27(3–4):190–2.
24. Kumpatla S, Kothandan H, Tharkar S, Viswanathan V. The costs of treating long-term diabetic complications in a developing country: a study from India. J Assoc Physicians India. 2013;61(2):102–9.
25. Viswanathan V, Rao VN. Managing diabetic foot infection in India. Int J Low Extrem Wounds. 2013;12(2):158–66.
26. Mohanan PP, Huffman MD, Baldridge AS, Devarajan R, Kondal D, Zhao L, et al. Microeconomic costs, insurance, and catastrophic health spending among patients with acute myocardial infarction in India. JAMA Netw Open. 2019;2(5):e193831.
27. Rajasulochana SR, Kar SS. Economic burden associated with stroke in India: insights from national sample survey 2017-18. Expert Rev Pharmacoecon Outcomes Res. 2022;22(3):455–63.
28. Kaur G, Prinja S, Ramachandran R, Malhotra P, Gupta KL, Jha V. Cost of hemodialysis in a public sector tertiary hospital of India. Clin Kidney J. 2018;11(5):726–33.
29. Gupta D, Jyani G, Ramachandran R, Bahuguna P, Ameel M, Dahiya BB, et al. Peritoneal dialysis—first initiative in India: a cost-effectiveness analysis. Clin Kidney J. 2021;15(1):128–35.
30. Ramachandran R, Jha V. Kidney transplantation is associated with catastrophic out of pocket expenditure in India. PLoS One. 2013;8(7):e67812.
31. Smith-Spangler CM, Bhattacharya J, Goldhaber-Fiebert JD. Diabetes, its treatment, and catastrophic medical spending in 35 developing countries. Diabetes Care. 2012;35(2):319–26.
32. Ramachandran A, Ramachandran S, Snehalatha C, Augustine C, Murugesan N, Viswanathan V, et al. Increasing expenditure on health care incurred by diabetic subjects in a developing country: a study from India. Diabetes Care. 2007;30(2):252–6.
33. Kapur A. Economic analysis of diabetes care. Indian J Med Res. 2007;125(3):473.
34. Shivane V, Lila A, Bandgar T. Type 2 diabetic Asian Indians and COVID-19: lessons learnt so far from the ongoing pandemic. J Postgrad Med. 2020;66(4):179–81.
35. Singh P, Bhaskar Y, Verma P, Rana S, Goel P, Kumar S, et al. Impact of comorbidity on patients with COVID-19 in India: a nationwide analysis. Front Public Health. 2023;10:1027312.
36. Kumar A, Arora A, Sharma P, Anikhindi SA, Bansal N, Singla V, et al. Is diabetes mellitus associated with mortality and severity of COVID-19? A meta-analysis. Diabetes Metab Syndr. 2020;14(4):535–45.
37. Novosad P, Jain R, Campion A, Asher S. COVID-19 mortality effects of underlying health conditions in India: a modelling study. BMJ Open. 2020;10(12):e043165.
38. Ghazi BK, Rackimuthu S, Wara UU, Mohan A, Khawaja UA, Ahmad S, et al. Rampant increase in cases of Mucormycosis in India and Pakistan: a serious cause for concern during the ongoing COVID-19 pandemic. Am J Trop Med Hyg. 2021;105(5):1144–7.
39. George TK, Sharma P, Joy M, Seelan G, Sekar A, Gunasekaran K, et al. The economic impact of a COVID-19 illness from the perspective of families seeking care in a private hospital in India. Dialogues Health. 2023;2:100139.
40. Cost of diabetes and its complications: results from a STEPS survey in Punjab, India—PMC [Internet]. 2023. https://www.ncbi.nlm.nih.gov/pmc/articles/PMC10080818/. Accessed 11 Dec 2023.
41. Singh K, Chandrasekaran AM, Bhaumik S, Chattopadhyay K, Gamage AU, Silva PD, et al. Cost-effectiveness of interventions to control cardiovascular diseases and diabetes mellitus in South Asia: a systematic review. BMJ Open. 2018;8(4):e017809.

2 Insulin Therapy and Glucose Monitoring Best Practices

Reena George and Urjitha Rajagopalan

2.1 Introduction

About 20–30% of all patients with type 1 or type 2 diabetes develop evidence of nephropathy. Once CKD develops, the primary goal of management is to slow down the progression of disease to ESKD by strict control of blood sugars and blood pressure, thus delaying requirement of kidney replacement therapy. Even for patients with diabetes who have progressed to ESKD and are receiving dialysis or renal transplant, strict glycemic control reduces morbidity and mortality. The United Kingdom Prospective Diabetes Study (UKPDS) showed that insulin was required in 50% of people with type 2 diabetes to keep HbA1C < 7% [1]. Although insulin therapy is safe and simple, the efficiency of therapy largely depends on the insulin administration technique and dose accuracy based on glucose monitoring. Yet this is often underemphasized in the routine patient care. Hence, it is imperative that all patients be offered training and advice on best practices in insulin administration techniques and glucose monitoring, in which nurses play the key role.

R. George (✉)
Nephrology Nursing, Christian Medical College, Vellore, Tamil Nadu, India
e-mail: reenarachel@cmcvellore.ac.in

U. Rajagopalan
MGM Healthcare, Chennai, Tamil Nadu, India
e-mail: urjitha.r@mgmhealthcare.in

G. Abraham et al. (eds.), *Management of Diabetic Complications*,
https://doi.org/10.1007/978-981-97-6406-8_2

2.2 Insulin Therapy

2.2.1 Insulin Syringes

- In India, conventional administration of insulin involves subcutaneous injection with strengths available as 40 units and 100 units. Syringes that match the concentration of U-40 and U-100 must be recommended to avoid dosing errors (Figs. 2.1 and 2.2).
- Each division of U-40 and U-100 syringe is equivalent to 1 unit of insulin and 2 units of insulin, respectively.
- Reuse of an insulin syringe and insulin pen needles are not recommended for the following reasons:
  - It compromises sterility.
  - Recapping requires manual dexterity and increases the risk for needle prick injury to caregivers.
  - With the advent of new, smaller needles (30/31G), the needle tips can become bent and can lacerate the tissue and may even leave needle fragments in the skin.
- Needles/syringes must be disposed as per the local protocol for disposal of medical waste.
- Avoid cleaning the needle with alcohol and reusing, as it will remove the silicon coating and makes the skin puncture more painful.
- *Syringe alternatives:* Pen-like devices and insulin-containing cartridges are available that deliver insulin subcutaneously through a needle. These devices improve the accuracy of dose and compliance of patients as they are not required to withdraw the medicine from the vial [2].

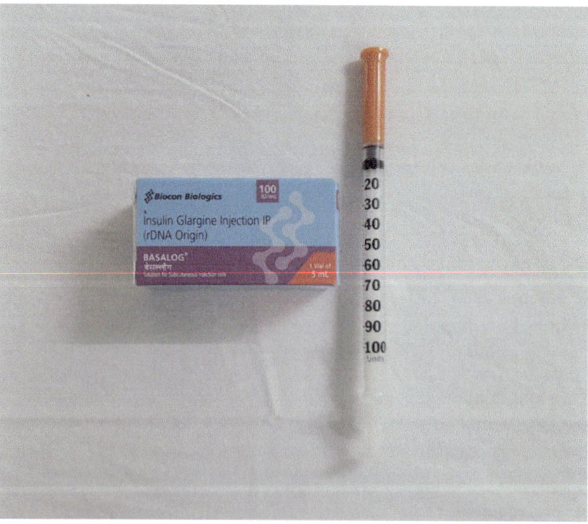

Fig. 2.1 Insulin syringe with capacity 100 units. (Original photographs from the department of Endocrinology, Christian Medical College, Vellore)

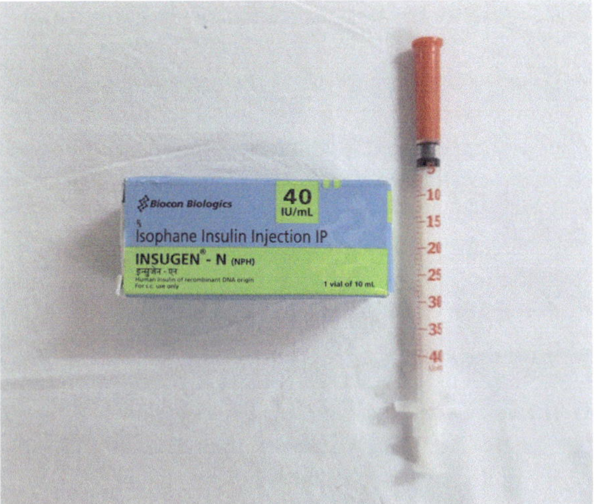

Fig. 2.2 Insulin syringe with capacity 40 units. (Original photographs from the department of Endocrinology, Christian Medical College, Vellore)

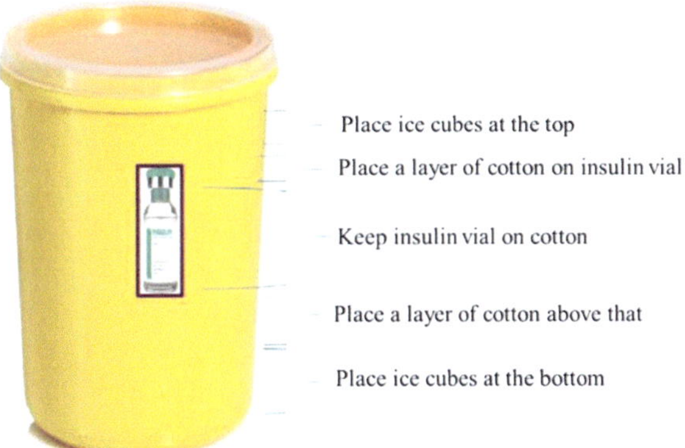

Fig. 2.3 Storage of insulin during long travel [3]. (https://link.springer.com/article/10.1007/s13300-019-0574-x)

2.2.2 Insulin Storage

- Insulin preparation is stable at room temperature, but can lose its potency in extremes of temperature. It is advisable to store unopened vials, cartridges, and pens of insulin in the refrigerator at 20 °C to 8 °C (36 °F to 46 °F) [2].
- Injecting cold insulin may cause pain and local irritation at the injection site, and hence is recommended that in-use vials be left at room temperature if room temperature is <30 °C, and to use the vial or pen within 1 month. At temperatures above 30 °C, insulin loses 1% potency over 30 days and 0.1% if refrigerated (Fig. 2.3) [3].
- If refrigerated, insulin can be left in room temperature for 10 min prior to administration and rolled between palms to normalize the temperature.
- Insulin can be stored in an earthen vessel if refrigerator is not available.
- During travel, insulin vials can be put in a polythene bag and submerged in cold water or ice in a thermos container [3].

2.2.3 Sites for Insulin Administration

- Anterior abdominal wall is the preferred site for subcutaneous administration of insulin considering the ease of self-administration, larger available surface area, and steady, rapid rate of absorption with less destruction by subcutaneous enzymes (Fig. 2.4a, b) [2].
- Sites of injection should be rotated at a distance of 0.5–1 in. away from the previous injection site to prevent lipohypertrophy, an abnormal subcutaneous fat accumulation that impairs vascular and nervous supply and reduces the rate of absorption. Making an anatomical "map" for injection rotation will be helpful (Fig. 2.5) [2, 3].
- Insulin must be injected at least four finger breadths away from the umbilicus.
- Insulin can be administered in the upper outer thighs in anterior and lateral aspects or in the upper outer arms, but not preferred for the following reasons:
  - There is very little subcutaneous tissue.
  - Privacy issue to expose thighs.
  - There is a higher risk of infection with poor hygiene when using the thighs for insulin administration.
  - Rate of absorption is not steady, varying with exercise or movement.
- Unhealthy sites as bruised or scarred areas are to be avoided for injection [3].

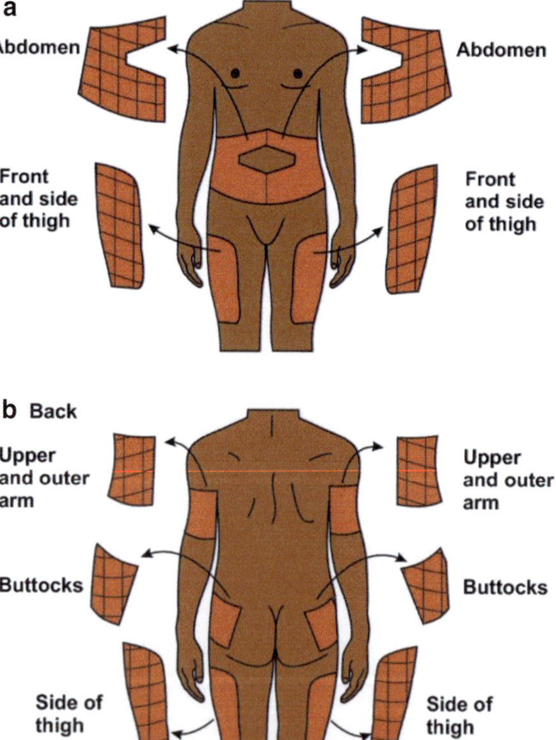

Fig. 2.4 (**a** and **b**) Sites for insulin administration [3]

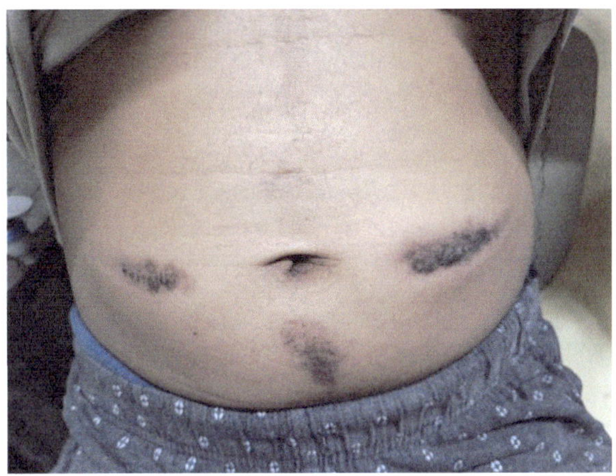

Fig. 2.5 Lipohypertrophy from administration of insulin in the same sites. (Original photographs from the department of Endocrinology, Christian Medical College, Vellore)

2.2.4 Mixing of Insulin

If a patient requires a mixture of different insulin formulations, they can be administered as two separate subcutaneous injections or can be mixed and administered as single injection. If mixing, the regular insulin must be drawn first and then the intermediate acting insulin so as to prevent contamination of regular insulin with neutral protamine Hagedorn (NPH). The mixed insulin is best if used immediately, but can be stored up to 24 h. Rapidly acting insulin analogs may be mixed safely with NPH or Ultralente, as the pharmacokinetics of either insulin does not alter on mixing. However, mixing regular insulin with lente or ultralente is not recommended, as the zinc in lente can bind with regular insulin and delay its onset of action. NPH when mixed with lente insulin produces zinc phosphate precipitates, converting long-acting insulin to short-acting, and therefore not recommended. Insulin glargine, being acidic, should not be mixed with any other insulin as it can produce precipitates. It is best to avoid mixing different brands of insulin [2, 4].

2.2.5 Factors That Affect the Rate of Absorption of Insulin

- Site of injection
- The rate of absorption is fastest when insulin is administered in the abdominal site, taking 60 min to reach the peak levels in blood as compared to arms and thighs which takes 75 min and 90–120 min, respectively.
- Site rotation
- Rotation of sites prevent lipohypertrophy, thus promoting insulin absorption.
- Temperature
- The warmer the area, faster the absorption of insulin into the blood stream.
- Exercise
- Exercise increases the blood circulation, thus promoting insulin absorption.

- Needle length
- Optimal needle length to ensure subcutaneous penetration and glycemic control even in obese patients is 4 mm [4].

2.2.6 Insulin Administration Technique: Using Syringe or Pen

Insulin administration technique is different as shown in Figs. 2.6, 2.7a, b, and 2.8.

2.2.7 Alternative Methods of Insulin Delivery

- Insulin pens.
  - Reusable.
  - Disposable.
- Insulin pump.
- Insulin port.

2.2.7.1 Insulin Pens

Insulin pens are designed to ease subcutaneous administration of insulin with dose accuracy and compliance, without having the need to withdraw insulin from the vial as in the conventional method. These are manufactured to fit cartridges of specific insulin type (Fig. 2.9).

Reusable insulin pens have small, prefilled cartridges (3 mL = 300 units) that are to be loaded into a pen-like holder. A 30–31G disposable needle is attached the device to give injection. Insulin is delivered by dialling a desired dose and pushing a button for every increment administered. A maximum of 60–70 units can be administered in

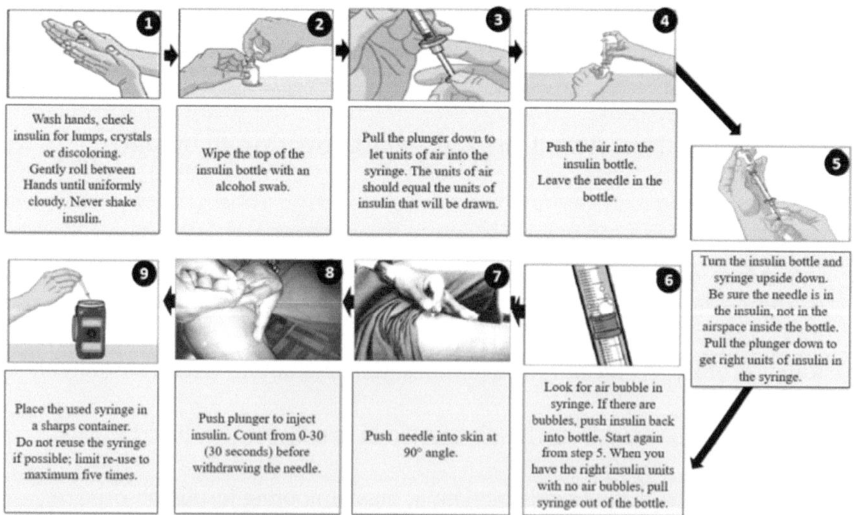

Fig. 2.6 Steps in insulin administration [3]

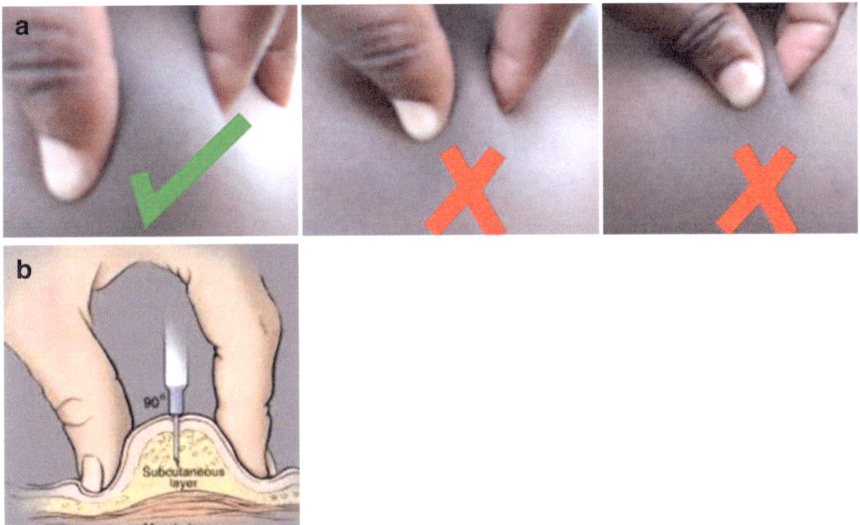

Fig. 2.7 (**a** and **b**) Pinching the skin and subcutaneous tissue for insulin injection [3]

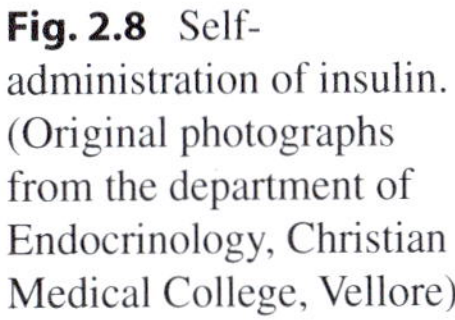

Fig. 2.8 Self-administration of insulin. (Original photographs from the department of Endocrinology, Christian Medical College, Vellore)

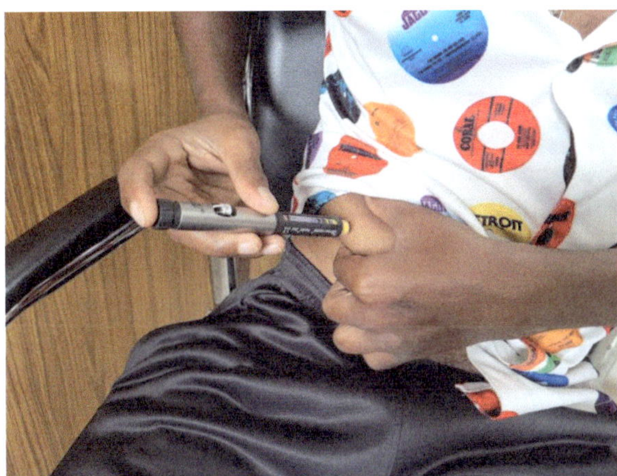

one single injection. They are durable and easy to use. Needle has to be changed after each injection. New cartridge can be loaded into the pen as it gets empty [5].

Disposable pens are compact and contain a built-in, single-use insulin cartridge. Patients do not have to load the pen with cartridge. But once the cartridge is empty, the pen has to be disposed. The needle is to be changed on each event of injection. These pens are compact, portable, durable, lightweight, and easy to handle.

Pen devices will not be ideal for those clients who take mixture of two kinds of insulin as this will require two pens and two injections. Similarly, those patients receiving different types of insulin with breakfast and dinner will also need to have two pens. Pen devices will not be a good option for those with visual or neurological impairment for independent use [2, 5, 6].

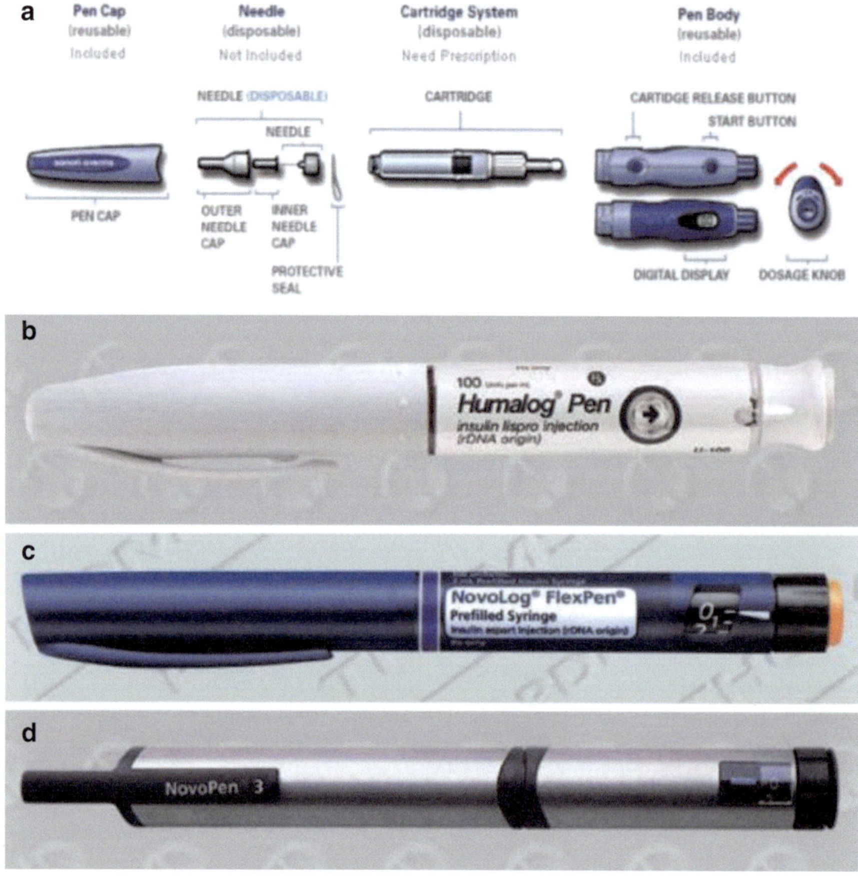

Fig. 2.9 Insulin pen devices [11]

2.2.7.2 Insulin Pump [2, 7]

An insulin pump is a small device, size of that of a cell phone that allows precise doses of continuous subcutaneous insulin infusion to closely match the body's insulin requirement (Fig. 2.10).

Basal rate is the steady dose of insulin that is delivered continuously to meet the demand for baseline insulin requirement due to endogenous hepatic glucose production, not associated with food intake. This constitutes 40%–50% of total daily insulin dose.

Bolus dose is the additional dose of insulin that is delivered by the pump "on demand," with meals to match the food intake or to correct high blood sugar levels.

Components of Insulin Pump

Insulin pump that has [7]

- A button to program the insulin dose delivery.
- A liquid crystal display (LCD) screen.

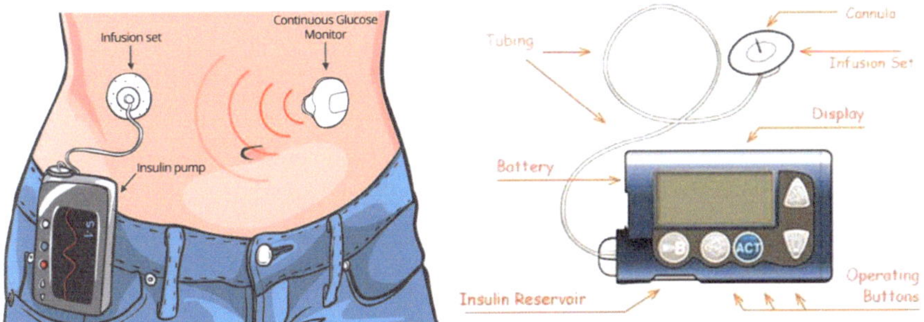

Fig. 2.10 Insulin pump. (https://www.umassmed.edu/dcoe/diabetes-education/pumps_and_cgm/; https://www.aliem.com/insulin-pumps-understanding-them-and-complications/)

- A battery compartment to hold one AAA battery.
- Reservoir compartment that holds insulin.

Reservoir—A plastic cartridge that can hold up to 300 units of insulin which need to be replaced with a new one depending on the dose requirement. It comes with a transfer guard that is to be removed before inserting the reservoir to the pump.

Infusion set includes a thin tube with a small needle and a cannula that goes from the reservoir to the infusion site in the body (anterior abdomen preferably). The needle is removed once the cannula is in place and secured so that the patients do not experience pain or discomfort.

Infusion set insertion device to place the infusion set with the push of a button.

Who will benefit from continuous subcutaneous insulin infusion?

Those patients with

- Type-1 DM.
- Uncontrolled blood sugar level on intensive management of type 2 DM, requiring more than or equal to four insulin injections.
- Equal to or more than four self-glucose monitoring (SGM) daily.
- High motivation to effectively operate the complex device.
- Erratic lifestyle and food habits.
- Wide fluctuations of blood sugars "dawn phenomenon."

2.3 Dose Adjustment for Normal Eating (DAFNE)

The Diabetes Control and Complications Trial compared intensive insulin therapy to conventional treatment, which showed reduced progression to complications and better HbA1C levels in the intensive group. However, there was a threefold increase in severe hypoglycemia and 33% increase in undesirable weight gain in the intensive group without any increase in the quality of life [8].

DAFNE program is a 5-day, skill based and client-centred group program to enable the client to eat freely and adjust the insulin to match their desired carbohydrate intake. DAFNE study, an RCT conducted in the United Kingdom involving 169

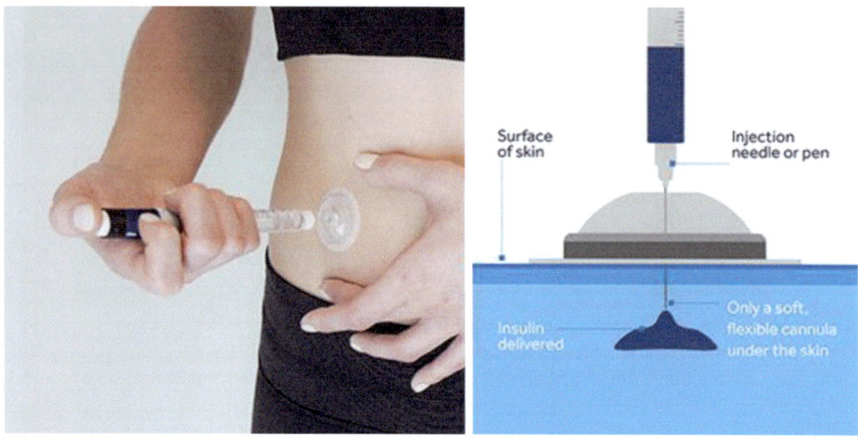

Fig. 2.11 Insulin port. (https://www.medtronic-diabetes.com/en-MENA/accessories/iport-advance-injection-port)

clients showed a reduction in HbA1C by 1% in 6 months in the study group, with no increase in hypoglycemia events or changes in weight, and better quality of life [9].

2.3.1 Insulin Port (I-Port)

Having to self-inject insulin on a regular, long-term basis is very dreading for most patients, especially children. I-Port Advance is a sterile, subcutaneous injection port that remains in place for up to 72 h to accommodate multiple injections without the discomfort of additional needle sticks. A needle longer than 8 mm or thicker than 28G should not be used in the port. I-Port can be used for pen devices [2] (Fig. 2.11).

2.4 Self-Monitoring of Blood Glucose (SMBG) [2, 10]

SMBG has an integral role in diabetes management, promoting good glycemic control, preventing diabetes-related complications, and enhancing quality of life. The American Diabetes Association (ADA) recommends SMBG for all patients taking insulin or oral glucose-lowering agents. SMBG is an empowering tool that helps patients and families become active partners in diabetes management. Training on SMBG requires significant time and effort from nurse educators or physicians.

2.4.1 Benefits and Barriers

- SMBG provides objective feedback of glycemic control achieved with treatment.
- The measured blood glucose values are used to adjust insulin dose, activity pattern, and food intake.

- Gives accurate record of daily glucose fluctuations and trends, thus helping to prevent episodes of hyperglycaemia hypoglycemia.
- Requires visual acuity, fine motor coordination, comfort with technology, and willingness to be consistent. Having to self-prick is a barrier perceived by many patients.

2.4.2 Frequency of Blood Glucose Monitoring [4]

The schedule for glucose monitoring varies between patients depending mainly on the type of diabetes and the acuity of illness.

Type 2 DM—it is measured once before breakfast, 2 h after breakfast, lunch, and dinner, and one–two times in a week.

Type 1 DM—monitor blood glucose pre- and post-breakfast, lunch, and dinner at least three times a week, and early morning glucose levels atleast once a week.

Pregnant women with diabetes—once before breakfast, 1 h after breakfast, lunch, and dinner, at least thrice a week.

Perioperative patients, kept nil by mouth—every 4–6 h or more depending on the glucose levels.

Acute phase of illness as in hypoglycemia, DKA—continuous glucose monitoring system (CGMS) will be beneficial.

2.4.3 SMBG Devices

2.4.3.1 Glucometers

It measures blood glucose by using colour reflectance or sensor technology. The accuracy of a glucometer is reflected by how close its readings are to the results generated by a reference method (plasma glucose levels measured by lab). According to FDA statement, the glucometer should have a difference of less than 15%. Some glucometers are automatically calibrated to provide the plasma glucose values though whole blood sample is used for testing. Patients must be taught to use calibration control solutions and interpret the results as part of the SMBG kit [2, 10] (Figs. 2.12a, b and 2.13).

2.4.3.2 Continuous Glucose Monitoring System (CGMS)

Glucometer readings obtained by finger pricks are snapshots of blood glucose levels at selected times over a 24-h period and will not capture fluctuations and trends. CGMS enables tracking of blood glucose levels automatically on a continuous basis over a 24-h period, thus capturing excursions in glucose levels, particularly during the nocturnal hours when hypoglycemia goes unnoticed. A two-week data of glucose readings can be stored in the monitor's memory, which can then be transferred to personal computer for analysis.

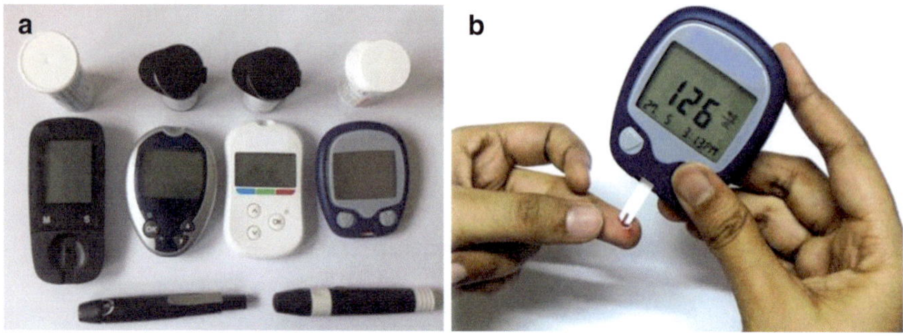

Fig. 2.12 (**a**) Different glucometers use different technologies to measure blood glucose. (**b**) Lancing devices with disposable lancets help to obtain a blood drop with minimal pain experience

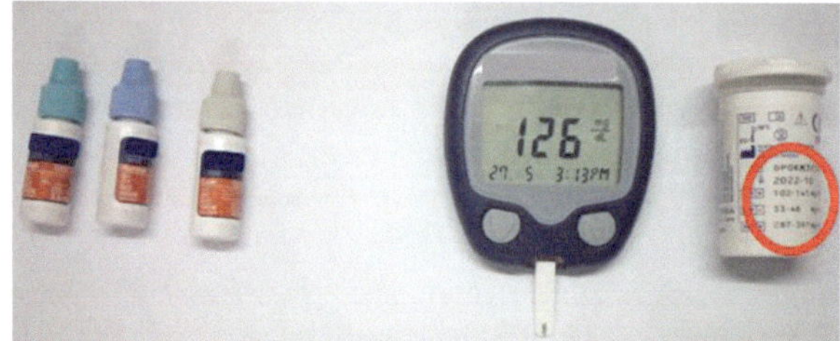

Fig. 2.13 Control solution for glucometer calibration and the range printed on the glucose strip box. (Original photographs from the department of Endocrinology, Christian Medical College, Vellore)

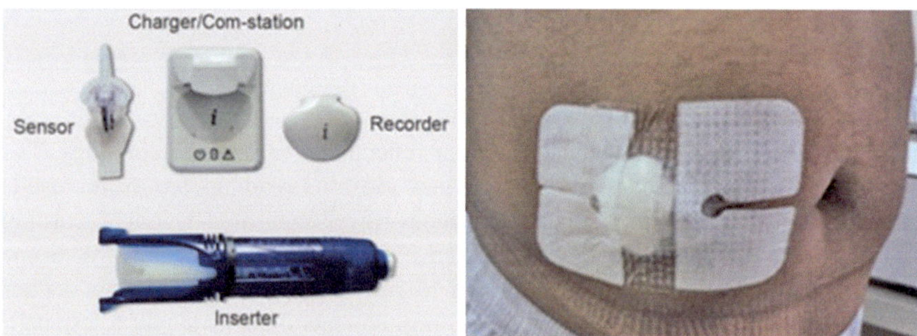

Fig. 2.14 Continuous glucose monitoring system (CGMS) devices collect glucose data and send the data wirelessly to the monitor for real-time use or the data can be downloaded to the computer for analysis. (Original photographs from the department of Endocrinology, Christian Medical College, Vellore)

Components of CGMS [2, 10]

Continuous glucose monitor—a portable, pager-sized device with a disposable glucose sensor that can be inserted subcutaneously. The monitor acquires and stores electronic signals from the sensors and converts them into clinical glucose values (Fig. 2.14).

Cable transmits electronic signals from the glucose sensor to the monitor.

Glucose sensor is a small, sterile, flexible electrode containing the enzyme glucose oxidase. It is attached to a connector, which adheres to the surface of the skin and is connected to the cable. The glucose sensor is inserted just under the skin using a rigid introducer needle. Then, the needle is removed, the and connector is secured against the skin with medical dressing.

Com station is a data downlink communication station to download the data into a database file which can be viewed and graphed using a utility program.

Continuous glucose monitoring devices are different, so familiarity with each one is necessary (Figs. 2.15 and 2.16).

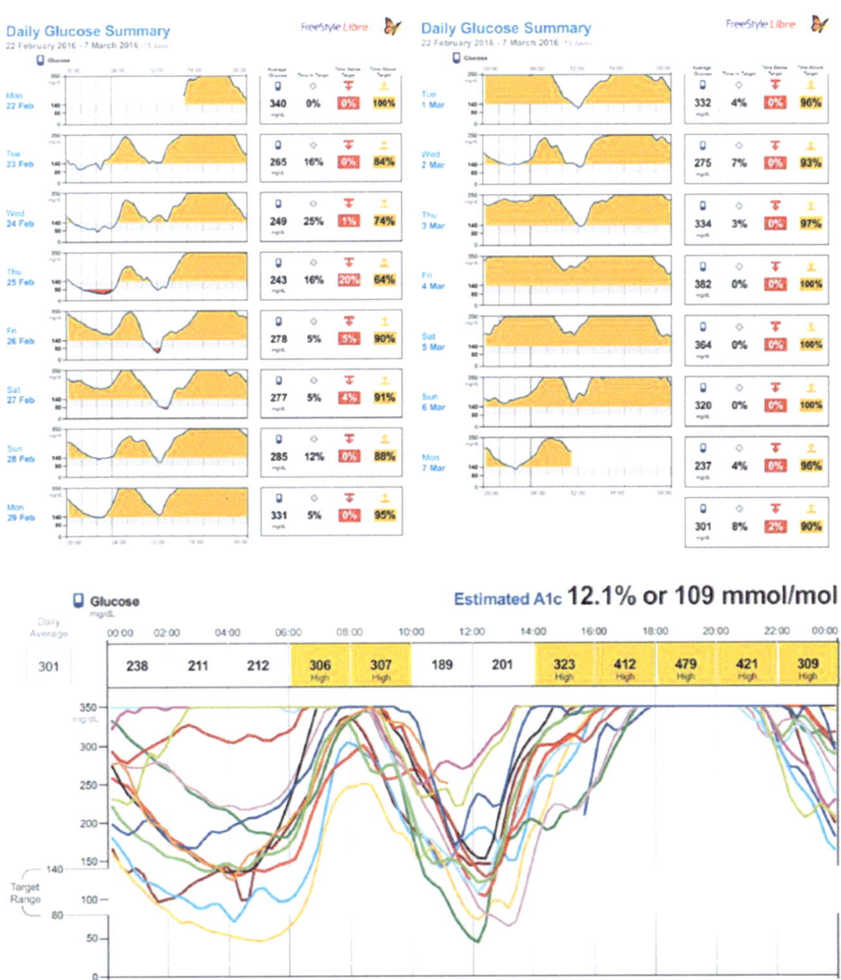

Fig. 2.15 Daily blood glucose summary from CGMS. (Original photographs from the department of Endocrinology, Christian Medical College, Vellore)

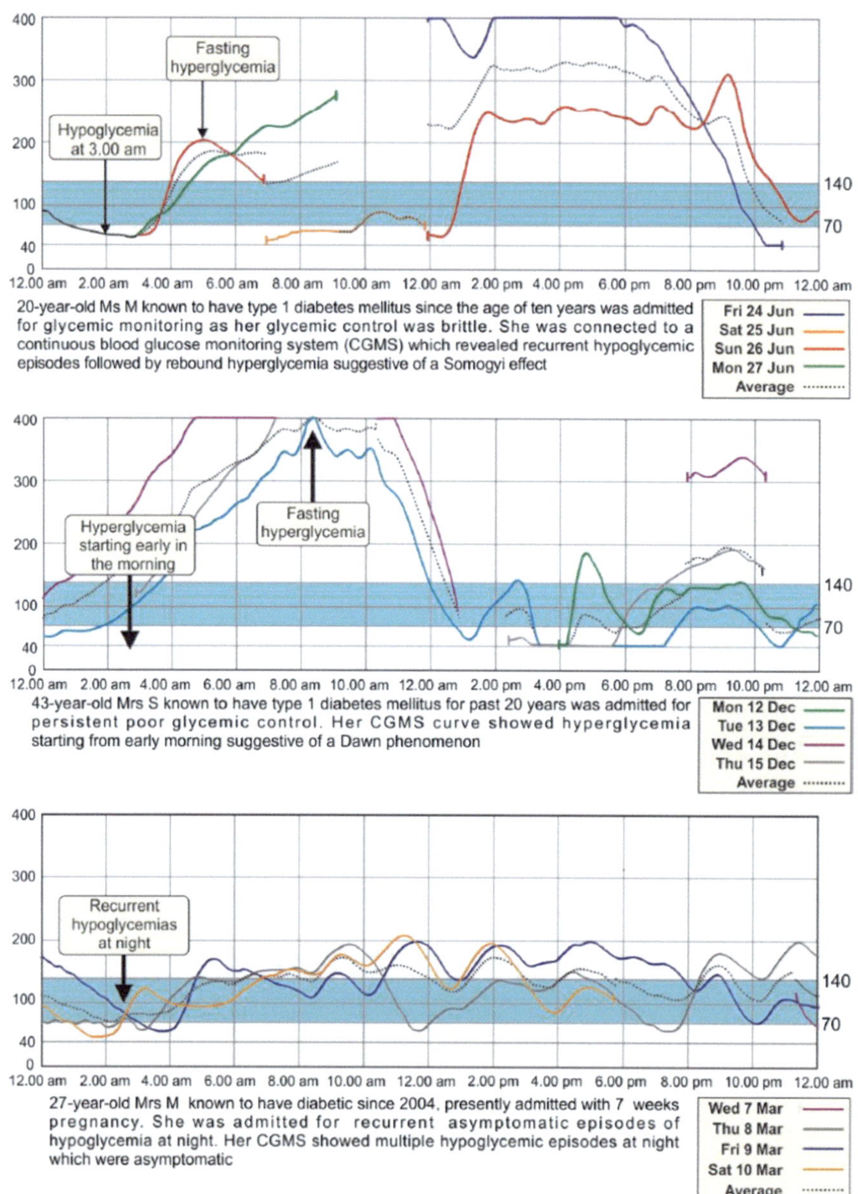

Fig. 2.16 Identifying blood glucose patterns from CGMS [4]. (Original photographs from the department of Endocrinology, Christian Medical College, Vellore)

2.4.3.3 Flash Glucose Monitoring System (FGMS) [2, 10]

FGMS is a very promising alternative to the CGMS and glucometer system though independent validation testing for its accuracy is not adequately studied yet. It has a

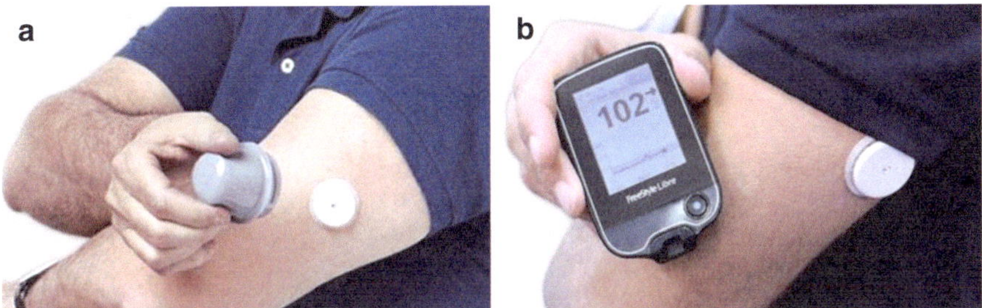

Fig. 2.17 Flash glucose monitoring system probe (**a**) in situ and (**b**) reader, respectively. (Original photographs from the department of Endocrinology, Christian Medical College, Vellore)

subcutaneous sensor with a button-like structure that firmly adheres to the skin which measures interstitial glucose every minute for up to 14 days after which it is disposed. A separate reader is used to scan the sensor and collect glucose measurements and trends for up to 8 h. Advantages of FGMS is that it is factory calibrated, spares finger pricks, is easy to use and cost-effective (Fig. 2.17a, b).

2.4.4 Training Needs

- Technique of insulin administration.
- Self-glucose monitoring.
- Use of gadgets for insulin administration.
- Use of gadgets for SGM.

It is very important that the patients are empowered to manage the disease and enjoy optimum quality of life without any complications. In patients with CKD, the focus of education shifts to renal diet, dialysis, and transplant, leading to the neglect of diabetes management. Diabetes management must become a component of patient education and training and the nurses and doctors in nephrology should be equipped with the necessary, evidence-based knowledge and skills to offer training.

References

1. King P, Peacock I, Donelly R. The UK prospective diabetes study (UKPDS): clinical and therapeutic implications for type 2 diabetes. Br J Clin Pharmacol. 1999;48(5):643.
2. Thomas N, Kapoor N, Velavan J, Vasan S. A practical guide to diabetes mellitus. 8th ed. Chennai: Jaypee Publishers; 2018. p. 147–89.
3. Bahendeka S, Kaushik R, Swai AB, Otieno F, Bajaj S, Kalra S, Bavuma CM, Karigire C. EADSG Guidelines: insulin storage and optimisation of injection technique in diabetes management. Diabetes Ther. 2019;10:341–66. Open access published: 27 February 2019.
4. ADA. Standards in medical care in diabetes—2017. Diabetes Care. 2016;40(1).
5. Frid AH, Kreugel G, Grassi G, et al. New insulin delivery recommendations. Mayo Clin Proc. 2016;91(9):1231–55.

6. Down S, Kirkland F. Injection technique in insulin therapy. Nurs Times. 2012;108(10):18–20.
7. George G, Bailey TS, Bode BW, et al. American Association of Clinical Endocrinologists and American College of endocrinology insulin pump management task force. Endocr Pract. 2014;20(5):463–89.
8. David M. Nathan the diabetes control and complications trial/epidemiology of diabetes interventions and complications study at 30 years: overview. Diabetes Care. 2014;37(1):9–16.
9. DAFNE Study Group. Training in flexible, Intensive insulin management to enable dietary freedom in people with type 1 diabetes: dose adjustment for normal eating (DAFNE) randomised controlled trial. BMJ. 2002;325:746.
10. Bailey TS, Grunberger G, Bode BW, et al. American Association of Clinical Endocrinologists and American College of Endocrinology 2016 outpatient glucose monitoring consensus statement. Endocr Pract. 2016;22(2):231–61.
11. Thurman JE. Insulin pen injection devices for management of patients with type 2 diabetes: considerations based on an Endocrinologist's Practical Experience in the United States. Endocr Pract. 2007;13(6):672–8.

Technologies for Prevention of Diabetes Mellitus and Complications

3

Jothydev Kesavadev, Anjana Basanth, and Krishnadev Jothydev

3.1 Introduction

3.1.1 Understanding Diabetes and Its Potential Complications

Diabetes is a progressive lifestyle disorder often associated with short-term and long-term complications. Not only are these a burden to the nation's economy, but they can have a tremendous impact on the quality of life (QoL) of people with diabetes. According to recent estimates published in *Lancet*, by the year 2050, more than 131 billion people worldwide may have diabetes [1]. The majority of people with diabetes were initially anticipated to reside in developing nations by 2025 as a result of aging populations, a rise in life expectancy, and growing urbanization. Therefore, the long-term effects of diabetes will continue to have an impact on people's personal and societal health in these regions [2].

Diabetes complications significantly contribute to morbidity and mortality rates. Chronic complications in diabetes can be categorized into two types: microvascular and macrovascular. Microvascular complications, which are more common, include conditions like neuropathy, nephropathy, and retinopathy. On the other hand, macrovascular complications encompass cardiovascular diseases, strokes, and peripheral artery diseases (PAD). A critical concern in diabetes care is the diabetic foot syndrome, characterized by foot ulcers combined with neuropathy, PAD, and infection, often leading to lower limb amputations. Additionally, diabetes leads to several other complications that do not fall strictly into these categories, such as dental

J. Kesavadev (✉) · K. Jothydev · A. Basanth
Jothydev's Diabetes Research Centre, Trivandrum, Kerala, India
e-mail: academics@jothydev.net; krishnadev@jothydev.net

G. Abraham et al. (eds.), *Management of Diabetic Complications*,
https://doi.org/10.1007/978-981-97-6406-8_3

diseases, a lowered resistance to infections, and complications during birth in cases of gestational diabetes [3].

Individuals with diabetes often experience a significant reduction in their QoL due to the extensive treatment requirements and complications associated with the disease. This reduction in QoL is notably more pronounced when compared to individuals without diabetes. Research has shown that a major contributing factor to this decreased quality of life is the impaired physical functionality resulting from diabetic complications. Additionally, the anxiety and depression often experienced due to fluctuating glucose levels further exacerbate the decline in QoL among people with diabetes [4].

3.1.2 Importance of Preventing Complications

The primary objective in preventing and managing diabetes complications is to reduce morbidity and mortality while enhancing the quality of life. Additionally, there is a significant focus on reducing the financial burden that diabetes imposes. This includes both direct costs, such as medical expenses, and indirect costs, like loss of productivity, which affect not only the individuals living with diabetes but also their families. The impact extends beyond personal finances to strain local, national, and global resources. Efficient management and preventive measures can lead to better health outcomes for patients and, in the long run, contribute to economic savings and resource optimization at multiple levels [5].

Effectively managing diabetes is key to minimizing the risk of its complications. Proper control of blood glucose levels can lower the likelihood of developing eye, kidney, and nerve diseases by up to 40%. Managing blood pressure (BP) is also crucial; it can diminish the risk of heart disease and stroke by approximately 33% to 50%. Moreover, maintaining optimal cholesterol levels can lead to a 20% to 50% reduction in cardiovascular complications.

Regular eye examinations and prompt treatments are vital as well, with the potential to prevent up to 90% of blindness caused by diabetes. Healthcare services that emphasize regular foot examinations and provide patient education can play a significant role in preventing up to 85% of amputations related to diabetes.

Additionally, early detection and treatment of diabetic kidney disease, particularly through kidney-protective medications that control BP, can slow the deterioration of kidney function by 33% to 37%. These statistics underscore the importance of comprehensive diabetes management in preserving the health and well-being of individuals with this condition (Table 3.1) [6].

In the context of preventing diabetes complications, the advent of digital tools and devices has been a game changer. These technological advancements are instrumental in each step of diabetes management and prevention.

Table 3.1 Landmark trials for the prevention of diabetes and its complications

Trial	Objectives	Outcomes
Action for Health in Diabetes (Look AHEAD)	Evaluated whether weight loss reduces the risk for cardiovascular disease events, such as heart attack, stroke, and other health problems in people who were overweight or had obesity and T2D	No significant effect on cardiovascular disease Significant benefits on blood pressure, blood glucose, blood cholesterol, fitness, QoL, sleep apnea, hospitalization frequency
Diabetes Prevention Program (DPP)	Evaluated whether the DPP Lifestyle Change Program or taking metformin would delay or prevent T2D	Satisfactory results were observed particularly in participants aged 60 years in lowering their chances of developing T2D
UK Prospective Diabetes Study (UKPDS)	Determined the effect of intensive blood glucose control on 21 predetermined clinical end points, using blood glucose control, sulphonylureas or insulin therapy, or in overweight patient, treatment with metformin Explored the impact of intensive blood pressure control on macro- and microvascular complications and compared captopril treatment with atenolol	Captopril and atenolol were found to be equally effective as antihypertensive agents, in preventing macrovascular complications and in reducing the progression of retinopathy and albuminuria
Action to Control Cardiovascular Risk in Diabetes (ACCORD)	Evaluated whether intensive therapy to control blood glucose levels in T2D would reduce CV events, compared to standard therapy	Intensive glucose lowering significantly increases the risk of CV and all-cause mortality
Action in Diabetes and Vascular Disease: Preterax and Diamicron MR Controlled Evaluation (ADVANCE)	Designed to assess whether intensifying glucose control to achieve an A1C of <6.5% would provide additional benefit in reducing the risk of both micro- and macrovascular disease	Intensive strategy with conventional agents contributes to a mean A1C levels of 6.5% safely with no rise in mortality has no significant effect in reducing macrovascular disease but reduces diabetic nephropathy by ~20%
LEADER (Liraglutide Effect and Action in Diabetes: Evaluation of CV Outcome Results)	Assessed the impact of liraglutide on CV outcomes in patients with type 2 diabetes and high CV risk	Liraglutide was associated with a significant reduction in CV mortality, nonfatal MI, or nonfatal stroke and a reduction in all-cause mortality
EMPA-REG OUTCOME Empagliflozin Cardiovascular Outcome Event Trial in type 2 diabetes mellitus patients—removing excess glucose	Evaluated the cardiovascular safety of empagliflozin in patients with T2D at high risk for CV events	Reduction of new onset or worsening of nephropathy, CV death and hospitalization for HF in CKD patients after treatment with empagliflozin

3.1.3 Technologies in Diabetes

Diabetes technology describes the hardware, devices, and software used by people with diabetes in managing the glycemic levels, avoiding the complications of diabetes, reducing the stress of living with diabetes, and making their lives better [4]. The evolution of diabetes technologies proffers patients with diabetes a wider arsenal of tools to achieve glycemic control and improve the quality of life. Interestingly, Bluetooth-enabled glucometers, continuous glucose monitoring (CGM) systems, and other devices are replacing conventional glucometers with a variety of novel features, including insulin-dosing facilitators and decision-support applications [7, 8]. In today's tech-world, insulin administration and blood glucose monitoring have transformed from multiple finger pricks in a day to a couple of swipes on a cell phone. Further, various CGM systems such as the real-time CGM has provided significant results to people with diabetes who, without a CGM, may have experienced potentially life-threatening complications. Majority of these devices are utilized in conjunction with comprehensive software systems and mobile applications [9].

The global uptake of wearable and mobile technologies paved the way for the healthcare sector to leverage treatment and related information in a portable and inexpensive manner [10]. Smart phones gained immense popularity owing to their robust processing capabilities and extensive use. Smart glucose and blood pressure monitors, activity trackers, and diet planners have become the most broadly accepted connected devices [11]. Wearable mini electrocardiographs, smart watches, smart clothing, etc. have arguably revolutionized the overall diabetes management ecosystem over the past 10 years [12]. Due to its ability to collect, store, transmit, and process data, these technologies have now become an inevitable part of diabetes management and care. Furthermore, the use of these technologies may help reduce the risk of acute complications and have a beneficial impact on psychosocial health by reducing the burden of diabetes.

Artificial intelligence (AI) is considered as the next cutting-edge technology in diabetes management [13]. Patients with diabetes may be overwhelmed with the thought of the extensive management strategies and may show a tendency toward skipping the prescribed methods. These circumstances can be prevented by the employment of AI. The combination of artificial intelligence approaches and advanced technologies enable hyper and hypoglycemia management, predict the value of blood glucose levels, predict insulin dosages, designing personalized management for each patient, and save them from early mortality risks [14].

Preventing complications associated with diabetes involves several key strategies:

- Early detection and treatment: Prompt identification of diabetes and adherence to prescribed treatment plans.
- Glycemic control: Effectively managing blood sugar levels to keep them within target ranges.

- BP management: Monitoring and maintaining blood pressure to avoid hypertension.
- Cholesterol management: Regulating cholesterol levels to prevent cardiovascular complications.
- Lifestyle management: This includes maintaining a healthy weight, engaging in regular physical activity, following a balanced diet, and ensuring adequate sleep.

3.1.3.1 Early Detection and Adherence to Treatment

Electronic solutions are revolutionizing patient and physician interactions in numerous ways. They facilitate the monitoring of physiological indicators, enhance patient status tracking, improve medication dosing, and boost treatment adherence. Self-management, an essential aspect of chronic illness prevention and management, needs to incorporate diverse techniques since it largely takes place outside traditional healthcare settings. Digital healthcare tools, including mobile apps, provide valuable benefits like informational messaging and prescription management. However, to be truly effective, they must be tailored to individual patient needs, offering support through all phases of medication and treatment, thereby optimizing adherence while still having scope for further enhancement [12].

- **Electronic health record (EHR):** EHR significantly streamlines the process of documenting, storing, and retrieving patient health information. This technological advancement is pivotal in early detection and effective management of diabetes, ensuring timely interventions and continuous monitoring of patient health.
- **Medication management applications:** These applications, designed to remind patients of their medication schedules, play a crucial role in enhancing adherence to treatment protocols. Adherence is a critical factor in the effective management of diabetes, as it ensures that patients consistently follow their prescribed treatment plans, for example, MyTherapy, Medisafe, Pill Reminder by Medisafe, Mango Health, Round Health, and Dosecast.
- **Telemedicine:** Telemedicine can be simply defined as the use of telecommunication equipment for delivering medical care; the simplest being via the telephone and most complex being via the connected devices and sophisticated telemedicine equipment. Tele ophthalmology, Tele podiatry, etc. are now becoming popular.

One example of a comprehensive diabetes care system that has been developed to harness the power of technology in diabetes care is the Diabetes Tele Management System (DTMS®). At Jothydev's Diabetes Research Centre, the use of telemedicine in diabetes care is embodied in DTMS®, which has been effectively utilized since 1997. DTMS® represents a comprehensive, multidisciplinary approach to diabetes management. It involves a team of experts, including physicians, nurses, dieticians, diabetes educators, pharmacists, and psychologists. The system employs customized software with a user-friendly interface to adjust medication dosages and provide personalized advice on diet and lifestyle. Unlike other telemedicine programs that might use fixed algorithms, DTMS® bases medication titration on various patient-specific characteristics.

Patients report their blood glucose values through phone, email, or a secure website. The DTMS® team then adjusts medication dosages based on these reports and individualized targets. Each teleconsultation also includes educational modules tailored to the patient's needs, covering topics like insulin injection techniques, diet, exercise, glucometer use, hypoglycemia, and medication compliance. This approach significantly reduces the need for frequent hospital visits, saving time and costs associated with travel, waiting, consultations, and lost work hours [15].

3.1.3.2 Glycemic Control

Glucose Meters

New Generation Blood Glucose Meters

New generation glucose meters are intended to monitor blood glucose (BG) with more reliability and accuracy as compared to conventional BG meters. They are accepted widely for BG monitoring with various beneficial features such as connectivity to the mobile phone, syncing data with websites and mobile apps via Bluetooth, data storage, and management in the cloud, color coding features that record and display readings as colored graphs, charts, and reminder alarms.

Following are some of the new generation BG meters, which are well established for their accuracy and available in most parts of the world (Table 3.2, Fig. 3.1).

Table 3.2 Diabetes management technologies

	Highlighted features	Software
Glucose meters		
OneTouch Verio®	ColorSure® technology	OneTouch Reveal®
CONTOUR®Plus ONE	smartLIGHT, second-Chance™, and sip-in sampling test strip, high accuracy	Contour™ Diabetes
Accu-Chek® instant	Synchronization with mySugr app	
Insulin delivery devices		
NovoPen® 6, NovoPen Echo Plus	Personal injection log	mySugr®, Glooko, and FreeStyle LibreLink
InPen	First FDA-cleared smart insulin pen system Only system that tracks active insulin	InPen™ App
Automated insulin delivery systems		
MiniMed™ 780G	Use in individuals with type 1 diabetes, aged ≥7 years SmartGuard technology, Guardian 4 sensor MiniMed™ Mio™ Advance infusion set	CareLink Connect
Omnipod 5	First and the only tubeless AID which got FDA approval Use in individuals with type 1 diabetes, aged ≥6 years SmartAdjust™ technology	SmartAdjust™ technology

(continued)

Table 3.2 (continued)

	Highlighted features	Software
Tandem t:slim X2	First interoperable insulin pump Can be used as a stand-alone insulin pump, or can be integrated with the Dexcom G6 CONTROL-IQ, BASAL-IQ technology for insulin delivery	t:connect® mobile app
Do-It Yourself Artificial Pancreas	"#WeAreNotWaiting" team initiative Self-designed hybrid closed-loop systems Not approved by FDA	
Diabetes management apps		
mySugr Glooko OneTouch Reveal	• Tracks blood glucose, meals, carbohydrates, physical activities, and medications • Personalized log-in screen which helps the individual-specific usage of app • Healthcare providers can use to remotely monitor patients, train patients, collect and monitor the remotely synced data ColorSure® technology	
CONTOUR DIABETES app	Collect, store, and analyze blood glucose readings from CONTOUR NEXT ONE meter	

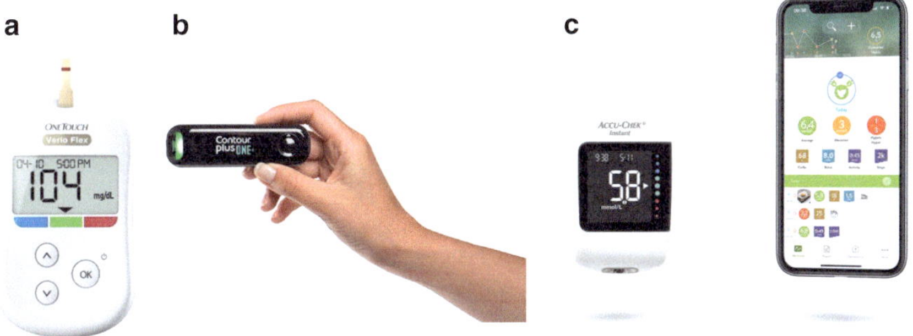

Fig. 3.1 Advanced glucose meters for diabetes management (**a**) OneTouch Verio® Meter, (**b**) CONTOUR®Plus ONE, (**c**) Accu-chek® Instant

- **OneTouch Verio® Meter:** OneTouch Verio® meter with its unique feature, the ColorSure® technology aids users to be aware of their current glycemic status in a more understandable color-coded manner. The results are displayed with a range indicator arrow pointing to a range indicating color bar, below the display as a visual reminder. The range indicator arrow and color bar can be together used to interpret the results. The meter can be synced to OneTouch Reveal® web app that collects data and creates simple, colorful reports to have meaningful interpretations of the data. The data will be instantly available in the cloud when the patients use the OneTouch Reveal® mobile app to wirelessly sync the OneTouch Verio®meter [16].

- **CONTOUR®Plus ONE:** CONTOUR®Plus ONE features data sharing via Bluetooth, smartLIGHT, second-Chance™, and Sip-in sampling test strip, which are designed to easily monitor the glycemic levels. The distinctive second-Chance™ sampling provides users a second chance sampling, that is, if in case the blood sample size is insufficient, subjects can apply more sample without wasting the test strip, if done within 60 s. The smartLIGHT feature offers users an instant indicator of the blood glucose results to know whether they are within (green), above (amber), or below (red) the target range. The system is simple to set up and easy to use, displaying results in 5 s. The Sip-in® sampling feature helps get the right amount of blood on the first try.
- The Contour®Plus ONE meter and Contour™ Diabetes app seamlessly connect via Bluetooth to capture the blood glucose readings that provides meaningful insights to the users to manage their diabetes easily. The device is compatible with Android or iOS device. Contour®Plus ONE is highly accurate and exceeds the ISO 15197: 2013 accuracy criteria, both in the laboratory and in clinical settings [17].
- **Accu-Chek® Instant:** Accu-Chek® Instant is intended to quantitatively measure glucose in fresh capillary whole blood from the conventional sites and also alternate sites such as palm, forearm, and upper arm. The salient features of the meter include effortless wireless synchronization with the mySugr diabetes management app, the easy-edge test strip, the intuitive target range indicator that provides visual reassurance and can be individualized to suit personal goals. The meter automatically stores at least 720 blood glucose results in memory, but only the last 7-, 30-, 90-day averages can be viewed. Users can view the stored blood glucose results after the transference of data to the Accu-Chek Connect Online diabetes management [18]. The users can also avail their estimated A1c or eA1c from mySugr app as the app syncs with the meter.

Noninvasive Blood Glucose Monitoring

Noninvasive BG monitoring refers to the detection of BG without drawing blood, puncturing the skin, or causing pain or trauma. Noninvasive BG detection includes optical methods, microwave methods, and electrochemical methods. Etouchus, GlucoTrack, DiamonTek, Eyva etc. are examples of noninvasive BG meters. The etouchus glucose meter uses sensor technology and has four touch type test points that read the results using the thumb and index fingers of both hands simultaneously. GlucoTrack is based on tracking the physiological effects of glucose variations in the earlobe tissue using three independent technologies: ultrasonic, electromagnetic, and thermal. D-base (which is a desktop device—roughly the size of a shoebox) intended for use by multiple people in a clinical setting), D-pocket (a hand-held device that fits in the user's pocket or handbag, and a finger press will provide glucose measurement), and D-sensor (an integrated sensor that can be worn as a bracelet) from Diamon-Tech are some of the other devices, which are awaiting FDA approval. Eyva is the world's first noninvasive glucose monitor and the world's first health-tech gadget designed by an Indian start-up called BlueSemi. This noninvasive gadget is capable of taking six biometric readings within just 60 s: blood glucose, temperature, ECG, heart rate, SpO_2 for blood oxygen, and blood pressure. Even though these devices possess potentially beneficial features, they still lack accuracy in the results which is a major limitation.

Insulin Delivery Systems

Connected Insulin Pens

Connected pens will integrate insulin injection data into certain apps/platforms and provide offer dosage advice/recommendations based on that information. There are two models of connected insulin pens: [19]

- Refillable insulin cartridges that feature built-in wireless communication abilities and sensors to track insulin delivery.
- Disposable pens with sensors in the form of a cap or a device that attaches to the side of the pen.

Types of Connected Insulin Pens:

- Tracking insulin pens (TIPs).
- Smart insulin pens (SIPs).
- Smart insulin caps.
  - **NovoPen® 6 & NovoPen Echo® Plus:** NovoPen® 6 and Novopen Echo® Plus automatically records the details of insulin dosing about each injection and can store the last 800 doses including flow check doses. These pens can be used with the prescribed Novo Nordisk insulin cartridges. The data on the effect of glucose levels as an outcome of insulin administration can be viewed side by side with glucose information from blood glucose meters and/or CGM. Patients can either bring the pen to the clinic, or if they have a smartphone, tablet, personal computer, blood glucose monitor, or another device that supports Near Field Communication (NFC), the insulin dosing information from these smart pens can be transferred to the device. The pens share compatibility with apps such as mySugr®, Glooko, and FreeStyle LibreLink [20].
  - **InPen:** InPen is the only FDA-cleared smart insulin pen that combines the Bluetooth® technology and intelligence through an easy-to-use smartphone app that helps patients administer correction and mealtime insulin doses. It is a home-use reusable pen injector for single-patient use by people with diabetes under the supervision of an adult caregiver, or by a patient aged seven and older for the self-injection of a desired dose of insulin under prescription. The pen injector is compatible with Humalog® U-100 3.0 mL cartridges, Novolog® U-100 3.0 mL cartridges, and Fiasp® U-100 3.0 mL cartridges and single-use detachable and disposable pen needles. The smart insulin injection system that collates a CGM and InPen™ can automatically log doses, provide mealtime and background insulin reminders, and reveals how diet and activities affects glucose levels. In addition, while using the i-Port Advance™ injection port, users can reduce needle pokes by 93% [21].

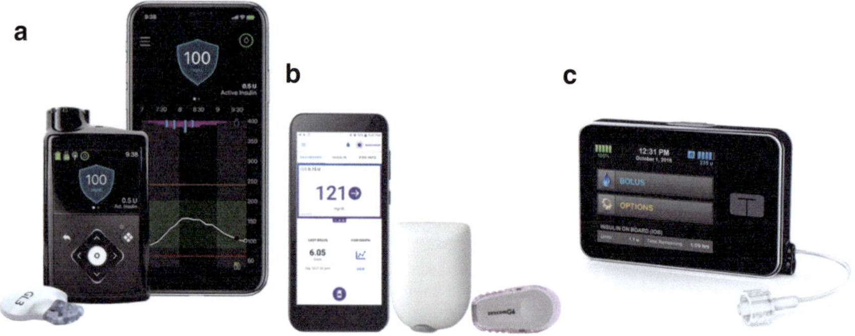

Fig. 3.2 Automated insulin delivery systems: (**a**) Medtronic 780G, (**b**) Omnipod 5, (**c**) Tandem tSlim X2

Automated Insulin Delivery Systems (AIDs)

Automated insulin delivery systems are automated or semi-automated systems automatically adjusts insulin delivery in response to blood glucose levels. The newer AID systems incorporate three components: the new generation insulin pumps, the continuous glucose monitoring device, and advanced control algorithm (Fig. 3.2) [22].

- **MiniMed™ 780G:** MiniMed™ 780G is the most advanced system from Medtronic approved by FDA for use in individuals with type 1 diabetes, aged 7 years and older. It continuously anticipates insulin needs, adjusts insulin delivery, automatically corrects highs, and prevents lows. It uses SmartGuard technology and the Guardian 4 sensor, which help achieve a Time-in-Range goal of >70% and an HbA1c goal of 7.0%. It has three major components: the Guardian 4 sensor, the MiniMed™ Mio™ Advance infusion set with a preloaded inserter, and a waterproof pump. The sensor measures the glucose levels every 5 min and sends the information to the waterproof pump. The pump gets glucose readings from the sensor and the transmitter automatically delivers a variable rate of insulin, 24 h a day based on individualized needs. 780G tracks the glucose levels and provides alarms, real-time glucose trends, and notifications on the connected smartphone via the CareLink Connect app. The system requires user-initiated meal announcements for optimal glycemic results. The auto correction feature compensates for occasionally missed meal doses. The MiniMed 780G system includes an Advanced Hybrid Closed Loop (AHCL) algorithm, which provides for both basal and correction bolus automated insulin delivery. The MiniMed™ 780G pump is now available in India [23].
- **Omnipod 5:** Omnipod 5 is the first and the only tubeless automated insulin delivery device which got FDA approval for use in people with type 1 diabetes aged 6 years and older. The system combines Omnipod patch pump with the Dexcom G6 CGM and a controller algorithm to automate insulin delivery.

Remarkably, Omnipod 5 makes history as the first system of its kind to get FDA clearance for mobile app control and insulin dosing directly from the user's smart phone, eliminating the need to always carry a separate controller unit. Omnipod 5 comprises three parts for the automated delivery of insulin: a tubeless, waterproof, wearable Pod, Dexcom G6 CGM system, and Omnipod 5 mobile app. The pod delivers insulin using built-in SmartAdjust™ technology, which receives a Dexcom CGM value and trend every 5 min and predicts the glucose value in the next 60 min. Individuals can place the pod on the arm, leg, back, abdomen, or buttocks. The system can also be controlled with the wireless Omnipod 5 Controller, which is provided at no additional cost with the first prescription [24].

- **Tandem t:slim X2:** Alternate controller-enabled (ACE) infusion pumps, unlike conventional stand-alone pumps, are interoperable. The first interoperable t:Slim X2 insulin pump got FDA authorization in 2019 for the subcutaneous insulin delivery in children and adults with diabetes. It can be used as a stand-alone insulin pump or integrated with the Dexcom G6 continuous glucose monitoring system. When used with CGM, users can choose either CONTROL-IQ technology or BASAL-IQ technology for insulin delivery. The pump can hold up to 300 units of insulin. The data can be uploaded wirelessly through the t:connect® mobile app, thus eliminating the need to plug the pump during in-patient visits [25].

Dual Hormone Closed-Loop Systems

Dual-hormone approaches intend to deliver two hormones: insulin and glucagon, or another hormone, to provide improved glycemic control. The major challenges in the dual-hormone closed-loop systems include increased system complexity, requirement of two separate infusion systems, and lack of approved room-temperature stable glucagon for subcutaneous delivery.

Do-It Yourself Artificial Pancreas (DIY-APs)

The developmental processes, clinical trials, and regulatory procedures mandatory for the commercialization of the AP systems are very complex and time-consuming. Frustrated by the slow pace and unaffordability of advanced insulin delivery systems, the Open APS, Loop, and Android APS communities, and caregivers gathered online in 2013 under the hashtag "#WeAreNotWaiting" to share knowledge of the open-source hardware and software solutions. This event marked the beginning of the DIY-APS movement. Patients with diabetes within this community initiated designing their own hybrid closed-loop systems from commercially available insulin pumps, CGM devices, and open-source algorithms. These automated insulin delivery systems developed by the tech-savvy diabetes enthusiasts of the #WeAreNotWaiting movement are generally known as a "Do-it-yourself" artificial pancreas. The lack of regulatory approvals for these systems still is the major hurdle to support the use of these devices by the diabetes care professionals even though the number of users of DIY-APs is increasing significantly worldwide [26].

3.1.3.3 Blood Pressure Management

Understanding blood pressure (BP) levels is crucial for assessing cardiovascular (CV) risk. Typically, a BP below 120/80 mmHg is considered normal. However, elevated BP levels are associated with increased risks of heart disease, heart attack, and stroke. Hypertension often coexists with other risk factors such as dyslipidemia, impaired glucose tolerance, and type 2 diabetes, amplifying CV risks.

Classification of Blood Pressure

The categorization of blood pressure is as follows:
Optimal: Systolic <120 mmHg and Diastolic <80 mmHg.
Normal: Systolic 120–129 mmHg and Diastolic 80–84 mmHg.
High-normal: Systolic 130–139 mmHg and/or Diastolic 85–89 mmHg.
Grade 1 hypertension: Systolic 140–159 mmHg and/or Diastolic 90–99 mmHg.
Grade 2 hypertension: Systolic 160–179 mmHg and/or Diastolic 100–109 mmHg.
Grade 3 hypertension: Systolic ≥180 mmHg and/or Diastolic ≥110 mmHg.
Isolated systolic hypertension: Systolic ≥140 mmHg and Diastolic <90 mmHg.
Isolated diastolic hypertension: Systolic <140 mmHg and Diastolic ≥90 mmHg.

Blood Pressure Measurement Devices

- Standard cuff-based devices: These devices, which have been in use for over a century, rely on indirect noninvasive methods. They include:
  - Manual auscultatory devices: Mercury sphygmomanometer, aneroid sphygmomanometer, and hybrid devices with digital displays.
  - Automated electronic devices: Automated oscillometric devices (including wrist cuff devices), automated auscultatory devices, and semi-automated devices.
- Cuffless blood pressure measuring devices: These modern devices, embedded in wearable technology and smartphones, address the dynamic nature of BP and are less intrusive than traditional methods.
- Standard office blood pressure measurement (OBPM).
  OBPM remains a widely used method for hypertension diagnosis despite its limitations and the growing use of out-of-office BP measurements. It is critical for establishing the diagnosis of hypertension, classifying BP, and determining BP-related CV risk.
- Home blood pressure monitoring (HBPM).
  HBPM offers multiple readings in a patient's usual environment, providing a more reproducible and predictive measure of cardiovascular outcomes and mortality compared to OBPM. For effective and reliable HBPM, it is recommended to use automated upper arm cuff devices. These devices, with features like automated data storage, averaging of multiple readings, and connectivity options (mobile phone, PC, or Internet), facilitate the physician's evaluation of BP values. The measurement conditions, including patient posture during HBPM, should align with those recommended for standard OBPM.
  A notable advantage of HBPM is its ability to minimize the white-coat effect, which refers to higher BP readings obtained in a clinical setting. As a result,

HBPM readings are generally lower than office BP values. In the absence of out-of-office BP data from randomized controlled trials (RCTs), the threshold for diagnosing hypertension at home is set slightly lower than in the clinical setting—at 135/85 mmHg, corresponding to the office BP threshold of 140/90 mmHg. Similarly, the target BP for home management is considered to be a few millimeters of mercury lower than the recommended office BP target.

- 24-h ambulatory BP monitoring (ABPM) and wearable BP devices.
  ABPM and HBPM, while effective, have limitations such as a finite number of measurements and potential discomfort. Wearable BP devices, such as the Omron HEM-6410 T and CareUp R Smartwatch, offer a convenient solution by providing continuous BP monitoring, thus improving hypertension management [27, 28].

3.1.3.4 Lifestyle Optimization

Lifestyle optimization plays a crucial role in both preventing diabetes and managing its complications. By adopting healthier habits and making conscious lifestyle choices, individuals can significantly reduce their risk of developing diabetes, and for those already diagnosed, such practices are key in controlling the disease and minimizing complications.

This includes maintaining a balanced diet, engaging in regular physical activity, achieving and sustaining a healthy weight, managing stress effectively, ensuring adequate and restful sleep, avoiding harmful habits like smoking and excessive alcohol consumption, and adhering to regular health checkups. These measures collectively contribute not only to better diabetes management but also to overall health enhancement. The use of digital tools enhances the effectiveness of these lifestyle changes.

- **Activity and fitness trackers:** By monitoring daily physical activity, these devices play a pivotal role in encouraging an active and healthy lifestyle. Example:
  - Fitbit: A popular wearable device that tracks daily steps, heart rate, and exercise intensity.
  - Garmin fitness trackers: Known for their durability and precision, ideal for outdoor activities.
  - Apple watch: Offers comprehensive fitness tracking, including workout detection and heart rate monitoring.
- **Nutritional tracking applications:** These tools assist in diet management by tracking food intake and offering nutritional insights. Example:
  - MyFitnessPal: A widely used app that tracks dietary intake and calories, with a large database of foods.
  - Lose It!: Focuses on calorie tracking and weight loss, with features for logging meals and snacks.
  - Cronometer: Offers detailed nutritional analysis, tracking not only calories but also micro- and macronutrients.

- **Sleep analysis tools:** Devices designed to monitor sleep patterns help in ensuring adequate and quality sleep, which is essential for overall health, especially in diabetes management. Example:
  - Fitbit (sleep tracking): Many Fitbit models include sleep tracking, analyzing sleep patterns and quality.
  - Sleep cycle: An app that analyzes sleep patterns and wakes you up during the lightest sleep phase.
  - Oura ring: A wearable device that provides detailed sleep analysis, including sleep stages and quality.

  Actigraphy employs a nonintrusive method to track the physical activity levels of individuals using a device similar to a wristwatch, capable of sensing motion. This device is designed for extended wear and is suitable for individuals of any age, whether used in a clinical lab or at home. By analyzing the patterns of rest and activity, actigraphy serves as an indirect indicator of sleep-wake cycles. As a result, it is highly beneficial in both research and clinical settings for the assessment of various sleep and movement-related disorders. Several actigraphy devices have gained FDA clearance, showcasing a range of options for monitoring physical activity and sleep patterns. These include ActGraph and Actiwatch® [29].
- **Weight management**: Sustained and modest weight loss emerges as a beneficial intervention, contributing to improvements in glycemia, blood pressure, and lipid profiles, potentially reducing the need for medications in individuals managing type 2 diabetes with overweight or obesity and experiencing inadequate control of various health parameters.

  In the era of modern technology, digital weighing machines have become indispensable tools for at-home weight monitoring. Ranging from smart scales to advanced bioelectrical impedance analysis machines, a variety of options are available in the market. With ongoing technological advancements, these digital weighing machines have evolved to become smarter and more intuitive, often seamlessly integrating with smartphones and fitness apps to provide real-time data and detailed insights into health and progress. Some contemporary models go beyond basic weight measurement and offer additional features such as assessing body fat percentage, muscle mass, and water weight. Important considerations when using a digital weighing machine at home include evaluating accuracy, weight capacity, body composition analysis capabilities, connectivity, and compatibility with other devices, as well as the display and user interface for ease of use [30].

3.1.4 Prevention of Diabetes Complications with the Use of Technologies

Diabetes can affect various organ systems in the body and, over time, can lead to serious complications that contribute substantially to morbidity and mortality.

- **Heart-related complications:** Cardiovascular disease (CVD) stands as the leading cause of death in individuals with diabetes, particularly type 2 diabetes.

Addressing multiple risk factors concurrently has shown considerable benefits, with notable improvements in the 10-year cardiovascular risk profile for diabetic patients. Key lifestyle interventions include adhering to a healthy diet, maintaining an optimal weight, engaging in regular physical activity, and managing the ABCs of diabetes—A1c, blood pressure, cholesterol, and smoking cessation. Additionally, managing stress is crucial in mitigating heart disease risks [31]. Incorporating technology into CVD prevention strategies, especially for individuals with diabetes, provides innovative and effective methods:

- Diet management applications: Tools like MyFitnessPal or Lose It! support users in adhering to diets that are low in saturated and trans fats, cholesterol, and sodium. These applications enable users to monitor their daily food consumption, offering valuable insights into nutritional content and aiding in maintaining a diet conducive to heart health.
- Weight management technologies: Integrating digital scales with smartphone applications aids in tracking weight fluctuations, assisting users in achieving and sustaining a healthy weight. These technologies often include motivational features and progress tracking.
- Activity and fitness tracking devices: Wearables, or smartphone-integrated applications, promote physical activity by monitoring steps, exercise activities, and providing movement reminders. These devices allow for the setting of personalized activity goals and track the user's advancement.
- Blood pressure monitoring devices: Smart blood pressure monitors or wearables facilitate regular home-based monitoring. They store and analyze blood pressure trends, providing valuable data that can be shared with healthcare providers for optimal management.
- Digital glucose monitoring systems: Technologies like continuous glucose monitoring systems (CGMs) and smart insulin pumps are pivotal in managing blood glucose levels (A1c), playing a key role in preventing cardiovascular complications in diabetes.
- Smoking cessation applications: Dedicated apps provide resources, support, and track progress in quitting smoking, a significant risk factor for heart disease.
- Stress management applications: These apps, offering meditation, mindfulness exercises, and stress management techniques, are beneficial in controlling stress, a known contributor to heart disease.
- Telehealth services: Virtual consultations and telemedicine platforms allow for regular communication with healthcare providers, ensuring treatment adherence and timely adjustments.

• **Kidney-related complications:** Kidney-related complications in diabetes, commonly known as "diabetic kidney disease" or previously termed "diabetic nephropathy," pose a significant health concern. Over time, this condition can progress to chronic kidney disease and potentially lead to kidney failure. To effectively manage and prevent diabetic kidney disease, it is essential to maintain blood glucose levels within target ranges, undergo regular A1C testing, monitor blood pressure, manage cholesterol, make dietary adjustments, engage in physical activity, and adhere to prescribed medications [32]. Incorporating technology can enhance the management of these factors:

- Digital glucose monitors and apps: Use continuous glucose monitoring systems (CGMs) or glucose tracking apps to maintain optimal blood glucose levels.
- Telehealth services: Regular virtual consultations can facilitate A1C test scheduling and medication reviews.
- Smart blood pressure monitors: These devices can track and record blood pressure readings over time, which can be shared with healthcare providers for better management.
- Nutritional tracking apps: Tools like MyFitnessPal, etc. assist in monitoring sodium intake and suggest healthier dietary choices.
- Fitness Trackers: Devices such as Fitbit, Apple watch, or other wearables encourage physical activity and track progress.
- Medication reminder apps: These apps ensure that medications are taken consistently and on time.

• **Nerve-related complications:** Diabetic neuropathy, a form of nerve damage, is a frequent complication arising from diabetes, often leading to decreased blood flow and sensation loss in the feet, thereby increasing the risk of severe foot complications like ulcers. Factors heightening the risk of nerve damage include poorly controlled blood glucose levels, prolonged diabetes duration, excess weight, being over 40, and having high blood pressure or cholesterol levels. To prevent or delay nerve damage, key strategies involve maintaining blood glucose levels within the target range, keeping blood pressure below 140/90 mmHg or as advised by a doctor, engaging in regular physical activity, weight management, limiting or avoiding alcohol, refraining from smoking, following a healthy diet, and adhering to prescribed medications [33]. Technological integration in these preventive measures includes:

- Digital blood glucose monitors: For accurate and regular monitoring of blood glucose levels.
- Smart blood pressure monitors: Enabling frequent home monitoring and data tracking of blood pressure.
- Fitness and activity trackers: To encourage and record regular physical activity.
- Digital scales and health apps: Assisting in weight management through monitoring and guidance.
- Mobile apps for alcohol moderation and smoking cessation: Offering support and tracking progress in limiting alcohol intake and quitting smoking, for example, Quit Tracker: Stop Smoking.
- Nutritional apps: For planning and tracking healthy eating habits.
- Medication reminder apps: To ensure adherence to prescribed drug regimens.

Diabetes foot care: For effective diabetic foot care, daily self-examination of the feet for any changes or injuries is essential, using a mirror or seeking assistance if needed. Daily foot washing with warm water, thorough drying, and careful application of lotion (excluding between the toes) is advised. It is important to always wear well-fitting shoes and socks, even indoors, to prevent injury, and to ensure shoes are free of objects and have a smooth lining. Toenails should be trimmed straight across and filed to avoid sharp edges, with a podiatrist consulted for any difficulties in self-care. Avoid self-removal of corns or calluses to prevent skin damage. Regular foot checkups should be part of healthcare visits, and an annual examination by a foot doctor is recommended, particularly for those with nerve damage. To maintain blood circulation, elevate feet when sitting and regularly wiggle toes. Engage in foot-friendly activities like walking, biking, or swimming, consulting with a doctor for suitable exercises [34].

- Technology can be incorporated into many of these steps to assist with foot care in diabetes:
  - Reminder apps: To ensure daily foot care routines are not missed, reminder apps can be set to prompt daily foot inspections and care activities.
  - Telehealth services: For patients who are unable to visit a podiatrist in person, telehealth services can be a valuable resource. Video consultations allow for remote evaluations of the feet, guidance on nail care, and advice on handling corns or calluses. Tele-podiatry is now among the most cost-effective solutions for remote detection and prevention of diabetic foot especially during the Covid pandemic. It is useful in referral of high-risk subjects for hospital/clinic visit, facilitating proper management. It also helps in the follow-up of the cases.
  - Activity tracking apps: These apps can be used to track and encourage feet-friendly activities like walking or swimming, as recommended by a healthcare provider.
- **Eye-related complications:** Diabetes can lead to a variety of eye-related issues, with diabetic retinopathy being the most prevalent. This condition involves abnormal growth and leakage of blood vessels in the retina, potentially leading to vision loss or blindness if untreated. Diabetic macular edema, glaucoma, and cataracts are also common eye problems in diabetic patients. Regular eye examinations are crucial for early detection and treatment of these conditions, helping to maintain vision. To prevent eye-related complications in diabetes, it is crucial to have annual dilated eye exams for early issue detection and maintain blood glucose levels within target ranges to protect eye blood vessels and vision. Additionally, managing blood pressure and cholesterol, quitting smoking, and staying physically active are essential [35]. Technology plays a significant role in these preventive measures:
  - Teleophthalmology: Offers remote eye exams and consultations, making it easier to access regular eye care.
  - Digital glucose monitoring devices: Continuous monitoring of blood glucose levels to prevent fluctuations that can affect eye health.
  - Mobile health apps: Track physical activities, blood pressure, and cholesterol levels, promoting lifestyle changes beneficial for eye health.
  - Smoking cessation apps: Provide support and resources for those trying to quit smoking.

3.2 Conclusion

Many complications arising from diabetes can be avoided through the meticulous maintenance of specific health targets. By keeping glucose levels within the recommended range, minimizing the occurrence of hypoglycemia, achieving, and sustaining a healthy body weight, meeting goals for blood pressure and lipid levels, ensuring consistent adherence to prescribed medications, and embracing a wholesome lifestyle, individuals can significantly reduce the risk of complications.

In the realm of modern health care, the integration of connected glucose meters, blood pressure apparatus, weighing scales, wearable sensors for monitoring sleep, heart rate, and glucose levels, as well as mobile health (mHealth) applications tailored for comprehensive diabetes care, coupled with the implementation of telemedicine, assumes a pivotal role. This technological synergy holds the promise of not only preventing complications but also adding life to the years of those living with diabetes.

References

1. The Lancet. Diabetes: a defining disease of the 21st century. Lancet. 2023;401:2087. https://www.thelancet.com/journals/lancet/article/PIIS0140-6736(23)01296-5/fulltext. Accessed 14 Nov 2023.
2. Ali J, Haider SMS, Ali SM, Haider T, Anwar A, Hashmi AA. Overall clinical features of type 2 diabetes mellitus with respect to gender. Cureus. 2023;15(3):e35771.
3. Papatheodorou K, Banach M, Bekiari E, Rizzo M, Edmonds M. Complications of diabetes 2017. J Diabetes Res. 2018;2018:3086167.
4. Pham TB, Nguyen TT, Truong HT, Trinh CH, Du HNT, Ngo TT, et al. Effects of diabetic complications on health-related quality of life impairment in Vietnamese patients with type 2 diabetes. J Diabetes Res. 2020;2020:4360804.
5. Prevention and Management of Diabetic Complications. PCORE. 2023. https://edblogs.columbia.edu/pcore/diabetes-prevention-and-management-of-diabetic-complications/. Accessed 14 Nov 2023.
6. Health and Economic Benefits of Diabetes Interventions. Power of Prevention. 2023. https://www.cdc.gov/chronicdisease/programs-impact/pop/diabetes.htm. Accessed 14 Nov 2023.
7. Didyuk O, Econom N, Guardia A, Livingston K, Klueh U. Continuous glucose monitoring devices: past, present, and future focus on the history and evolution of technological innovation. J Diabetes Sci Technol. 2021;15(3):676–83.
8. Daly A. Technology in the management of type 2 diabetes: present status and future prospects. Diabetes Obes Metab. 2021;23:1722. Accessed 14 Nov 2023. https://doi.org/10.1111/dom.14418.
9. Doupis J, et al. Smartphone-based technology in diabetes management. Diabetes Ther. 2020;11:607. Accessed 14 Nov 2023. https://doi.org/10.1007/s13300-020-00768-3.
10. Wright R, Keith L. Wearable technology: if the tech fits, wear it. J Electron Resour Med Libr. 2014;11(4):204–16.
11. Dankwa-Mullan I, Rivo M, Sepulveda M, Park Y, Snowdon J, Rhee K. Transforming diabetes care through artificial intelligence: the future is here. Popul Health Manag. 2019;22(3):229.
12. Fagherazzi G, Ravaud P. Digital diabetes: perspectives for diabetes prevention, management and research. Diabetes Metab. 2019;45(4):322–9.
13. Ellahham S. Artificial intelligence: the future for diabetes care. Am J Med. 2020;133(8):895–900.

14. Makroum MA, et al. Machine learning and smart devices for diabetes management: systematic review. Sensors. 2022;22:1843. https://www.ncbi.nlm.nih.gov/pmc/articles/PMC8915068/. Accessed 14 Nov 2023.
15. Kesavadev J, Saboo B, Shankar A, Krishnan G, Jothydev S. Telemedicine for diabetes care: an Indian perspective—feasibility and efficacy. Indian J Endocrinol Metab. 2015;19(6):764–9.
16. OneTouch Verio Flex®. Blood Glucose Meter. OneTouch®. https://www.onetouch.com/products/glucose-meters/onetouch-verio-flex. Accessed 14 Nov 2023.
17. CONTOUR PLUS ONE. Your diabetes, illuminated. https://www.diabetes.ascensia.in/products/contour-plus-one/. Accessed 14 Nov 2023.
18. Accu-Chek® [Internet]. Accu-Chek instant S. https://www.accu-chek.in/meter-systems/instant-s. Accessed 14 Nov 2023.
19. What is a smart insulin pen? ADA. https://diabetes.org/about-diabetes/devices-technology/smart-insulin-pen. Accessed 14 Nov 2023.
20. Novo Nordisk [Internet]. NovoPen® 6 and NovoPen Echo® Plus. https://www.novonordisk.com/content/nncorp/global/en/our-products/smart-pens/novopen-6.html. Accessed 14 Nov 2023.
21. InPen™ Smart Insulin Pen. Medtronic Diabetes [Internet]. https://www.medtronicdiabetes.com/products/inpen-smart-insulin-pen-system. Accessed 14 Nov 2023.
22. Sherr JL, Heinemann L, Fleming GA, Bergenstal RM, Bruttomesso D, Hanaire H, et al. Automated insulin delivery: benefits, challenges, and recommendations. A consensus report of the joint diabetes technology working Group of the European Association for the study of diabetes and the American Diabetes Association. Diabetologia. 2023;66(1):3–22.
23. MiniMed™ 780G System. Medtronic [Internet]. https://www.medtronicdiabetes.com/products/minimed-780g-insulin-pump-system. Accessed 14 Nov 2023.
24. Omnipod® 5 Automated Insulin Delivery System | Omnipod [Internet]. https://www.omnipod.com/what-is-omnipod/omnipod-5. Accessed 14 Nov 2023.
25. Diabetes Management. Insulin Pumps. Tandem Diabetes Care [Internet]. https://www.tandemdiabetes.com/home. Accessed 14 Nov 2023.
26. The Do-It-Yourself Artificial Pancreas. https://pubmed.ncbi.nlm.nih.gov/34264792/. Accessed 14 Nov 2023.
27. Mancia G, Kreutz R, Brunström M, Burnier M, Grassi G, Januszewicz A, et al. 2023 ESH guidelines for the management of arterial hypertension the task force for the management of arterial hypertension of the European Society of Hypertension: endorsed by the International Society of Hypertension (ISH) and the European Renal Association (ERA). J Hypertens. 2023;41(12):1874.
28. Konstantinidis D, Iliakis P, Tatakis F, Thomopoulos K, Dimitriadis K, Tousoulis D, et al. Wearable blood pressure measurement devices and new approaches in hypertension management: the digital era. J Hum Hypertens. 2022;36(11):945–51.
29. Krishna J, Mashaqi S. Actigraphy. In: Aminoff MJ, Daroff RB, editors. Encyclopedia of the neurological sciences. 2nd ed. Oxford: Academic Press; 2014. p. 36–40. https://www.sciencedirect.com/science/article/pii/B9780123851574005479. Accessed 16 Nov 2023.
30. ElSayed NA, Aleppo G, Aroda VR, Bannuru RR, Brown FM, Bruemmer D, et al. 8. Obesity and weight management for the prevention and treatment of type 2 diabetes: standards of care in diabetes—2023. Diabetes Care. 2023;46(Suppl 1):S128–39.
31. CDC. Centers for Disease Control and Prevention. Diabetes and your heart. 2022. https://www.cdc.gov/diabetes/library/features/diabetes-and-heart.html. Accessed 14 Nov 2023.
32. CDC. Centers for Disease Control and Prevention. Make the connection. 2021. https://www.cdc.gov/diabetes/managing/diabetes-kidney-disease.html. Accessed 14 Nov 2023.
33. CDC. Centers for Disease Control and Prevention. Diabetes and nerve damage. 2022. https://www.cdc.gov/diabetes/library/features/diabetes-nerve-damage.html. Accessed 14 Nov 2023.
34. CDC. Centers for Disease Control and Prevention. Diabetes and your feet. 2023. https://www.cdc.gov/diabetes/library/features/healthy-feet.html. Accessed 14 Nov 2023.
35. CDC. Centers for Disease Control and Prevention. Diabetes and vision loss. 2022. https://www.cdc.gov/diabetes/managing/diabetes-vision-loss.html. Accessed 14 Nov 2023.

Cardiovascular Diseases Caused by Diabetes: An Overview of Pathogenesis and Treatment

4

A. B. Gopalamurugan and L. Srichandran

4.1 Introduction

Diabetes mellitus (DM) is one of the major risk factors associated with cardiovascular disease (CVD) [1–4]. Its prevalence and associated complications including coronary artery disease, cardiac autonomic neuropathy (CAN), and hypertension are higher in diabetic patients compared to nondiabetics. CVD is the leading cause of mortality and morbidity in diabetic populations [1–4]. The death rates in the United States are 1.7 times higher in adults with DM than those without, mainly due to an increased risk of stroke and a twofold risk of death from myocardial infarction. Here, the pathogenesis and treatment of two conditions are discussed: cardiac autonomic neuropathy and coronary artery disease.

CVD risk factors such as obesity, dyslipidemia, and hypertension are more common in patients with T2DM. These patients also present with factors such as increased coagulability, increased oxidative stress, and endothelial dysfunction that contribute to the development of CVD and increased prevalence of myocardial infarction, revascularization, and stroke. Atherosclerosis and atherothrombosis happen in earlier ages, progress quicker, and are associated with more complications among diabetic patients. T2DM is a prothrombotic and hypercoagulable state predisposing to increased thrombin generation by platelets, thrombus formation, and impaired fibrinolysis. This is due to increased levels of plasminogen activator inhibitor-1. Diabetic patients not only have an increased risk of atherosclerosis but can also have an accelerated progression of stable plaques to unstable or ruptured plaques.

A. B. Gopalamurugan (✉) · L. Srichandran
MGM Healthcare, Chennai, Tamil Nadu, India
e-mail: secretary@gopalamurugan.com; srichandran.l@mgmhealthcare.in

G. Abraham et al. (eds.), *Management of Diabetic Complications*,
https://doi.org/10.1007/978-981-97-6406-8_4

Due to obesity and the production of advanced glycation end products (AGE), patients with diabetes also have higher levels of subclinical inflammation and develop endothelial dysfunction [5, 6] (Fig. 4.1). Hypercholesterolemia, inflammation, and endothelial dysfunction are some of the key mechanisms involved in the progression of atherosclerotic coronary artery disease.

The best treatment for coronary artery disease for patients with diabetes mellitus is prevention. It is essential to make therapeutic lifestyle changes as well as taking medications such as SGLT2 inhibitors and statins. Aspirin is commonly used in patients with DM to prevent CVD. In comparison to other antiplatelet medications, aspirin has the lowest risk of bleeding. Clopidogrel has also shown a reduction in CVD in patients. Avoiding episodes of hypoglycemia is also essential in preventing any arrhythmias and acute coronary syndrome. It is important to reduce insulin resistance through weight management plans, exercise, and surgery, if required.

Cardiac autonomic neuropathy (CAN) is a type of diabetic neuropathy that happens when autonomic nerve fibers responsible for the innervation of the heart and blood vessels become damaged (Fig. 4.2).

It is a common microvascular complication of T2DM with a multifactorial etiology not entirely understood. CAN causes dysfunction of the autonomic nervous system and disrupts the balance between the sympathetic and parasympathetic branches responsible for regulating important cardiovascular functions including

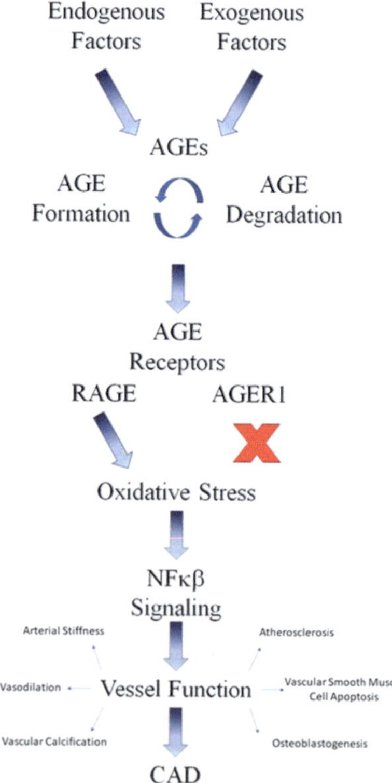

Fig. 4.1 Consequences of AGE formation

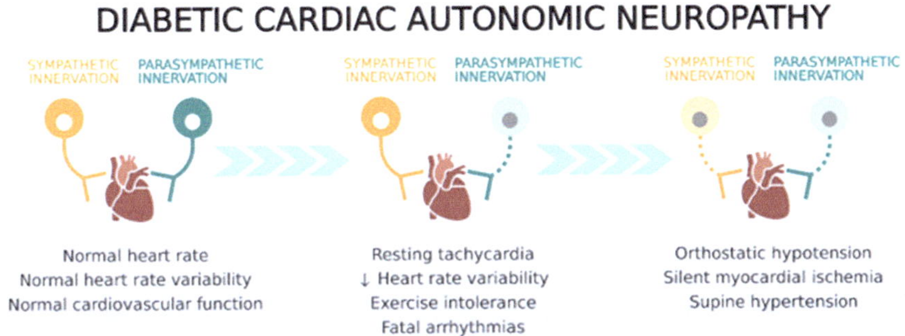

Fig. 4.2 CAN symptoms as progressive denervation occurs

heart rate and blood pressure. Risk factors for developing CAN include increased age, increased duration of T2DM, female sex, and smoking. Clinical manifestations of CAN include resting tachycardia, postural hypotension, and asymptomatic myocardial ischemia, among others. CAN increases with the duration of disease, and therefore manifestations appear in the later stages.

It is thought that the primary driver of CAN is persistent hyperglycemia which ultimately causes oxidative stress. One of the causative mechanisms is the activation of the polypol pathway, which uses NADPH as a cofactor. As NADPH continuously is depleted, the production of reactive oxygen species increases, exceeding antioxidant levels and causing oxidative stress. Oxidative stress is further increased by the nonenzymatic glycosylation of lipids and proteins resulting in the formation of AGEs. AGEs and oxidative stress can both lead to nerve hypoxia and axonal degeneration.

The longest nerves are affected first by neuropathy, which is why often the first manifestation seen in this complication is resting tachycardia [7, 8]. The vagus nerve, which is responsible for the parasympathetic innervation of the heart is one of the first to be affected. The parasympathetic nervous system acts to decrease heart rate; thus, damage to it causes the sympathetic nervous system to dominate, leading to an increase in heart rate. As the disease progresses and other fibers become affected, the sympathetic nerves become damaged and the tachycardia reduces. To combat resting tachycardia, beta-1 adrenergic antagonists may be prescribed, reducing sympathetic function to the heart and balancing out the two autonomic branches.

Orthostatic hypotension can develop as a result of CAD in patients with DM. It is defined as a drop of 20 mmHg systolic or 10 mmHg diastolic pressure after standing. Upon standing, gravity will cause the pooling of blood to lower body parts. Following the Frank–Starling curve, this leads to a drop in venous return and subsequently a reduced end-diastolic volume, ultimately reducing stroke volume and so cardiac output. In people unaffected by CAD, baroreceptors in the carotid sinus sense this drop in arterial pressure and increase sympathetic drive, causing compensatory vasoconstriction and increased vascular resistance, all with the aim of increasing venous return to the heart. In contrast, denervation to efferent sympathetic fibers in those with CAD results in a loss of this compensatory response, and may experience pre-syncopal symptoms such as lightheadedness, blurred vision, diaphoresis, and weakness, followed by syncope. To treat this condition, lifestyle methods can be employed including increased water intake, avoiding quick postural changes, as well as the use of compression stockings. Pharmacological management includes the prescription of fludrocortisone, a mineralocorticoid which causes increased plasma volume, or midodrine, a peripheral alpha-1 agonist, causing increased blood pressure via vasoconstriction. Good glycemic control is essential in preventing the progression of CAN and will reduce further complications. Difficulties can arise as certain medications used to treat DM and associated conditions, for example, insulin or tricyclic antidepressants, can cause orthostatic hypotension.

On top of previously discussed factors surrounding coronary artery disease, the higher rates of myocardial infarction-related morbidity and mortality seen in diabetics may be in part due to asymptomatic myocardial ischemia seen in CAN. With no warnings, patients are not alerted to any morbidity and so do not seek medical attention and the disease is allowed to progress, and complications including heart failure and arrhythmias can occur.

To conclude, there are multiple pathophysiological mechanisms by which DM can cause CVD, notably the formation of AGEs. Additionally, multiple risk factors for CVD in the general population are seen in higher rates in those with DM. As discussed, the management of CVD in patients with DM includes lifestyle modifications, glycemic control, pharmacological approaches, as well as surgical intervention; however, it is also worth noting that some medications used to treat DM can provoke additional cardiovascular symptoms. Addressing CVD risk factors such as obesity and smoking is necessary to reduce the morbidity and mortality seen in those with DM.

4.2 Heart Failure Management

Four pillars of heart failure therapy are:

1. ARNI.
2. Beta-blockers.
3. SGLT-2 inhibitors.
4. Mineralocorticoid receptor antagonist.

In patients with HfrEF with symptoms, a combination of these four agents as shown in trials to reduce morbidity and mortality compared with placebo [9–11]. Meta-analysis of trials of the above therapy for patients with HfrEF suggest that the addition of these four molecules reduced the risk of all-cause mortality compared to placebo (HR −0.39, 95% CI 0.31–0.49) (Fig. 4.3).

The treatment of heart failure with preserved ejection fraction (HFpEF) is given in Fig. 4.4.

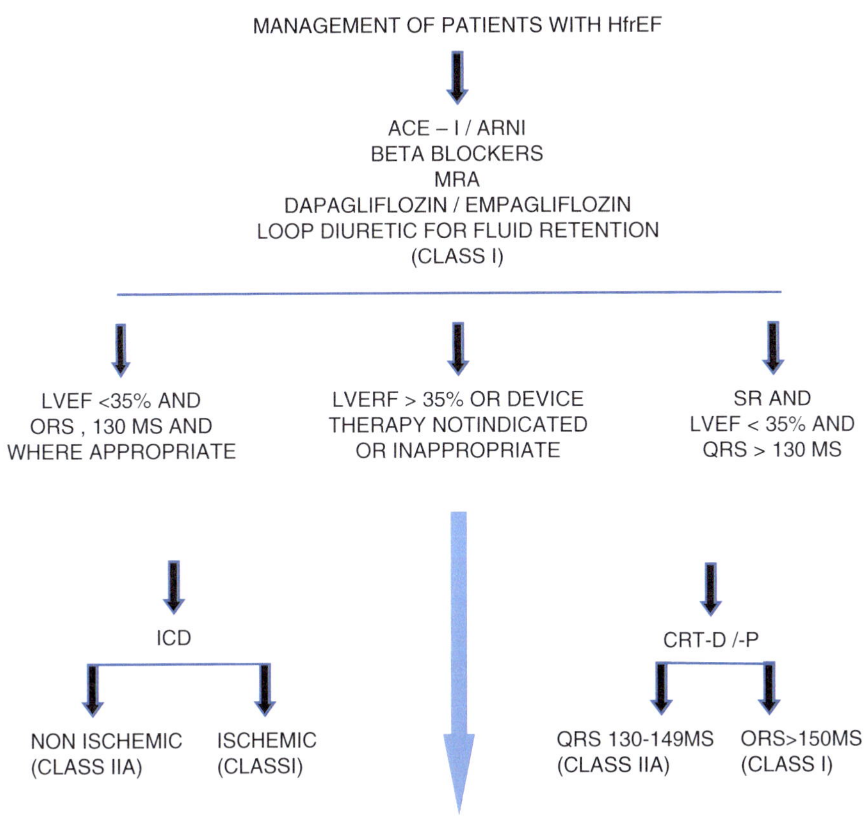

Fig. 4.3 Therapeutic algorithm of class i therapy indications for a patient with heart failure with reduced ejection fraction

1. **Angiotensin-Converting Enzyme Inhibitors**

   ACE-Is were the first class of drugs shown to reduce mortality and morbidity in patients with HfrEF. They have also been shown to improve symptoms. They are recommended in all patients unless contraindicated or not tolerated. They should be uptitrated to the maximum tolerated recommended doses.

2. **Beta-Blockers**

   Beta-blockers have been shown to reduce mortality and morbidity in patients with HFrEF, in addition to treatment with an ACE-I and diuretic. They also improve symptoms by decreasing sympathetic over activity, decreasing heart rate, and optimizing myocardial oxygen demand. There is consensus that ACE-I and beta-blockers can be commenced together as soon as the diagnosis of symptomatic HFrEF is established. There is no evidence favoring the initiation of a beta-blocker before an ACE-I and vice versa. Beta-blockers should be initiated in clinically stable, euvolemic, patients at a low dose and gradually uptitrated to

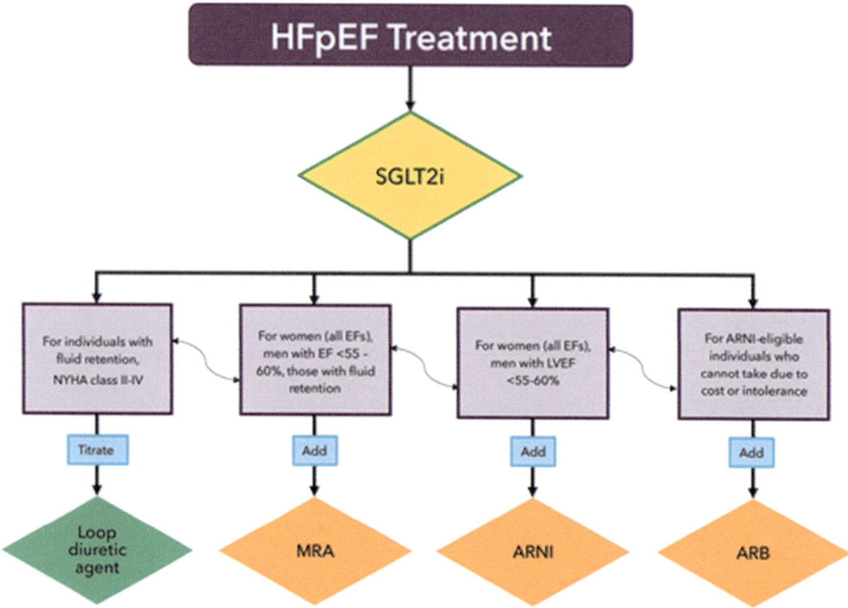

Fig. 4.4 Heart failure with preserved EF treatment [1]

the maximum tolerated dose. In patients admitted with AHF, beta-blockers should be cautiously initiated in hospital, once the patient is hemodynamically stabilized.

3. **Mineralocorticoid Receptor Antagonists**

   MRAs (spironolactone or eplerenone) are recommended, in addition to an ACE-I and a beta-blocker, in all patients with HFrEF to reduce mortality and the risk of HF hospitalization. They improve symptoms by reducing ventricular remodelling in HF. MRAs block receptors that bind aldosterone and, with different degrees of affinity, other steroid hormones (e.g., corticosteroid and androgen) receptors. Eplerenone is more specific for aldosterone blockade and, therefore, causes less gynecomastia. Caution should be exercised when MRAs are used in patients with impaired renal function and in those with serum potassium concentrations >5.0 mmol/L. Dose: Spironolactone—12.5 mg/25 mg. Finerenone—increases outcome in heart failure and CKD patients. Dose: Finerenone if eGFR >60 = 20 mg, if eGFR >25 to <60 = 10 mg, if eGFR >25 = not indicated).

4. **Angiotensin Receptor-Neprilysin Inhibitor**

   In the PARADIGM-HF trial, sacubitril/valsartan, an ARNI, was shown to be superior to enalapril in reducing hospitalizations for worsening HF, CV mortality, and all-cause mortality in patients with ambulatory HFrEF with LVEF $\leq$40% (changed to $\leq$35% during the study). Patients in the trial had elevated plasma NP concentrations, an eGFR $\geq$30 mL/min/1.73 m^2 and were able to tolerate enalapril and then sacubitril/valsartan during the run-in period. Additional benefits of sacubitril/valsartan included an improvement in symptoms and QOL, a reduction in the incidence of diabetes requiring insulin treatment, and a reduction in the decline in eGFR, as well as a reduced rate of hyperkalemia. Additionally, the use of sacubitril/valsartan may allow a reduction in loop diuretic requirement. Symptomatic hypotension was reported more commonly in patients treated with sacubitril/valsartan as compared to enalapril, but despite developing hypotension, these patients also gained clinical benefits from sacubitril/valsartan therapy. Therefore, it is recommended that an ACE-I or ARB is replaced by sacubitril/valsartan in ambulatory patients with HFrEF, who remain symptomatic despite optimal treatment outlined above. Two studies have examined the use of ARNI in hospitalized patients, some of whom had not been previously treated with ACE-I. Initiation in this setting appears safe and reduces subsequent CV death or HF hospitalizations by 42% compared to enalapril. As such, initiation of sacubitril/valsartan in ACE-I naive (i.e., de novo) patients with HFrEF may be considered (class of recommendation IIb, level of evidence B). Patients being commenced on sacubitril/valsartan should have an adequate blood pressure (BP), and an eGFR ≥30 mL/min/1.73 m^2. A washout period of at least 36 h after ACE-I therapy is required in order to minimize the risk of angioedema.

5. **Sodium-Glucose Cotransporter 2 Inhibitors**

   The DAPA-HF trial investigated the long-term effects of dapagliflozin (SGLT2 inhibitor) compared to placebo in addition to optimal medical therapy (OMT), on morbidity and mortality in patients with ambulatory HfrEF (Fig. 4.5). Patients participated in the trial if they were in NYHA class II–IV, and had an LVEF ≤40% despite OMT. Patients were also required to have an elevated plasma NT-proBNP and an eGFR ≥30 mL/min/1.73 m^2. Therapy with dapagliflozin resulted in a 26% reduction in the primary end point: a composite of worsening HF (hospitalization or an urgent visit resulting in i.v. therapy for HF) or CV death. Both of these components were significantly reduced. Moreover, dapagliflozin reduced all-cause mortality, alleviated HF symptoms, improved physical function, and QOL in patients with symptomatic HfrEF. Benefits were seen early after the initiation of dapagliflozin, and the absolute risk reduction was large. Survival benefits were seen to the same extent in patients with HFrEF with and without diabetes, and across the whole spectrum of HbA1c values. Subsequently, the EMPEROR-reduced trial found that empagliflozin reduced the combined primary end point of CV death or HF hospitalization by 25% in patients with NYHA class II–IV symptoms, and an LVEF ≤40% despite OMT. This trial included patients with an eGFR >20 mL/min/1.73 m^2 and there was also a reduction in the decline in eGFR in individuals receiving empagliflozin. It was also associated with an improvement in QOL. Although there was not a significant reduction in CV mortality in the EMPEROR-reduced trial, a recent meta-analysis of the DAPA-HF and EMPEROR-reduced trials found no heterogeneity in CV mortality. Therefore, dapagliflozin or empagliflozin are recommended, in addition to OMT with an ACE-I/ARNI, a beta-blocker and an MRA, for patients with HFrEF regardless of diabetes status. The diuretic/natriuretic properties of SGLT2 inhibitors may offer additional benefits in reducing

Drug Class	Contraindications	Cautions
SGLT2i	Type 1 diabetes mellitus (limitation to use) Lactation On dialysis Known hypersensitivity	Kidney impairment: For dapagliflozin, eGFR <25 mL/min/1.73 m^2 For empagliflozin, eGFR <20 mL/min/1.73 m^2 Pregnancy Increased risk of mycotic genital infections May contribute to volume depletion or hypotension Ketoacidosis (including euglycemic) in individuals with poorly controlled diabetes, dehydration, or fasting Acute kidney injury Necrotizing fasciitis of the perineum (Fournier's gangrene) is rare but can be serious and life-threatening
MRA	Potassium ≥5.0 mmol/L Addison disease Pregnancy Known hypersensitivity	Kidney impairment: Avoid if eGFR <30 mL/min/1.73 m^2 or serum creatinine ≥2.5 mg/dL Initiate at half dose if eGFR 30 to 50 mL/min/1.73 m^2 Concomitant use with drugs and supplements that increase serum potassium, such as: Potassium supplementation ACE inhibitors, ARBs, or ARNIs NSAIDs Trimethoprim Gynecomastia (consider use of eplerenone) Lactation
ARNI	Coadministration within 36 h of ACE inhibitor use History of any angioedema Pregnancy/lactation Severe (Child-Pugh C) hepatic impairment Known hypersensitivity Use of aliskiren in individuals with diabetes mellitus	Reduce the starting dose to half the usually recommended starting dose if: Not currently taking an ACE inhibitor or ARB or taking a low dose of an ACE inhibitor or ARB Moderate (Child-Pugh B) hepatic impairment Renal artery stenosis Hypotension
ARB	Pregnancy/lactation Avoid concomitant use with an ACE inhibitor, aliskiren, or ARNI Known hypersensitivity Renal artery stenosis	History of any angioedema Hyperkalemia Hypotension Acute kidney injury

Fig. 4.5 Contraindications and cautions for SGLT2i, MRAs, ARNIs, and ARBs

congestion and may allow a reduction in loop diuretic requirement. The combined SGLT-1 and 2 inhibitor, sotagliflozin, has also been studied in patients with diabetes who were hospitalized with HF. The drug reduced CV death and hospitalization for HF. Therapy with SGLT2 inhibitors may increase the risk of recurrent genital fungal infections. A small reduction in eGFR following initiation is expected and reversible, and it should not lead to premature discontinuation of the drug.

6. **Hydrazaline and Nitrates**
   Can be considered in patients with intolerance to ACE, ARB, or ARNI (hypotension, hyperkalemia, worsening renal insufficiency). Target dose: Hydrazaline—75 mg, ISD—40 mg thrice a day.
7. **Digoxin**
   Not indicated as primary therapy. Mainly for patients with heart failure with reduced EF with controlled symptoms (Fatigue, dyspnea, reduced exercise tolerance) and in patients with Atrial fibrillation to control ventricular rate. Dose: 0.125 mg or less—based upon renal function. To monitor serum digoxin level between 0.5 to 0.8 ng/mL.
8. **Ivabradine**
   Specifically binds the funny channel. Reduces the slope for diastolic depolarization—prolongs diastolic duration. Does not alter ventricular repolarization, myocardial contractibility, and blood pressure. Indications: Patients with chronic HFrEF, LVEF <35%, sinus rhythm, and resting heart rate of >70 bpm.

4.2.1 Investigational Drugs

VERCIGUAT

Initial dose of 2.5 mg to maximum dose of 10 mg.

Soluble guanylate cyclase activator.

The incidence of primary outcome of death of cardiovascular causes or first hospitalization for heart failure are significantly lower with Verciguat than with placebo.

Side effects—hypotension, anemia, embryo fetal toxicity.

OMNECAMTIV MECARBI

Direct activation of cardiac myosin.

Dose 50 mg 1–0-1.

RT 100

Human AC 6 gene therapy-single dose via intra coronary injection [11].

4.2.2 Heart Transplant and Assisted Devices

The primary indication for heart transplant is severe, very symptomatic heart failure despite optical medical therapy [12, 13]. When there are no alternate options are contraindications. Heart transplantation is essentially rationed to those patients who have the greatest chance of durable benefit. An LVAD may be used as a bridge to transplant until a new heart becomes available or as a destination therapy. The goal is to alleviate signs and symptoms of heart failure and extend life.

4.3 Acute Coronary Syndrome

The algorithm for acute coronary syndrome (ACS) management is given in Fig. 4.6.

The management of ST elevation myocardial infarction (STEMI) and non-ST elevation are given in Figs. 4.7 and 4.8.

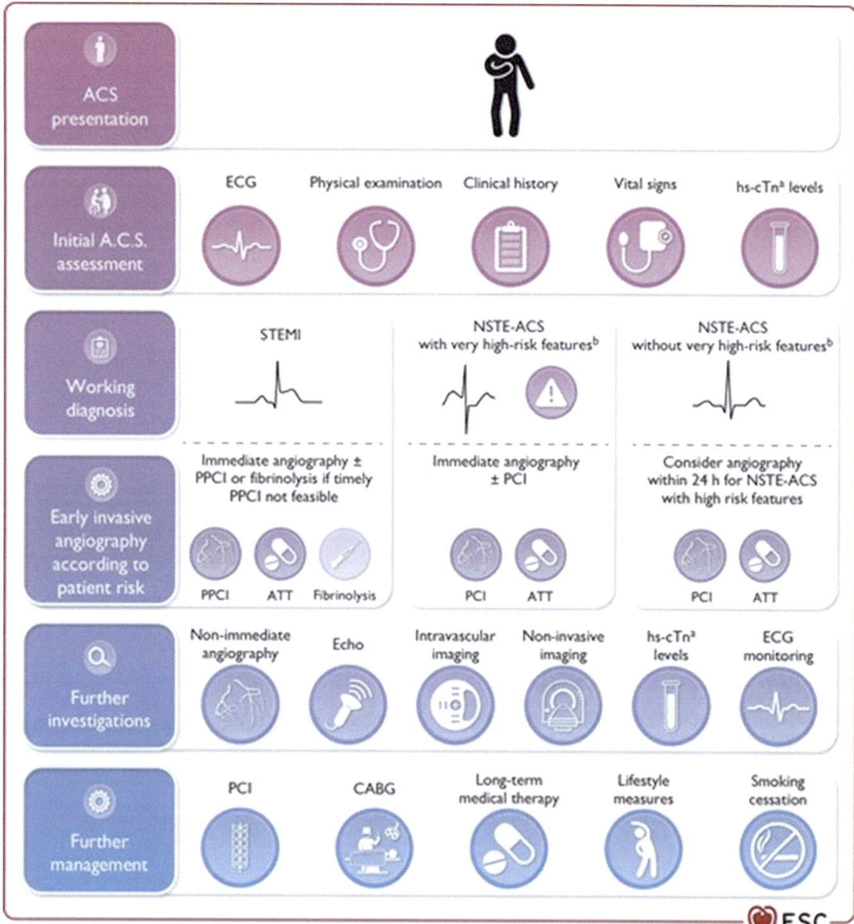

Fig. 4.6 Acute coronary syndrome

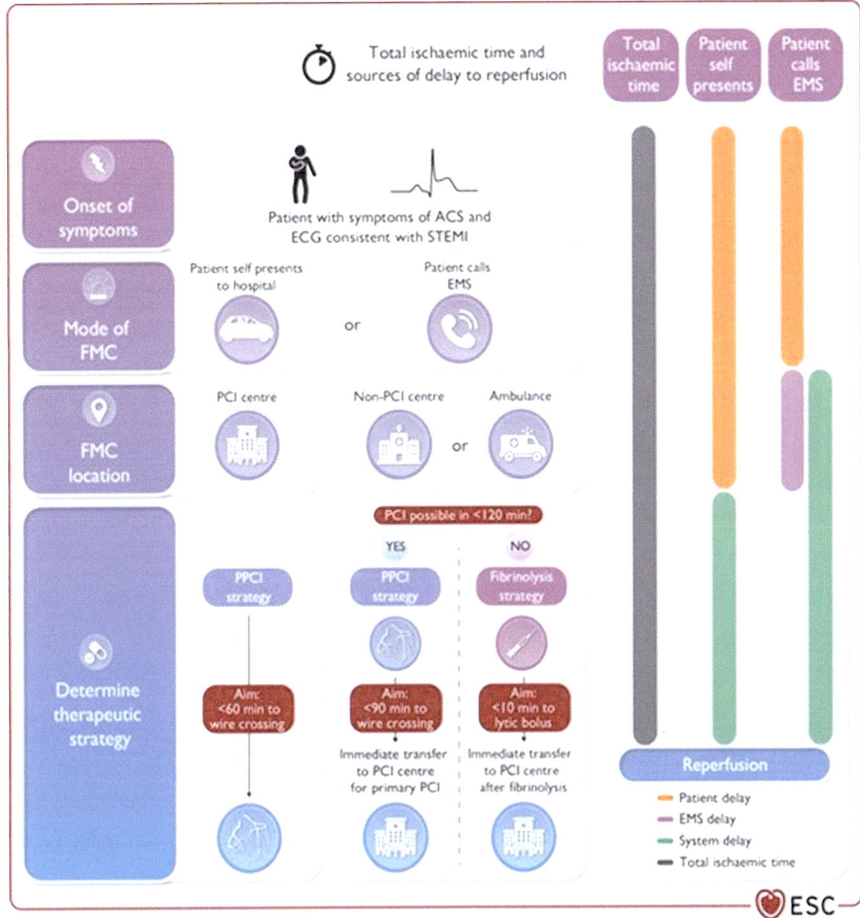

Fig. 4.7 Management of STEMI

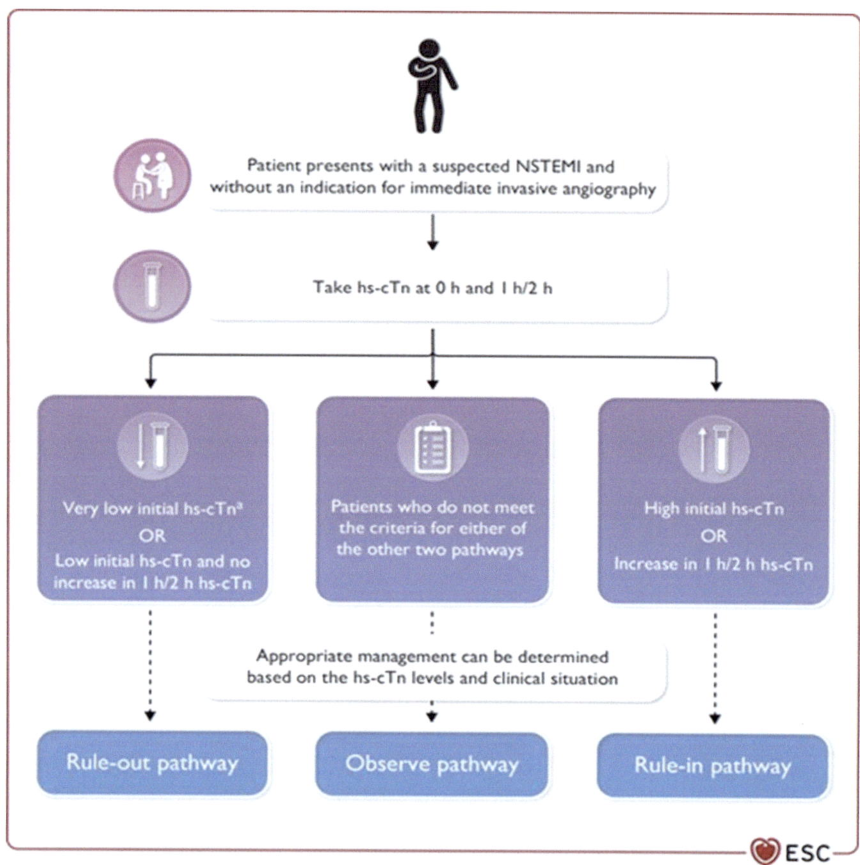

Fig. 4.8 Management of NSTEMI

Antiplatelet drugs	
Aspirin	LD of 150–300 mg orally or 75–250 mg i.v. if oral ingestion is not possible, followed by oral MD of 75–100 mg o.d.; no specific dose adjustment in CKD patients
P2Y12 receptor inhibitors (oral or i.v.)	
Clopidogrel	LD of 300–600 mg orally, followed by an MD of 75 mg o.d.; no specific dose adjustment in CKD patients Fibrinolysis: at the time of fibrinolysis an initial dose of 300 mg (75 mg for patients older than 75 years of age)
Prasugrel	LD of 60 mg orally, followed by an MD of 10 mg o.d. in patients with body weight < 60 kg, an MD of 5 mg o.d. is recommended. In patients aged ≥75 years, prasugrel should be used with caution, but an MD of 5 mg o.d. should be used if treatment is deemed necessary. No specific dose adjustment in CKD patients. Prior stroke is a contraindication for prasugrel
Ticagrelor	LD of 180 mg orally, followed by an MD of 90 mg b.i.d.; no specific dose adjustment in CKD patients

Cangrelor	Bolus of 30 μg/kg i.v. followed by 4 μg/kg/min infusion for at least 2 h or the duration of the procedure (whichever is longer) In the transition from cangrelor to a thienopyridine, the thienopyridine should be administered immediately after discontinuation of cangrelor with an LD (clopidogrel 600 mg or prasugrel 60 mg); to avoid a potential DDI, prasugrel may also be administered 30 min before the cangrelor infusion is stopped. Ticagrelor (LD 180 mg) should be administered at the time of PCI to minimize the potential gap in platelet inhibition during the transition phase
GP IIb/IIIa receptor inhibitors (i.v.)	
Eptifibatide	Double bolus of 180 μg/kg i.v. (given at a 10-min interval) followed by an infusion of 2.0 μg/kg/min for up to 18 h For CrCl 30–50 mL/min: first LD, 180 μg/kg i.v. bolus (max 22.6 mg); maintenance infusion, 1 μg/kg/min (max 7.5 mg/h). Second LD (if PCI), 180 μg/kg i.v. bolus (max 22.6 mg) should be administered 10 min after the first bolus. Contraindicated in patients with end-stage renal disease and with prior ICH, ischemic stroke within 30 days, fibrinolysis, or platelet count <100,000/mm^3
Tirofiban	Bolus of 25 μg/kg i.v. over 3 min, followed by an infusion of 0.15 μg/kg/min for up to 18 h For CrCl ≤60 mL/min: LD, 25 μg/kg i.v. over 5 min followed by a maintenance infusion of 0.075 μg/kg/min continued for up to 18 h Contraindicated in patients with prior ICH, ischemic stroke within 30 days, fibrinolysis, or platelet count <100,000/mm^3
II. Anticoagulant drugs	
UFH	Initial treatment: i.v. bolus 70–100 U/kg followed by i.v. infusion titrated to achieve an aPTT of 60–80 s During PCI: 70–100 U/kg i.v. bolus or according to ACT in case of UFH pretreatment
Enoxaparin	Initial treatment: for treatment of ACS 1 mg/kg b.i.d. subcutaneously for a minimum of 2 days and continued until clinical stabilization. In patients whose CrCl is below 30 mL per minute (by Cockcroft–Gault equation), the enoxaparin dosage should be reduced to 1 mg per kg o.d. During PCI: For patients managed with PCI, if the last dose of enoxaparin was given less than 8 h before balloon inflation, no additional dosing is needed. If the last s.c. administration was given more than 8 h before balloon inflation, an i.v. bolus of 0.3 mg/kg enoxaparin sodium should be administered
Bivalirudin	During PPCI: 0.75 mg/kg i.v. bolus followed by i.v. infusion of 1.75 mg/kg/h for 4 h after the procedure In patients whose CrCl is below 30 mL/min (by Cockcroft–Gault equation), maintenance infusion should be reduced to 1 mg/kg/h
Fondaparinux	Initial treatment: 2.5 mg/d subcutaneously During PCI: A single bolus of UFH is recommended Avoid if CrCl <20 mL/min

Strategies to reduce bleeding risk related to percutaneous coronary intervention
• Anticoagulant doses adjusted to body weight and renal function, especially in women and older patients
• Radial artery approach as default vascular access
• Proton pump inhibitors in patients on dual antiplatelet therapy at higher-than-average risk of gastrointestinal bleeds (i.e. history of gastrointestinal ulcer/hemorrhage, anticoagulant therapy, chronic nonsteroidal anti-inflammatory drug/corticosteroid use), or two or more of: • Age ≥ 65 years • Dyspepsia • Gastro-esophageal reflux disease • *Helicobacter pylori* infection • Chronic alcohol use
• In patients on OAC: • PCI performed without interruption of VKAs or NOACs • In patients on VKAs, do not administer UFH if INR >2.5 • In patients on NOACs, regardless of the timing of the last administration of NOACs, add low-dose parenteral anticoagulation (e.g., enoxaparin 0.5 mg/kg i.v. or UFH 60 IU/kg)
• Aspirin is indicated but avoid pre-treatment with P2Y12 receptor inhibitors
• GP IIb/IIIa receptor inhibitors only for bailout or peri-procedural complications.

4.4 Anti Thrombotic Therapy as an Adjunct to Fibrinolysis [2]

- Anti coagulation is recommended in all patients treated with fibrinolysis until revascularisation.
- Enoxaparin IV followed by S.C is recommended as preferred anticoagulant.
- When Enoxaparin is not available, UFH is recommended as weight adjusted IV Bolus followed by infusion.
- In patients treated with streptokinase, IV Bolus of Fondaparinux followed by SC dose 24 h later should be considered.

4.5 Fibrinolytic Therapy

- When fibrinolysis is the reperfusion strategy, it is recommended to initiate this treatment as soon as possible after diagnosis in the prehospital setting (aim for target of <10 min to lytic bolus).
- A fibrin-specific agent (i.e., tenecteplase, alteplase, or reteplase) is recommended.
- A half dose of tenecteplase should be considered in patients >75 years of age.

4.6 Descalation of Anti Platelet

De-escalation of antiplatelet therapy in the first 30 days is not recommended, but de-escalation of P2Y12 receptor inhibitor therapy may be considered as an alternative strategy beyond 30 days after an ACS, in order to reduce the risk of bleeding events. DAPT abbreviation strategies (followed preferably by P2Y12 inhibitor monotherapy within the first 12 months post-ACS) should be considered in patients who are event-free after 3–6 months of DAPT and who are not high ischemic risk, with the duration of DAPT guided by the ischemic and bleeding risks of the patient. For HBR patients, aspirin or P2Y12 receptor inhibitor monotherapy after 1 month of DAPT may be considered. Adding a second anti thrombotic agent to aspirin for extended long term secondary prevention should be considered in patients with high ischemic risk and without high bleeding risk. Adding a second antithrombotic agent to aspirin for extended long-term secondary prevention should be considered in patients with moderate ischemic risk and without high bleeding risk. P2y 12 inhibitor monotherapy may be considered as an alternative to aspirin monotherapy for long term treatment.

References

1. Management of Acute coronary syndrome. https://academic.oup.com/eurheartj/article/44/38/3720/7243210?login=false-.
2. Balcıoğlu AS. Diabetes and cardiac autonomic neuropathy: clinical manifestations, cardiovascular consequences, diagnosis and treatment. World J Diabetes. 2015;6(1):80. https://doi.org/10.4239/wjd.v6.i1.80.
3. Gupta N, Elnour AA. Diabetes and the heart: coronary artery disease, European Society of Cardiology. https://www.escardio.org/Journals/E-Journal-of-Cardiology-Practice/Volume-22/diabetes-and-the-heart-coronary-artery-disease. Accessed 14 Oct 2023.
4. Management of stable coronary artery disease in patients with diabetes mellitus. American College of Cardiology. https://www.acc.org/Latest-in-Cardiology/Articles/2020/08/18/07/41/Management-of-Stable-Coronary-Artery-Disease-in-Patients-with-DM. Accessed 14 Oct 2023.
5. Fishman SL, Sonmez H, Basman C, et al. The role of advanced glycation end-products in the development of coronary artery disease in patients with and without diabetes mellitus: a review. Mol Med. 2018;24:59. https://doi.org/10.1186/s10020-018-0060-3.
6. Leon B. Diabetes and cardiovascular disease: epidemiology, biological mechanisms, treatment recommendations and future research. World J Diabetes. 2015;6(13):1246. https://doi.org/10.4239/wjd.v6.i13.1246.
7. Serhiyenko VA, Serhiyenko AA. Cardiac autonomic neuropathy: risk factors, diagnosis and treatment. World J Diabetes. 2018;9(1):1–24. https://doi.org/10.4239/wjd.v9.i1.1.
8. Sharma J, Rohatgi A, Sharma D. Diabetic autonomic neuropathy: a clinical update. J R Coll Physicians Edinb. 2020;50(3):269–73. https://doi.org/10.4997/jrcpe.2020.310.
9. Teerlink JR, et al. Omecamtiv Mecarbil in chronic heart failure with reduced ejection fraction: rationale and design of GALACTIC—HF. JACC Heart Fail. 2020;8:329–40.
10. Management of Heart failure. https://www.escardio.org/Guidelines/Clinical-Practice-Guidelines/Acute-and-Chronic-Heart-Failure. (Figure 3, Figure 4).
11. Hammond HK, et al. Intracoronary gene transfer of Adenylyl Cyclase 6 in patients with heart failure—a randomized clinical trial. JAMA Cardiol. 2016;1(2):163–71. https://doi.org/10.1001/jamacardio.2016.008.
12. https://www.escardio.org/Journals/E-Journal-of-Cardiology-Practice/Volume-22/diabetes-and-the-heart-coronary-artery-disease.
13. https://www.acc.org/Latest-in-Cardiology/Articles/2020/08/18/07/41/Management-of-Stable-Coronary-Artery-Disease-in-Patients-with-DM.

Management of Oral Complications of Diabetes Mellitus

5

Nandita Shenoy

5.1 Oral Health in Renal Disease

The oral mucosa is a membrane lining the mouth, with layers of tissue that vary depending on their location. Some areas have more protection against mechanical stress, while others have more taste buds. The mucosa also senses pressure, temperature, and pain to protect the digestive tract and provide a barrier function. Its structure and protein expression are unique to its functions.

5.1.1 Macroscopy of the Oral Cavity

The oral mucosa lines the oral cavity and is anatomically divided into three parts: the vestibule (between the lips and teeth), the oral cavity proper (within the teeth), and the oropharyngeal isthmus (the transition zone to the oropharynx). The oral cavity is essential for food ingestion, mastication, phonation, and ventilation. The lips are the transition zone from the external skin to the oral mucosa and are supported by the orbicularis oris muscle. Under normal conditions, the lips fully cover the incisors, and the upper incisors are located below the upper border of the lower lip. Moisture for the lips comes from saliva within the mouth or minor salivary glands located within the lips.

A close-up look at the mouth reveals several distinct areas. The lips mark where the skin meets the inner lining of the mouth, called the labial mucosa, at the vermilion zone. The alveolar mucosa and gingiva cover the alveolar bone and teeth, respectively. The transition between these two areas is called the mucogingival junction

N. Shenoy (✉)
Department of Oral Medicine and Radiology, Manipal College of Dental Sciences, Mangalore, Karnataka, India

Manipal College of Dental Sciences Mangalore, Manipal Academy of Higher Education, Manipal, Karnataka, India

G. Abraham et al. (eds.), *Management of Diabetic Complications*,
https://doi.org/10.1007/978-981-97-6406-8_5

zone, while the point where the gingiva attaches to the teeth is called the dentogingival junction. When the mouth is open, three distinct areas can be seen: the vestibulum oris, the oral cavity proper, and the oropharyngeal isthmus. In the retromolar region, there is a connection between the vestibulum oris and the cavities oris proper.

The adjoining vestibulum oris is a narrow space reaching from the lips and cheeks on the outer side to the teeth on the internal side. The mucosa of the distinct parts turns over at the fornix vestibule. A labial frenulum is present in the upper fornix, which is tightly attached to the alveolar crest. When teeth are closed, the vestibulum is adequately separated from the oral cavity except for the retromolar region. Alveolar mucosa and gingiva cover the alveolar bone and the neck of the teeth, respectively.

The moist surface of the oral cavity needs to be maintained by saliva produced by major and minor salivary glands. Whereas minor salivary glands are labial, palatal, lingual, and buccal in the oral mucosa, major salivary glands can be found outside the oral mucosa and oral cavity. The saliva reaches the oral cavity through ducts.

The serous parotid gland is located between the mandible and sternocleidomastoid below the external acoustic meatus and reaches the masseter surface. The duct runs through the cheek and ends in the oral vestibule opposite the maxillary second permanent molar tooth. The seromucous submandibular gland has a superficial part in the digastric triangle and a deep part extending to the sublingual gland's posterior end. The sublingual gland is mucoserous and lies on the mylohyoid. It has 8–20 excretory ducts opening to the sublingual fold or fuse to a sublingual duct that combines with the submandibular duct. The submandibular duct ends at the caruncula sublingualis.

The oral cavity comprises lymphoid tissue regions characterized as crypts invading the epithelium into the lamina propria.

5.1.2 Histology of the Oral Mucosa

The oral mucosa consists of an epithelium and a lamina propria which is undermined from a submucosa in many regions before reaching the underlying structure, bone at the palate, and muscle at the cheeks and lips. The thickness and keratinization of the epithelium and its melanin pigments, as well as the vascularization of the connective tissue, determine the color of the respective area of the oral mucosa. All mentioned factors differ in several areas of the oral mucosa and contribute to their respective function. The lining of the oral cavity can be roughly divided into areas covered by masticatory mucosa and those covered by lining or specialized mucosa.

5.1.3 Functions of the Oral Mucosa

The oral mucosa fulfills various functions, like protecting deeper tissues from mechanical forces like compression and stretching during everyday activities, including eating and chewing. Further, the oral mucosa is an essential barrier for normal resident bacteria in the oral cavity and against thermal and chemical stresses. The constant renewal of the oral mucosal cells enables the superficial cells to be scaled off due to mechanical stress without causing trauma to the tissue or loss of barrier function—functions of the oral mucosa. The oral mucosa fulfills a plethora of functions crucial for the organisms. They provide a proper nutritive function and protect adjoining parts of the gastrointestinal tract from ingested noxious substances.

The oral mucosa is mainly responsible for sensation. Connective tissue receptors detect temperature, pressure, and pain, while Merkel cells in the epithelium sense pressure. This function protects various parts of the gastrointestinal system from potential harm. Additionally, taste buds identify the classic sweet, salty, sour, and bitter tastes, but recent data suggest that fat and water can also be detected. Reflex arcs rely on receptor integration, including swallowing, gagging, retching, and salivation.

5.1.4 Saliva

Saliva is uniquely adapted to the functions it needs to perform in the oral cavity. It continually bathes the hard and soft tissues to maintain the healthy tissues of the oral cavity, oropharynx, and larynx. Saliva is formed by three pairs of major salivary glands, namely parotid, submandibular, and sublingual, and hundreds of minor salivary glands, with some of the gingival crevicular fluid (GCF) being secreted from the gingival sulcus. Saliva in the oral cavity is vital for maintaining healthy teeth and oral tissues, the parasympathetic and sympathetic nerve supply mediates its secretion, and the autonomic nervous system controls its type and volume. The accessible and noninvasive collection and diagnosis of saliva have facilitated extensive research into carrier susceptibility, physiological and pathological changes, and monitoring levels of hormones, drugs, ions, antibodies, and microorganisms. Saliva is considered an ideal diagnostic bio-medium and provides an excellent alternative to other body fluids for investigation. It is easily collected, stored, and transported, while being safe to handle compared to other biological media.

5.1.5 Gingival Crevicular Fluid

The gingival crevicular fluid (GCF) is a type of exudate that is found in the space between the tooth and the marginal gingiva known as the gingival sulcus. In a healthy gingival sulcus, the GCF is a small amount of interstitial fluid that passes through it. Under stimulated or inflamed conditions, the GCF flow rate increases, which reflects the concentration of metabolites in the serum.

GCF comprises serum components, inflammatory cells, connective tissue, epithelium, and microbial flora in the gingival sulcus. It acts as a defence mechanism by flushing out particles and bacteria from the sulcus while possessing antimicrobial properties and antibodies that improve inflammation resistance.

5.2 Oral Changes in Kidney Disorders

Good oral health is crucial for overall health, well-being, and quality of life. According to WHO, oral health means being free from chronic pain in the mouth and face, oral and throat cancer, oral infections and sores, periodontal disease, tooth decay, tooth loss, and other disorders that limit an individual's ability to bite, chew, smile, speak, and experience positive mental health. Oral diseases are the most common noncommunicable diseases (NCDs) and can cause pain, discomfort, disfigurement, and even death. The Global Burden of Disease Study 2016 found that oral diseases affected at least 3.58 billion people worldwide.

The World Oral Health Report (2003) stated clearly that the relationship between oral health and general health is proven by evidence. Oral and general health are related in four significant ways: (1) Poor oral health is significantly associated with major chronic diseases, (2) Poor oral health causes disability, (3) Oral health issues and significant diseases share common risk factors, and (4) General health problems may cause or worsen oral health conditions.

As technology and medicine progress, oral healthcare professionals must take a holistic approach when treating patients with complex medical issues. This means looking at the person's physical, mental, emotional, and social well-being. Of all the systemic disorders, diseases affecting the renal system are a leading cause of morbidity and mortality worldwide. The kidneys are essential for maintaining homeostasis and a stable internal environment. India is facing an increasing burden of chronic diseases like diabetes and hypertension, which can lead to chronic kidney disease (CKD) and end-stage renal disease (ESRD) in 25% to 40% of affected individuals. As a result, healthcare professionals must be prepared to manage these conditions effectively in the future.

Various diseases can lead to chronic renal failure, but diabetes mellitus (DM) is the most common and significant cause. So, when a patient with DM presents to a dental clinic, it becomes essential to rule out CKD, which refers to any abnormalities in the structure or function of the kidneys, with or without a decrease in GFR. This can be shown through pathological abnormalities or markers of kidney damage, such as changes in blood or urine composition or imaging test results. Renal diseases can be classified as acute or chronic based on their onset. Dentists are most likely to encounter patients with CKD and occasionally deal with nephrotic syndrome and renal transplants. The gradual loss of kidney function can result in uremia, a clinical syndrome. Dental practitioners should know the systemic signs of renal failure and uremia, including hematologic, bone metabolism, and immune system changes.

As the condition progresses, the glomerular filtration rate drops below 15 mL/min, causing an accumulation of metabolic by-products like urea and creatinine in the bloodstream and an imbalance of electrolytes. This makes renal replacement therapy (RRT) necessary to prevent severe complications that could lead to death. Regular hemodialysis at proper intervals can be a life-sustaining alternative to RRT for CKD patients.

Dialysis is a procedure that removes toxic waste products and nitrogenous substances from the blood. Essentially, it washes out waste products from the blood through mechanical means. However, dialysis can cause systemic changes and oral complications. Monitoring metabolic by-products, including creatinine, urea, and potassium levels in the bloodstream, is essential.

CKD is a condition that affects the balance of calcium and phosphorus in the body, leading to an increase in calcium levels due to the use of calcium-based phosphate binders. This results in cardiovascular problems which are the leading cause of illness and death among CKD patients, especially those in end-stage renal disease (ESRD).

CKD patients may experience gingival inflammation, gingival enlargement, and attachment loss, changes in salivary composition and reduced salivary flow rate, mucosal lesions, oral malignancies, dental anomalies, bone lesions, and malocclusions. Increased dental calculus and lower caries rates have also been reported. Many studies have been conducted on this subject. Neglecting oral care is linked to poor oral hygiene, increased plaque, and gingival inflammation in end-stage renal disease (ESRD) patients. Chronic diseases are associated with poorer oral health and more significant unmet dental needs, including untreated dental disease, self-reported poor oral health, and tooth loss.

Research on dental caries occurrence among individuals with CKD has yielded conflicting results when compared to healthy individuals. Some studies indicate that CKD patients may have a lower prevalence of dental caries due to higher saliva pH and buffer capacity, which may offer protection. However, other studies have found no significant difference in dental caries occurrence between CKD patients and those without CKD.

Patients with CKD undergoing treatment with calcium channel blockers and calcineurin inhibitors are at risk of developing gingival hyperplasia. This condition can cause severe overgrowth of the gums, affecting the interdental papilla, and marginal gingiva. Typically, surgical resection is necessary to treat this issue, although improved oral hygiene practices have been shown to reduce the incidence or delay the onset of gingival hyperplasia. Additionally, CKD patients may experience platelet dysfunction, which can lead to gingival bleeding, petechiae, and ecchymosis, as well as periodontal issues such as attachment loss, recession, and deep pockets.

Periodontitis is a bacterial infection that affects the tissues supporting the teeth, causing both local and systemic inflammation. This condition has been linked to an increased risk of CKD. Patients with poor oral health may experience delays in medical procedures due to the risk of infection after surgery, which can be life-threatening. Saliva is a blood filtrate containing molecules that reach it through different routes, reflecting the body's physiological state. Research has indicated differences in the amounts of urea, creatinine, calcium, phosphorus, and potassium found in the saliva of patients with kidney failure. The classic signs of altered calcium metabolism in the mandible and maxilla are bone demineralization, loss of trabeculation, ground-glass appearance, total or partial loss of lamina dura, giant cell lesions or brown tumors, and metastatic calcification.

High plasma creatinine levels can increase the salivary glands' permeability. Urea, which has a low molecular weight, can also filter from the blood into the saliva. Studies have shown that patients with CKD have higher creatinine and urea levels in their saliva than healthy people of the same age. The creatinine and urea concentration in the saliva was also positively correlated with the levels found in the patient's blood. Patients with more severe kidney damage also had even higher creatinine and urea levels in their saliva than those with less severe damage. Overall, there is a positive correlation between the severity of kidney disease and the concentration of creatinine and urea in the patient's saliva.

Unlike people with normal kidney function, who only get rid of 5%–10% of their daily potassium through the gut, CKD patients can eliminate as much as 25% through this route. Salivary potassium levels are also higher in CKD patients, likely because swallowing saliva can help remove potassium from the body. This information comes from a study that found this extra-renal method of potassium disposal in CKD patients.

Regular dental care is essential for preventing CKD progression. Several studies have shown that individuals with significant periodontal disease have a higher risk of CKD, even after accounting for diabetes, tobacco use, and socioeconomic status.

Regular oral examinations are essential for patients with CKD as they can help identify multisystem diseases at an early stage. Thus, it is recommended that such patients undergo regular evaluations for oral lesions and receive appropriate treatment. Dental care for patients with renal disease can be challenging due to the systemic effects of renal failure, including anemia, bleeding, and cardiovascular, or endocrine diseases. However, dental management can be safe and effective with suitable treatment protocols. All clinicians caring for renal patients should make routine oral examinations a standard practice before undergoing hemodialysis or transplantation, as this can prevent endocarditis and septicemia.

5.3 Oral Manifestations in Patients with CKD

The oral healthcare professional should recognize these oral symptoms as part of the patient's systemic disease rather than as isolated occurrences. In studies of renal patients, up to 90% were found to have oral symptoms of uremia. Some presenting signs were an ammonia-like taste, smell, stomatitis, gingivitis, decreased salivary flow, xerostomia, and parotitis.

As the disease progresses, one of the early symptoms may be a sour taste and odor in the mouth, particularly in the morning. This uremic fetor, an ammonia odor, is typical of any uremic patient and is caused by the high concentration of urea in the saliva and its subsequent breakdown into ammonia.

Due to multiple drug intake, patients can present with oral lichenoid reactions. Additionally, because of their immunocompromised state, oral lichen planus is also a common finding in these patients.

Salivary levels of urea are closely related to BUN levels, but the correlation is not strictly linear. A sudden increase in BUN levels can lead to uremic stomatitis, which may manifest as a red patch on the mucosa covered with thick exudate and a pseudomembrane, or as ulcerations with redness. All reported cases of intraoral lesions have been linked to BUN levels exceeding 150 mg/dL, and these lesions typically disappear after medical treatment reduces BUN levels. Uremic stomatitis is believed to be caused by chemical burns or a general loss of tissue resistance, making regular and traumatic influences challenging to withstand (Fig. 5.1).

Although uncommon, white patches called "uremic frost" can sometimes appear on the skin and inside the mouth. This frost forms when urea crystals are left on the skin or mouth surfaces after sweat evaporates or due to decreased saliva production. Dry mouth, or xerostomia, is a more frequent oral condition caused by inflammation, dehydration, breathing through the mouth (Kussmaul's respiration), or problems with the salivary glands.

Sometimes, there may be swelling in the salivary glands. In children, a low occurrence of cavities has been linked to increased salivary urea nitrogen. Even with high sugar intake and subpar oral hygiene, the urea breakdown process can better neutralize acids.

Calcium metabolism changes can significantly impact the mandibular molar region above the mandibular canal. Generalized osteoporosis can lead to rarefaction in both the mandible and maxilla. Over time, the finer trabeculae can disappear, leaving behind a coarser pattern. In some cases, small lytic lesions may develop that are later found to be giant cell or brown tumors. The compact bone in the jaws may also become thinner and eventually disappear, resulting in the loss of the lower border of the mandible, cortical margins of the inferior dental canal and floor of the antrum, and lamina dura.

Studies have shown that decreasing cortical bone thickness at the mandible angle correlates well with the degree of RO.

Spontaneous and pathologic fractures may occur with the thinning of these areas of compact bone and may complicate dental extractions. Although the skeleton may undergo decalcification, fully developed teeth are not directly affected; however, in the presence of significant skeletal decalcification, the teeth will appear more radiopaque.

Other clinical manifestations of RO include tooth mobility, malocclusion, and metastatic soft tissue calcifications. Increasing mobility and drifting of teeth with no apparent pathologic periodontal pocket formation may be seen. Periapical radiolucencies and root resorption also may be associated with this gradual loosening of

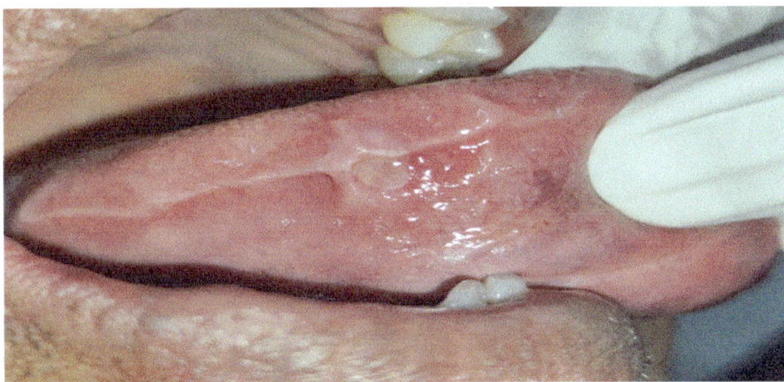

Fig. 5.1 Ulcer on right lateral border of the tongue

the dentition. Malocclusion may result from the advanced mobility and drifting of the dentition.

Patients with renal disease may experience abnormal bone repair after tooth extraction, which is known as "socket sclerosis." This condition is characterized by the deposition of sclerotic bone within the lamina dura without any resorption. Enamel hypoplasia, a discoloration of white or brownish hue, is commonly observed in patients with renal disease who developed the condition at a young age. The location of hypoplastic enamel on permanent teeth corresponds to the onset of advanced renal failure. It should be noted that socket sclerosis and enamel hypoplasia are not unique to patients with renal disease.

5.4 Oral Health Considerations

For dental management, patients with renal disease can be categorized into two groups: patients with AKI and patients with chronic progressing renal failure or end-stage renal failure who are undergoing dialysis.

Improving periodontal health, endothelial function, and reducing inflammation markers have been proven possible through nonsurgical periodontal therapy. A recent study has indicated that CKD does not affect the osseointegration quality of titanium implants. Both in quality and quantity, platelet defects are responsible for bleeding tendencies in such patients, leading to common hemorrhagic episodes in the gingiva. Patients may also show ulcerations, petechial or purpural lesions in the oral mucosa. Hematoma formation and bruising after alveolectomy or periodontal surgery can be expected. Patients at risk should consider adjunctive hemostatic measures. DDAVP, a synthetic analog of the antidiuretic hormone vasopressin, has shown effectiveness in bleeding management in renal failure patients in the short term. Tranexamic acid, an antifibrinolytic agent, administered through mouthwash or soaked gauze, can significantly reduce operative bleeding following surgical procedures.

When it comes to dental care for patients undergoing dialysis, there is some debate about the timing of treatment. Ideally, non-dialysis days should be chosen for elective dental procedures, extractions, and other surgeries. A dental practitioner should consult the patient's platelet count and complete blood count to manage bleeding tendencies and anemia. Generally, peritoneal dialysis does not present any contraindications for dental treatment, except during acute peritoneal infections when elective care should be postponed. It is essential to identify and note the arm with vascular access on the patient's chart and instruct them to avoid blood pressure measurements and IV injections of medication in that arm. Additionally, the access site should not be used as an injection site.

Infective endocarditis is a severe concern in hemodialysis patients after receiving dental treatment. The incidence of infective endocarditis in patients undergoing hemodialysis is 2.7%. Streptococcus viridans account for almost one-third of the cases of infective endocarditis, whereas staphylococcal species such as *Staphylococcus epidermidis* and *Staphylococcus aureus* account for most cases.

CKD patients are usually immunocompromised and prone to oral candidiasis, which prevents as a curdy white precipitate that is usually scrapable (Fig. 5.2).

Preventing excessive stress when undergoing dental procedures is crucial, and it is advisable to use sedatives beforehand. Dentists need to be cautious with pharmacotherapeutic treatments for patients with renal disease. As most medications are eliminated, at least partially, through the kidneys, dentists should take safety measures to avoid drug reactions and prevent further renal damage. NSAIDs may induce sodium retention, impair the action of diuretics, prevent aldosterone production, affect renal artery perfusion, and cause acidosis. Tetracyclines and steroids are anti-anabolic, increasing urea nitrogen to approximately twice the baseline levels. Other drugs, such as phenacetin, are nephrotoxic and put added strain on an already damaged kidney.

5.5 Summary of Dental Considerations and Management of the Patient with Renal Disease

5.5.1 Before Treatment

When planning dental treatment for hemodialysis patients, scheduling appointments for the day after dialysis is crucial. This concern does not apply to patients undergoing peritoneal dialysis.

It is recommended to consult with the patient's nephrologist to review recent laboratory tests and discuss the possibility of antibiotic prophylaxis if the patient has a history of infective endocarditis.

Please identify the arm with vascular access and note the type in the patient's chart. Please avoid taking blood pressure measurements or injecting medication into this arm. Routinely check the patient for any signs of hypertension or hypotension.

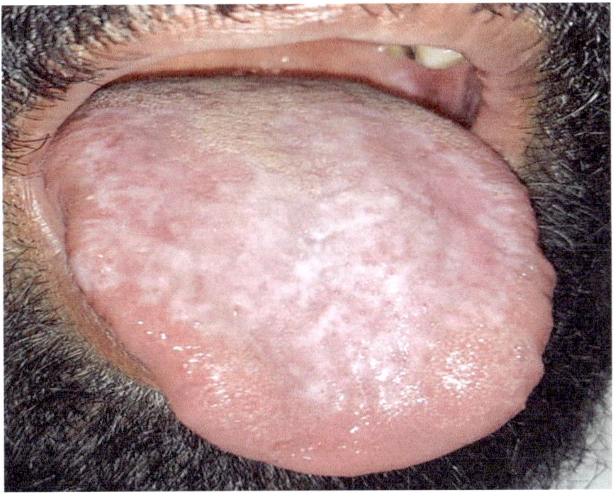

Fig. 5.2 Candidiasis of tongue

Institute preoperative hemostatic aids (DDAVP, conjugated estrogen) when appropriate.

Obtain routine annual dental radiographs to establish the presence and follow manifestations of renal osteodystrophy.

Consider routine serology for HBV, HCV, and HIV antibody.

Consider antibiotic prophylaxis when appropriate according to current AHA guidelines.

Consider sedative premedication for patients with dental anxiety.

5.5.2 During Treatment

Perform a thorough history and physical examination for the presence of oral manifestations.

Aggressively eliminate potential sources of infection/bacteremia.

Use adjunctive hemostatic aids during oral/periodontal surgical procedures.

Maintain the patient in a comfortable uncramped position in the dental chair.

Allow the patient to walk or stand intermittently during long procedures.

5.5.3 After Treatment

Use postsurgical hemostatic agents.

Encourage meticulous home care and hygiene.

Institute therapy for xerostomia/salivary gland hypofunction when appropriate.

Consider the use of postoperative antibiotics for traumatic procedures if uremic.

Cautious use of respiratory-depressant drugs in the presence of severe anemia.

Adjust dosages of postoperative medications according to the extent of renal failure.

Ensure routine recall maintenance.

Further Reading

Collins AJ, Kasiske B, Herzog C, et al. Excerpts from the United States renal data system 2004 annual data report: atlas of end-stage renal disease in the United States. Am J Kidney Dis. 2005;45(1 suppl 1):A5–7.

de Francisco AL. Medical therapy of secondary hyperparathyroidism in chronic kidney disease: old and new drugs. Expert Opin Pharmacother. 2006;7:2215–24.

De Rossi SS, Glick M. Dental considerations for patients with renal disease receiving hemodialysis. J Am Dent Assoc. 1996;127:211–9.

Dembowska E, Jaroń A, Gabrysz-Trybek E, Bladowska J, Trybek G. Oral mucosa status in patients with end-stage chronic kidney disease undergoing hemodialysis. Int J Environ Res Public Health. 2023;20(1):835.

El-Kishawi AM, El-Nahas AM. Renal osteodystrophy: review of the disease and its treatment. Saudi J Kidney Dis Transpl. 2006;17:373–82.

Fishbane S. Iron supplementation in renal anemia. Semin Nephrol. 2006;26:319–24.

Ganesh SK, Hulbert-Shearon TE, Port FK, et al. Mortality difference by dialysis modality among incident ESRD patients with and without coronary artery disease. J Am Soc Nephrol. 2003;14:415–28.

Gupta M, Gupta M, Abhishek. Oral conditions in renal disorders and treatment considerations - a review for pediatric dentist. Saudi Dent J. 2015;27(3):113–9.

Ledebo I, Lamiere N, Charra B, et al. Improving the outcome of dialysis—opinion vs scientific evidence. Nephrol Dial Transplant. 2000;15:1310–6.

Lee J, Nicholl DD, Ahmed SB, et al. The prevalence of restless legs syndrome across the full spectrum of kidney disease. J Clin Sleep Med. 2013;9(5):455–9.

Levey AS, Bosch JP, Lewis JB, et al. A more accurate method to estimateglomerular filtration rate from serum creatinine: a new prediction equation. Modification of diet in renal disease study group. Ann Intern Med. 1999;130(6):461–70.

Liu J, Kalantarinia K, Rosner MH. Management of lipid abnormalities associated with end-stage renal disease. Semin Dial. 2006;19:391–401.

Maggiore Q, Pizzarelli F, Dattolo P, et al. Cardiovascular stability during hemodialysis, hemofiltration, and hemodialfiltration. Nephrol Dial Transplant. 2000;15(suppl 1):68–73.

Orth SR. Effects of smoking on systemic and intrarenal hemodynamics: influence on renal function. J Am Soc Nephrol. 2004;15(suppl1):S58–63.

Pereira BJ. Optimization of pre-ESRD care; the key to improved dialysis outcomes. Kidney Int. 2000;57:351–65.

Singh AK, Szczech L, Tang KL, et al. Correction of anemia with epoetin alfa in chronic kidney disease. N Engl J Med. 2006;355(20):2085–98.

St Peter WL, Obrador GT, Roberts TL, Collins AJ. Trends in intravenous iron use among dialysis patients in the United States (1994–2002). Am J Kidney Dis. 2005;46:650–60.

Strippoli GF, Palmer SC, Ruospo M, et al. Oral disease in adults treated with hemodialysis:prevalence, predictors, and association with mortality and adverse cardiovascular events: the rationale and design of the ORAL diseases in hemodialysis (ORAL-D) study, a prospective, multinational, longitudinal, observational, cohort study. BMC Nephrol. 2013;14:90.

Gastrointestinal Manifestations in Diabetes Mellitus and Management

6

Arulprakash Sarangapani

6.1 Introduction

Diabetes mellitus (DM) is a complex and multisystemic chronic disease that has become an epidemic over the past decades. International Diabetic Federation reports that 10.5% of the adult population is affected by diabetes, with half of these population undiagnosed. By 2045, 783 million will be living with diabetes. The gastrointestinal (GI) system is one of the main systems affected by DM, and up to 75% of patients with the disease report some kind of long-term GI symptom, including oesophageal symptoms.

6.2 Esophagus

The esophagus, a muscular tube connecting the pharynx to the stomach, enables propulsion of swallowed food, with a sphincter at both end (the upper and lower esophageal sphincters) to prevent esophago-pharyngeal and gastroesophageal reflux, respectively.

Two common esophageal symptoms include heartburn and dysphagia. Techniques to evaluate esophageal symptoms include gastroscopy, high-resolution esophageal manometry (HREM), and 24-h pH impedance. Gastroscopy helps in mucosal changes like erosions and ulcers, while manometry helps to diagnose motility disorder and laxity of lower oesophageal sphincter. pH impedance confirms both acid and nonacid reflux along with bolus transit. Barium swallow and scintigraphy are investigations not widely useful in current clinical practice.

A. Sarangapani (✉)
MGM Health Care, Chennai, Tamil Nadu, India
e-mail: arulprakash.s@mgmhealthcare.in

G. Abraham et al. (eds.), *Management of Diabetic Complications*,
https://doi.org/10.1007/978-981-97-6406-8_6

Acute hyperglycemia inhibits esophageal motility, and reduces the basal lower esophageal sphincter pressure [1]. It has been postulated that the major mechanism underlying esophageal dysmotility is a reduction of cholinergic activity and vagal parasympathetic dysfunction [2]. The pathological abnormalities associated with gastroparesis, such as a reduction in interstitial cells of Cajal and inhibitory intrinsic neurons, have also been postulated to be relevant to esophageal dysmotility [3]. Diffuse esophageal muscular hypertrophy was reported in two-thirds of people with diabetes in one case series [4].

General measures for managing esophageal symptoms include lifestyle modifications (improved glycemic control, weight reduction, dietary changes, and physical activity). Prokinetic agents have tried with no significant evidence to support efficacy. The latter include dopaminergic agents (metoclopramide, domperidone), serotonin receptor agonists, and motilin agonists [5]. Functional heartburn and noncardiac chest pain can be managed with SSRI and SNRI.

Gastroesophageal reflux disease (GERD) is extremely common in the general population and also frequently seen in diabetes. In nonerosive GERD, treatment involves lifestyle measures (bed elevation of 30° at headend) and use of proton-pump inhibitors.

Disordered esophageal motility, especially the elderly, increases the risk of "pill-induced esophagitis," with mucosal injury due to prolonged exposure to impacted medications [3]. Diabetes is an independent risk factor, and the condition usually presents as chest pain with or without odynophagia. Treatment involves withdrawal of the offending agent and use of proton-pump inhibitors (Fig. 6.1) [4].

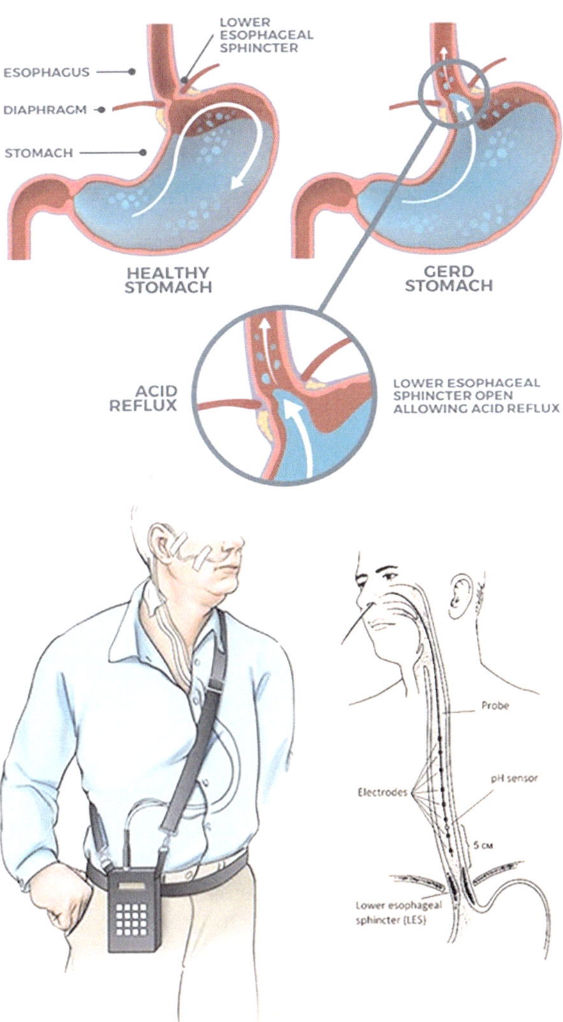

Fig. 6.1 Gastroesophageal reflux disease

6.3 Stomach

Common gastric symptoms include epigastric discomfort, bloating, belching, pain, nausea, and vomiting. Conditions like gastric ulcers, erosions, and *Helicobacter pylori* gastritis are more common in diabetic patients. More frequent and complicated and clinical challenge is delayed gastric emptying. Assisting in diagnosis of gastric problems are contrast imaging, upper GI endoscopy, gastric emptying studies (nuclear scintigraphy), and the latest electrogastrography (EGG). Gastroparesis: Delayed gastric emptying in diabetes was reported by Kassander, in 1958, and coined the term "gastroparesis diabeticorum" [6]. Gastroparesis occurs in both type 1 and 2 diabetes and may not, necessarily, be indicative of a poor prognosis (Fig. 6.2) [7].

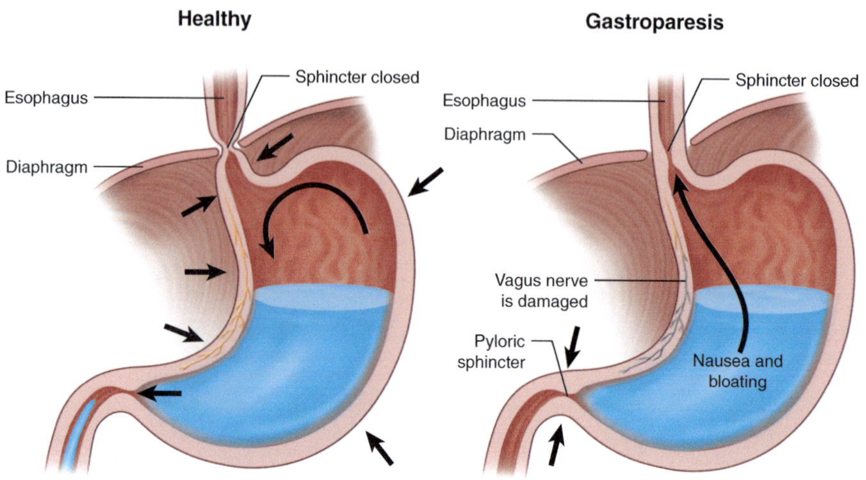

Fig. 6.2 Gastroparesis in diabetic neuropathy

The rate of gastric emptying is a major determinant of postprandial glycemia in both healthy individuals and those with diabetes. Newer antidiabetic medications, such as short-acting GLP-1 receptor agonists, are widely used to diminish postprandial glycemic excursions predominantly by slowing gastric emptying. Gastric emptying is a complex, coordinated process by which chyme is delivered to the small intestine at a regulated rate and involves the GI smooth muscles, enteric nerves, gastric "pacemaker" (interstitial cells of Cajal or ICC), and immune cells.

Delayed gastric emptying of a solid meal occurs in 47% of patients with diabetics [8]. Risk factors for gastroparesis include a long duration of diabetes, the presence of other microvascular complications, female gender, obesity, and smoking [7]. Incidence of diabetes is around 5% in type 1 and 1% in type 2 diabetic patients [9].

Clinical symptoms include, bloating, nausea, and vomiting. American Neurogastroenterology and Motility defines gastroparesis as intragastric retention of >60% of a standardized meal at 2 h and/or >10% at 4 h [10]. General measures include small frequent meals, less in fat and fiber, most of calories as liquid. Prokinetics are the mainstay of treatment. Major limitations of these prokinetics include adverse effects and tachyphlaxis. Metaclopramide and domperidone are dopamine receptor antagonist, which improves gastric emptying. Erythromycin, a motilin receptor agonist, is effective for acute treatment and is relatively inexpensive. However, it needs to be administered frequently and may also prolong the QT interval. Newer medications like pruclopride, 5 HT4 agonist appears promising [11].

Gastroparesis that is refractory to diet and medications can be treated with tube feeding to bypass the stomach. Gastric electrical stimulation (GES) using the "Enterra" device appeared to be a promising therapeutic option. Pyloric botulinum toxin injections, surgical and endoscopic interventions, such as pyloroplasty and pyloromyotomy have been described in literature [12].

6.4 Gallbladder

Gallstones are more common with type 2 diabetic patients with accompanied, obesity and hypertriglyceridemia [13]. Gallbladder symptoms include right upper quadrant pain, nausea, vomiting, dyspeptic symptoms and jaundice. Altered lipid metabolism with gallbladder dysmotility leads to formation of gallstones. Diagnosis is made by abdominal ultrasound, MRI or CT, rarely gallbladder scintigraphy is required to look for gallbladder dyskinesia. Symptomatic complications such as cholecystitis, cholangitis, or biliary pancreatitis may require surgery or endoscopic treatment. Newer antidiabetic medications, like GLP-1 agonists, are prone for gallbladder disease related to drug-induced delayed gallbladder refilling time [14].

6.5 Pancreas

Prevalence of pancreatic exocrine insufficiency in diabetes has been reported to be greater in type 1 (25–75%) compared to type 2 (25–50%) diabetes [15]. Autoimmunity, autonomic neuropathy, and microvascular damage are proposed to be the pathogenesis. Common symptoms are variable and include diarrhea (steatorrhea), abdominal pain, and failure to thrive in children. Diagnostic tests can be direct or indirect. Direct tests involve stimulation with exogenous hormones or nutrients while simultaneously collecting pancreatic secretions via duodenal intubation. Direct tests are too expensive, invasive, and requires high-end techniques. These factors limit its clinical utility despite being the most sensitive and specific. Indirect tests include the 3-day fecal fat, fecal elastase measurement, and breath tests (14C-triolein). Of these, the most common indirect and noninvasive (as well as relatively inexpensive) test in clinical practice is measurement of fecal elastase. It has been suggested that a fecal elastase-1 level less than 200 μg/g stool is indicative of mild pancreatic exocrine insufficiency, and a level of 100 μg/g stool of severe pancreatic exocrine insufficiency [16]. The sensitivity (55%) and specificity (60%) of fecal elastase-1 in diagnosing pancreatic exocrine insufficiency is not impressive. Fat-soluble vitamin level estimation is another indirect but less-specific test. General principle in managing pancreatic exocrine insufficiency include consumption of smaller, frequent meals, abstinence from alcohol, and specific diet. Pancreatic enzyme replacement therapy is regarded as the cornerstone of treatment [16]. Proton-pump inhibitor or H2 blockers are prescribed with enzyme replacement to avoid inactivation of enzymes by acidic environment of stomach.

6.6 Small Intestine

Diabetic enteropathy is less-studied compared to diabetic gastroparesis. Vagal dysfunction has been regarded as the major impairment in diabetic enteropathy. Evidence has suggested a critical role of both interstitial cells of Cajal and nNOS in pathogensis of enteropathy [17]. Acute hyperglycemia also has a major effect on postprandial small intestinal motility in healthy individuals and in those with diabetes. It reduces the amplitude of duodenal and jejunal pressure waves as well as retards duodenal-cecal transit. Small intestinal bacterial overgrowth (SIBO), probably secondary to altered small intestinal motility, is commonly encountered in diabetes. Estimates range between 15% and 40% in type 1 diabetics. Enteropathy is often a diagnosis of exclusion. It is essential to exclude underlying nondiabetes-related etiologies like testing for celiac disease as it commonly associated with type 1 diabetic patients. Clinicians should be aware that commonly used antidiabetic medications (metformin, GLP-1RAs, SGLT2 inhibitors, and particularly alpha-glucosidase inhibitors like acarbose) are commonly associated with intestinal symptoms. Small bowel manometry, wireless capsule, and scintigraphy are limited to specialized centers, and their diagnostic utility remains uncertain. Small intestinal bacterial overgrowth can be diagnosed by aspiration and culture of intestinal fluid or breath tests, but both have substantial limitations. Managing enteropathy is mostly symptomatic, SIBO is managed with antibiotics like Rifaximin, Amoxicillin clavulanate, and Metronidazole. Prokinetics used for gastroparesis may help in motility issues.

6.7 Large Intestine

Most common lower gastrointestinal symptoms are constipation, diarrhea, abdominal pain, and distention. Function of the colon is to reabsorb water and electrolytes from the intraluminal contents, to concentrate and solidify the fecal matter, and prepare for its evacuation. Studies have reported the presence of chronic constipation in up to 25% of people with type 1 and 2 diabetes, while that of chronic diarrhea is up to 5% [18]. Various population-based survey has demonstrated that the prevalence of diarrhea and constipation is significantly higher in diabetic patients.

Among multiple factors, autonomic neuropathy and slow colonic transit have been proposed as reasons for constipation. Evaluation of constipation includes colonoscopy, imaging of abdomen, colonic transit studies with radiopaque markers, or nuclear scan (scintigraphy)/wireless motility capsule. Management of diabetic constipation must include a medication history review and looking for drug-induced constipation and avoiding such medications. Mild constipation can be managed with increased physical exercise and dietary fiber. Over-the-counter laxatives (bulk, osmotic, or stimulatory), such as senna, bisacodyl, and water-soluble fiber supplements, are commonly prescribed. Osmotic laxative medications like lactulose and pegylated glycol are also prescribed. Stimulant laxatives can help for moderate constipation, which includes bisacodyl, sodium picosulphate. Lubiprostone, chloride channel which acts by direct activation of CIC-2 chloride channels on enterocytes, has been reported to improve both spontaneous bowel movements and accelerate colon transit in a randomized controlled trial in a cohort with diabetes [19]. The 5HT-4 agonist prucalopride is a new promising colokinetic useful in diabetic patients. Linoclotide results in the generation of cyclic guanosine monophosphate (cGMP), which stimulates chloride secretion, resulting in increased luminal fluid secretion and an acceleration of intestinal transit.

"Diabetic diarrhea" is considered a manifestation of autonomic neuropathy. The typical symptom is large volume, painless, nocturnal, diarrhea with or without fecal incontinence. Diagnosis is by exclusion of other common aetiologies and it is important to distinguish diarrhea from fecal incontinence. Antidiabetic medications like metformin (malabsorptive), acarbose (osmotic), and GLP-1 receptor agonists, commonly cause diarrhea. It is likely that optimizing glycemic control is important in the management of diabetic diarrhea. Dietary strategies include a low FODMAP (fermentable oligosaccharides, disaccharides, monosaccharides, and polyols) diet helps in reducing bloating and stool frequency. Loperamide, a mu-opioid receptor agonist, is used widely in refractory patients. Ramosetron is a newer 5-HT3 receptor antagonist bile acid sequestrants, such as cholestyramine and colesevelam, are used when bile salt malabsorption is suspected, and have the added advantage of reducing LDL cholesterol and glycated hemoglobin. Other agents include clonidine, diphenoxylate, octreotide, and ondansetron. Incidence of inflammatory bowel disease, including ulcerative colitis, is more with type 1 diabetic patients. Also, diabetic patients are more often affected by Clostridium difficile infection. Fecal incontinence occurs more frequently in people with diabetes and is associated with the duration of disease, and the presence of microvascular complications, including autonomic and peripheral neuropathy [20]. Both internal anal sphincter tone and anal squeeze pressures are reduced in those with diabetes compared to healthy individuals [21]. A key step in management is to exclude important differential diagnoses, such as colorectal malignancy and irritable bowel disease. Evaluation includes sigmoidoscopy, high-resolution anorectal manometry, MRI defecography, which are useful to detect rectal motor, sensory, and structural abnormalities [22].

Management of fecal incontinence is challenging, as its rarely curative. The main focus of management is to improve symptoms and quality of life. Fecal impaction with overflow incontinence can be managed by initial manual removal of stool from the rectum and enemas (promoting evacuation) and the subsequent prescription of bulk laxatives, increasing fiber intake, and toilet training. Biofeedback training can be useful in treating fecal, as well as urinary, incontinence. The technique involves visual demonstration of voluntary contraction of external anal sphincter (EAS) contraction to the patient and training to improve the quality of the response (both strength and duration). Biofeedback training is effective in the longer term in only about 60% of patients in clinical trials [23].

6.8 Liver

6.8.1 Glycogenic Hepatopathy

Glycogenic hepatopathy is a rare clinical condition that develops due to excessive accumulation of glycogen in the hepatocytes predominantly seen in pediatric patients and young adults with poorly controlled type 1 diabetes mellitus (T1DM), and rarely observed in a patient with type 2 diabetes mellitus (T2DM). This underrecognized liver condition characterized by transient liver dysfunction with elevated liver enzymes and associated hepatomegaly caused by a reversible accumulation of excess glycogen in hepatocytes. The collection of glycogen seen on a liver biopsy is critical for the diagnosis. In 2006, Torbenson and colleagues proposed the term "glycogenic hepatopathy" due to hepatocyte glycogen overload. Recurrent fluctuations in glucose level with hyperglycemia, hypoglycemia, and hyperinsulinization are proposed to be the reasons for this unique condition. Mostly, asymptomatic elevated liver enzymes or with symptoms of hyperglycemia like polyuria, polydipsia, weight loss, and lethargy. Occasional hepatomegaly can cause abdomen pain. Ultrasound is not helpful. CT liver is hyperdense compared to NAFLD where its hypodense. Hence, CT and MRI can help in differentiating liver biopsy is the gold standard for diagnosis of glycogenic hepatopathy, typical features are swollen hepatocytes, due to the accumulation of glycogen in the cytoplasm. The hematoxylin and eosin (HE) stain shows pale and enlarged hepatocytes with numerous glycogenated nuclei. PAS staining shows empty hepatocytes (ghost cells). In T2DM, metformin is typically the first-line of treatment maintaining glycemic control is the key. Glycogenic hepatopathy (GH) is a benign and potentially reversible condition within few days to weeks with good glycemic control unlike NAFLD which progress to fibrosis and cirrhosis [24].

6.8.2 Hepatogenous Diabetes

Hepatogenous diabetes appears to be the most prevalent form of diabetes in patients with liver cirrhosis. The prevalence rates have been reported to vary from 21% to 57%. Naunyn first coined the term "hepatogenous diabetes" in 1906. The pathophysiological basis of hepatogenous diabetes seems to involve insulin resistance (IR) and pancreatic β-cell dysfunction. The neurohormonal changes, endotoxemia, and chronic inflammation of LC initially create insulin resistance; however, the toxic effects eventually lead to β-cell dysfunction, which marks the transition from impaired glucose tolerance to hepatogenous diabetes. Distinguishing HD from T2DM can be challenging, especially in early cirrhosis, because both DM and cirrhosis have a long, indolent, and clinically silent course, making it difficult to determine which condition appeared first. However, the characteristics of hepatogenous diabetes include occurrence after onset of cirrhosis. Low prevalence of metabolic risk factors or family history of DM, normal fasting but abnormal GTT, low prevalence of microvascular complications, associated with higher insulin resistance/risk of hypoglycemia and remission after transplant. The presence of both DM and liver cirrhosis is associated with numerous complications and poor outcomes. Currently, there are no standardized guidelines for managing diabetes in cirrhosis patients. T2DM and HD are generally treated in a similar manner, with insulin recommended atn all stages of liver disease [25]. Treatment should be individualized.

6.8.3 Nonalcoholic Fatty Liver Disease

Nonalcoholic fatty liver disease (NAFLD) is a range of liver disorders that includes hepatic steatosis, steatohepatitis, and hepatic fibrosis. This may further progress to cirrhosis and hepatocellular carcinoma (HCC) (Fig. 6.3) [26].

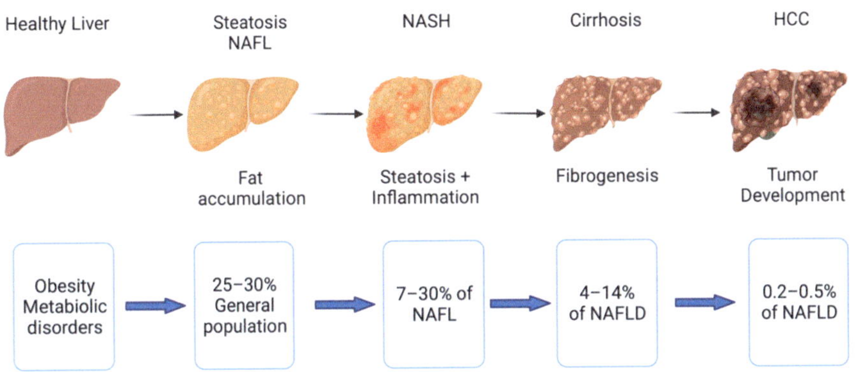

Fig. 6.3 Nonalcoholic fatty liver diseases

NAFLD is an overarching term that includes all disease grades and stages and refers to a population in which ≥5% of hepatocytes display macrovesicular steatosis in the absence of a readily identified alternative cause of steatosis (e.g., medications, starvation, and monogenic disorders) in individuals who drink little or no alcohol (defined as <20 g/d for women and <30 g/d for men). The spectrum of disease includes NAFL, characterized by macrovesicular hepatic steatosis that may be accompanied by mild inflammation, and NASH, which is additionally characterized by the presence of inflammation and cellular injury (ballooning), with or without fibrosis, and finally cirrhosis, which is characterized by bands of fibrous septa leading to the formation of cirrhosis. Approximately, 25% of the global population has been affected by NAFLD [27]. Prevalence of NAFLD has been increasing progressively over the past years due to the higher prevalence of obesity, physical inactivity, metabolic syndromes, and type 2 diabetes mellitus (T2DM), which represent the major risk factors of NAFLD. It was found that more than half the patients with T2DM are diagnosed with NAFLD, which shows a strong relationship between them. Proposed mechanism of fatty liver is the multihit theory. According to this, the first hit involves the buildup of triglycerides in the liver, causing steatosis. This increases the susceptibility of the liver to undergo second hits caused by oxidative stress, endoplasmic reticulum stress, mitochondrial dysfunction, inflammatory cytokines, adipokines, gut microbiota, and glucocorticoids. Free fatty acids (FFA) in causing liver injury through direct lipotoxicity. FFA influx into the liver leads to lysosomal destabilization, activating inflammatory pathways such as the nuclear factor kappa B-dependent tumor necrosis factor-alpha pathway [27]. The third hit is proposed to be initiated by the death of hepatocytes. The progression from nonalcoholic fatty liver to NASH occurs when the protective mechanisms of FFA-mediated lipotoxicity become exhausted, and the rate of hepatocyte death exceeds the rate of hepatocyte regeneration. This triggers the activation of myofibroblasts, which produce liver progenitor cells. These cells induce inflammatory immune responses and differentiate to replace the dead hepatocytes, causing variable degrees of hepatic architecture distortion. Insulin resistance results in hyperinsulinemia which has been shown to cause hepatocellular ballooning and lobular inflammation.

NAFLD is a well-defined risk factor for diabetes mellitus. Meta-analysis have shown the increased risk of diabetes in patients with NAFLD, as diagnosed by different diagnostic modalities including liver enzymes and imaging studies [28].

Diabetes mellitus is considered a well-known risk factor for NAFLD. Studies have shown a higher prevalence of NAFLD in diabetic patients. A recent meta-analysis published in 2017 showed that the pooled prevalence of NAFLD in diabetic patients is around 60%. In addition, patients who presented with NAFLD and diabetes have shown a greater risk of chronic liver disease, fibrosis, and cirrhosis compared to nondiabetic patients. Moreover, NAFLD in diabetic patients increases the risk of cardiovascular disease and other diabetic complications like kidney diseases.

Diabetes plays an important role in the progression of NAFLD and has been proven to augment the risk of NASH by approximately two to threefold. Based on liver histology, studies reveal that about 80% of patients with diabetes exhibit NASH, and 30–40% of them exhibit advanced fibrosis [29]. Furthermore, the risk of developing HCC increases by two to threefold with the presence of diabetes. Therefore, it is clear that advancement of NAFLD is driven by the presence of diabetes.

Diabetes augments NAFLD by multiple pathways. Fatty-acid release from adipose tissue is increased by insulin resistance. Liver inflammation and fibrosis are induced by direct lipotoxicity caused by excessive hepatic FFA influx in diabetics. Further damage is caused to the liver by the oxidative stress induced by oxidation and metabolism of excessive FFAs in the liver, which consequently elicits hepatocellular damage and apoptosis. Hepatocyte apoptosis and necrosis are then activated by hepatocellular injury. Consequently, this causes stimulation of hepatic stellate cells, and ultimately hepatic fibrosis. There has been further evidence that liver fibrosis can be promoted by IR because of the stimulation of lysyl oxidase-like 2, independent of hepatic stellate cell activity.

Diagnosis of fatty liver is through blood investigations, imaging, and histology. Initial evaluation of patient having suspicion of NAFLD is looking for other associated comorbidities like obesity, dyslipidemia, diabetes, hypothyroidism, polycystic ovary syndrome, and sleep apnea. History and details of alcohol intake, medications, and family history of fatty liver or liver disease should be considered. Clinical evaluation includes anthropometry and looking for peripheral signs of metabolic syndrome, such as acanthosis. Blood investigations include lipid profile, thyroid test, HBA1C, ANA, and hepatitis serology. Imaging tools like ultrasound of liver, MRI spectroscopy, MR elastography, or MRI-proton density fat fraction are useful for assessing fatty liver and steatohepatitis. Although standard ultrasound can detect hepatic steatosis, it is not recommended as a tool to identify hepatic steatosis due to low sensitivity across the NAFLD spectrum. Serum biomarker for fibrosis are worth to mention but not widely practised.

Noninvasive techniques include APRI (AST to platelet ratio index), Fib-4, the enhanced liver fibrosis panel, and the NFS NAFLD fibrosis score. Transient elastography includes FibroScan or ARFI (acoustic radiation force impulse imaging). Among the noninvasive test, FIB-4 and NFS are widely used in clinical practice (Fig. 6.4).

Fig. 6.4 Liver biopsy procedures

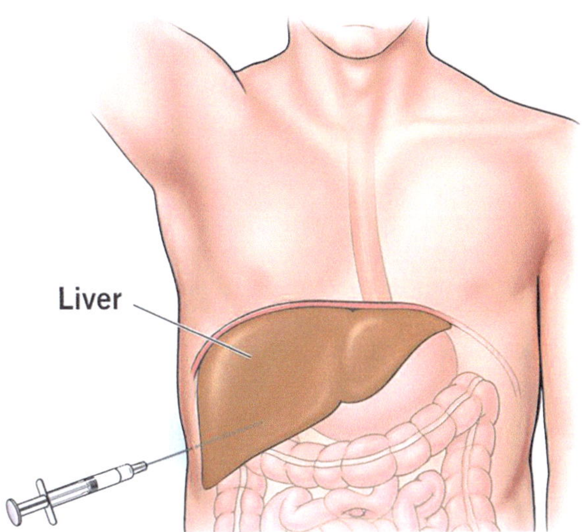

Liver stiffness is a physical characteristic that increases with fibrosis severity, infiltration, and inflammation. Liver stiffness measurement by FibroScan between 8 and 12 kPa may be associated with fibrotic NASH, and LSM >12 kPa is associated with a high likelihood of advanced fibrosis. Current guidelines suggest using the FIB-4 in suspicious scenario, followed by transient elastography. Histology remains the gold standard for diagnosing and assessing the grading of necroinflammation and severity of fibrosis.

A healthy diet and regular exercise form the foundation of treatment for the vast majority of those with NAFLD. Weight loss of 3%–5% improves steatosis, but greater weight loss (>10%) is generally required to improve NASH and fibrosis. Sustained weight loss reduces adipose tissue stress and improves peripheral insulin sensitivity, which can reduce the drive for liver injury in NASH. A diet containing excess calories, particularly excess saturated fats, refined carbohydrates, and sugar-sweetened beverages, is associated with obesity and NAFLD. Excessive fructose consumption in particular increases the risk of NAFLD, NASH, and advanced fibrosis independent of calorie intake. Changes in dietary composition (e.g., low-carbohydrate vs. low-fat diets, saturated vs. unsaturated fat diets, intermittent fasting, and Mediterranean diet) and different intensities of caloric restriction appear comparable in their ability to improve NAFLD/NASH. The Mediterranean diet is often recommended to patients with NAFLD based on its associated improvement in cardiovascular health and reduction in liver fat. Coffee consumption, independent of caffeine content, may also be beneficial. Drinking three or more cups per day could be recommended.

Exercise, independent of weight loss, has hepatic and cardiometabolic benefit and should be routinely recommended and tailored to the patient's preferences and physical abilities. Studies demonstrate that regular moderate exercise at least five times per week for a total of 150 min per week or an increase in activity level by more than 60 min per week can prevent or improve NAFLD. Though the optimal duration and intensity of exercise need to be individualized, patients should be encouraged to exercise as much as possible. Exercise can also improve frailty, sarcopenia, and quality of life in patients with chronic liver disease. NAFLD/NASH is increasingly accepted as a comorbid condition benefitting from bariatric surgery. Bariatric surgery can resolve NASH, improve hepatic fibrosis, induce sustained weight loss of up to 30%, cure diabetes, and decrease all-cause morbidity and mortality. Restrictive surgical procedures result in substantially less weight loss than malabsorptive procedures and are more likely to be associated with persistent NASH [30]. Bariatric surgery currently cannot be considered a primary therapy for the treatment of compensated NASH cirrhosis; however, it seems to be safe in carefully selected patients.

Currently, there are no FDA-approved drugs for the treatment of NASH at any disease stage. However, some medications approved for other indications have shown benefits for NASH in clinical trials.

Vitamin E: PIVENS, a multicenter, randomized controlled trial (RCT), pioglitazone versus vitamin E versus placebo for the treatment of nondiabetic patients with NASH, treatment with α-tocopherol (the natural form of vitamin E) 800 IU daily for 96 weeks improved histology (≥2-point reduction in NAS) compared with placebo. Indicated in patients with NASH without diabetes of cirrhosis. There are conflicting reports on potential risks like hemorrhagic stroke and prostate cancer are linked with high-dose vitamin E.

Thiazolidinediones: These are ligands for peroxisome proliferator-activated receptor γ, approved for the treatment of T2DM. In patients with NASH with or without pre-DM or T2DM, treatment with pioglitazone improves histology and insulin resistance and lipid profile [31]. Potential side effects associated with pioglitazone include weight gain, osteoporosis in postmenopausal women, a debated risk of bladder cancer, and potential risk for worsening heart failure in those with preexisting cardiac dysfunction. Its use in clinical practice has been overtaken by newer antidiabetic agents such as glucagon-like peptide-1 receptor agonist (GLP-1RA) and sodium glucose cotransporter-2 (SGLT-2) inhibitors (SGLT-2i) with more metabolic benefits, like weight loss and reduction in cardiovascular mortality.

GLP-1R agonist: Its effects on lipids, glucose metabolism, weight loss, and cardiovascular outcomes make them attractive agents for the treatment of NASH. RCT of daily s.c. semaglutide, 320 patients with NASH (F1–3) were randomized to 0.1, 0.2, or 0.4 mg or placebo daily for 72 weeks, NASH resolution was dose-dependent and occurred in 59% in the treatment group versus 17% in the placebo group ($p < 0.001$). Tirzepatide, a recently approved glucagon-like peptide-1/ glucose-dependent insulinotropic polypeptide receptor agonist for the treatment of T2DM, demonstrates weight loss as high as 20.9% in nondiabetics compared with 3.1% in the placebo group and an absolute reduction in liver fat content of 8.1%, suggesting a possible benefit in NASH.

SGLT-2 inhibitor: Target renal glucose resorption from the glomerular filtrate and are approved for the treatment of T2DM. Reduction in steatosis, improvement in insulin sensitivity, and benefits in cardiovascular and renal outcomes, along with modest weight loss, are observed. Potential risks of genitourinary yeast infection, volume depletion, bone loss have been reported.

Metformin, ursodeoxycholic acid, dipeptidyl peptidase-4, statins, and silymarin are well studied in NASH and should not be used as a treatment for NASH as they do not offer a meaningful histological benefit. Semaglutide can be considered for its approved indications (T2DM/obesity) in patients with NASH, as it confers a cardiovascular benefit and improves NASH. Statins are safe and recommended for CVD risk reduction in patients with NAFLD across the disease spectrum, including compensated cirrhosis. Limited data exist on the safety and efficacy of statins in patients with decompensated cirrhosis, although statin use could be considered in patients with high CVD risk with careful monitoring.

In summary, pioglitazone improves NASH and can be considered for patients with NASH in the context of patients with T2DM. Vitamin E can be considered in select individuals as it improves NASH in some patients without diabetes. Available data on semaglutide, pioglitazone, and vitamin E do not demonstrate an antifibrotic benefit, and none has been carefully studied in patients with cirrhosis [30].

Flint trial and regenerate trial have studied the usefulness of obitocholic acid in significant reduction of ALT, FIB-4, and transient elastography.

References

1. De Boer SY, Masclee AA, Lam WF, Lamers CB. Effect of acute hyperglycemia on esophageal motility and lower esophageal sphincter pressure in humans. Gastroenterology. 1992;103:775–80.
2. Lam WF, Masclee AA, de Boer SY, Lamers CB. Hyperglycemia reduces gastric secretory and plasma pancreatic polypeptide responses to modified sham feeding in humans. Digestion. 1993;54:48–53.
3. Monreal-Robles R, Remes-Troche JM. Diabetes and the esophagus. Curr Treat Options Gastroenterol. 2017;15:475–89.
4. Iyer SK, Chandrasekhara KL, Sutton A. Diffuse muscular hypertrophy of esophagus. Am J Med. 1986;80:849–52.
5. Tack J, Zaninotto G. Therapeutic options in oesophageal dysphagia. Nat Rev Gastroenterol Hepatol. 2015;12:332–41.
6. Kassander P. Asymptomatic gastric retention in diabetics (gastroparesis diabeticorum). Ann Intern Med. 1958;48:797–812.
7. Camilleri M, Chedid V, Ford AC, et al. Gastroparesis. Nat Rev Dis Primers. 2018;4:41.
8. Bharucha AE, Batey-Schaefer B, Cleary PA, et al. Delayed gastric emptying is associated with early and long-term hyperglycemia in type 1 diabetes mellitus. Gastroenterology. 2015;149:330–9.
9. Jung HK, Choung RS, Locke GR 3rd, et al. The incidence, prevalence, and outcomes of patients with gastroparesis in Olmsted County, Minnesota, from 1996 to 2006. Gastroenterology. 2009;136:1225–33.
10. Camilleri M, Parkman HP, Shafi MA, Abell TL, Gerson L. Clinical guideline: management of gastroparesis. Am J Gastroenterol. 2013;108:18–37.

11. Carbone F, Van den Houte K, Clevers E, et al. Prucalopride in gastroparesis: a randomized placebo-controlled crossover study. Am J Gastroenterol. 2019;114:1265–74.
12. Phillips LK, Deane AM, Jones KL, Rayner CK, Horowitz M. Gastric emptying and glycaemia in health and diabetes mellitus. Nat Rev Endocrinol. 2015;11:112–28.
13. Pazzi P, Scagliarini R, Gamberini S, Pezzoli A. Review article: gall-bladder motor function in diabetes mellitus. Aliment Pharmacol Ther. 2000;14(Suppl 2):62–5.
14. Marso SP, Daniels GH, Brown-Frandsen K, et al. Liraglutide and cardiovascular outcomes in type 2 diabetes. N Engl J Med. 2016;375:311–22.
15. Piciucchi M, Capurso G, Archibugi L, Delle Fave MM, Capasso M, Delle FG. Exocrine pancreatic insufficiency in diabetic patients: prevalence, mechanisms, and treatment. Int J Endocrinol. 2015;2015:595649.
16. Toouli J, Biankin AV, Oliver MR, et al. Management of pancreatic exocrine insufficiency: Australasian pancreatic Club recommendations. Med J Aust. 2010;193:461–7.
17. Kashyap P, Farrugia G. Diabetic gastroparesis: what we have learned and had to unlearn in the past 5 years. Gut. 2010;59:1716–26.
18. Lysy J, Israeli E, Goldin E. The prevalence of chronic diarrhea among diabetic patients. Am J Gastroenterol. 1999;94:2165–70.
19. Christie J, Shroff S, Shahnavaz N, et al. A randomized, double-blind, placebo-controlled trial to examine the effectiveness of Lubiprostone on constipation symptoms and colon transit time in diabetic patients. Am J Gastroenterol. 2017;112:356–64.
20. Epanomeritakis E, Koutsoumbi P, Tsiaoussis I, et al. Impairment of anorectal function in diabetes mellitus parallels duration of disease. Dis Colon Rectum. 1999;42:1394–400.
21. Sun WM, Katsinelos P, Horowitz M, Read NW. Disturbances in anorectal function in patients with diabetes mellitus and faecal incontinence. Eur J Gastroenterol Hepatol. 1996;8:1007–12.
22. Carrington EV, Scott SM, Bharucha A, et al. Expert consensus document: advances in the evaluation of anorectal function. Nat Rev Gastroenterol Hepatol. 2018;15:309–23.
23. Narayanan SP, Bharucha AE. A practical guide to biofeedback therapy for pelvic floor disorders. Curr Gastroenterol Rep. 2019;21:21.
24. Sherigar JM, De Castro J, Yin YM, Guss D, Mohanty SR. Glycogenic hepatopathy: a narrative review. World. J Hepatol. 2018;10(2):172–85.
25. Kumar R, García-Compeán D, Maji T. Hepatogenous diabetes: knowledge, evidence, and skepticism. World J Hepatol. 2022;14(7):1291–306.
26. Smith BW, Adams LA. Non-alcoholic fatty liver disease. Crit Rev Clin Lab Sci. 2011;48:97–113.
27. Feldstein AE, Werneburg NW, Canbay A, et al. Free fatty acids promote hepatic lipotoxicity by stimulating TNF-alpha expression via a lysosomal pathway. Hepatology. 2004;40:185–94.
28. Mantovani A, Byrne CD, Bonora E, Targher G. Nonalcoholic fatty liver disease and risk of incident type 2 diabetes: a meta-analysis. Diabetes Care. 2018;41:372–82.
29. Sanyal A, Poklepovic A, Moyneur E, Barghout V. Population-based risk factors and resource utilization for HCC: US perspective. Curr Med Res Opin. 2010;26:2183–91.
30. Rinella ME, Neuschwander-Tetri BA, Siddiqui MS, et al. AASLD Practice Guidance on the clinical assessment and management of nonalcoholic fatty liver disease. Hepatology. 2023;77(5):1797–835.
31. Aithal GP, Thomas JA, Kaye PV, Lawson A, Ryder SD, Spendlove I, et al. Randomized, placebo-controlled trial of pioglitazone in nondiabetic subjects with nonalcoholic steatohepatitis. Gastroenterology. 2008;135:1176–84.

Role of Imaging in Managing Diabetic Complications

7

Georgi Abraham, Preetha Nethaji, and Aarthi Deepesh

7.1 Introduction

As successful management of diabetic complications embraces imaging technologies, a multidisciplinary approach with treating diabetologists, radiologists, and sub-speciality physicians and surgeons are mandatory. Here, we describe various imaging techniques involved in the care of diabetics with complications.

7.2 CNS

A 75-year old woman with a long history of diabetes and dementia shows diffuse atrophy of the cerebral parenchyma, with prominent sulcal spaces and dilated ventricles, diffuse periventricular hypoattenuation suggestive of small vessel ischemic changes. Incidentally, choroid plexus calcification is observed within the occipital horns of bilateral lateral ventricles, in the axial sections of NCCT brain (Fig. 7.1).

Microvascular and macrovascular complications develop in long-standing diabetics with poor glycemic control. This will lead to lacunar infarcts and subtle neurological deficits in older diabetic patients. The management consists of glycemic control with diet, lifestyle management, oral hypoglycemic drugs, and insulin. However, blood pressure control with calcium channel blockers and RAAS blockade, along with antiplatelet agents, are useful means. It may be worthwhile doing a color doppler of carotid and vertebral circulation for atheromatous vessel wall changes.

G. Abraham (✉)
Department of Nephrology, MGM Healthcare, Chennai, Tamil Nadu, India

P. Nethaji · A. Deepesh
Division of Imaging Sciences, MGM Healthcare, Chennai, Tamil Nadu, India

G. Abraham et al. (eds.), *Management of Diabetic Complications*,
https://doi.org/10.1007/978-981-97-6406-8_7

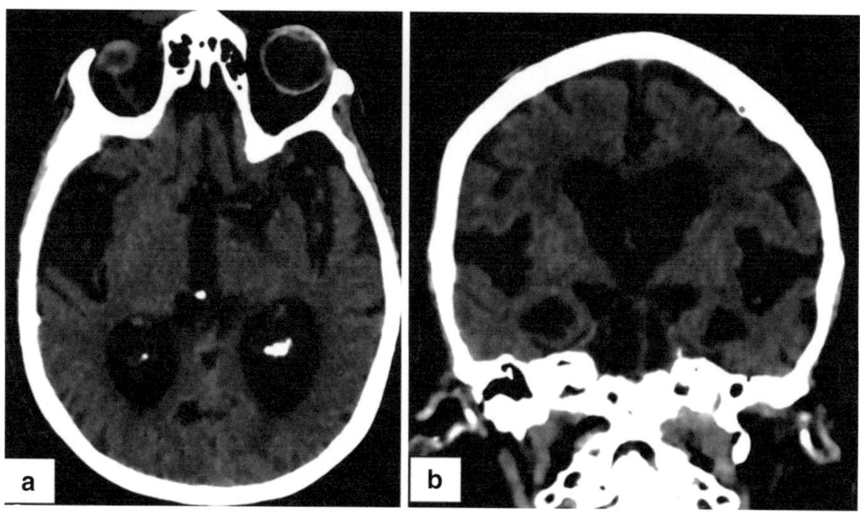

Fig. 7.1 (**a**) Axial and (**b**) coronal reformatted images of noncontrast CT (NCCT) brain

A 59-year-old male with a history of type 2 DM came with complaints of altered sensorium and slurring of speech.

MRI of the brain with MR angiogram was done. The diffusion-weighted sequences showed multiple acute nonhemorrhagic internal and external watershed infarcts. Acute evolved infarcts were seen involving bilateral occipital cortices (Fig. 7.2).

MR angiogram showed complete occlusion of the left internal carotid artery (ICA). Severe narrowing (80% to 90% stenosis) of the cavernous and clinoid segments of right internal carotid artery, severe attenuation of left M1 MCA seen with nonvisualization of distal cortical branches. There is attenuated caliber and faint flow involving the bilateral PCA-P3 and P4 segments.

These large infarcts are probably due to uncontrolled hypertension, and we should always perform a 2D echocardiogram to rule out a left ventricular clot in addition to color Doppler of the neck vessels [1]. As it involves multiple territories, revascularisation is not a preferable option.

7.2.1 Revascularisation and Recovery

A 48-year-old T2DM male presented with a history of sudden onset progressive decrease in sensorium. MRI brain showed acute nonhemorrhagic infarcts in the right hemi-pons. MR angiogram showed occlusion of the basilar artery. Coronal reformatted and 3D volume rendered images of CT angiogram (Fig. 7.3a, b) show complete occlusion of the basilar artery. Digital subtraction angiography (DSA) of the cerebral vessels (Fig. 7.3c) was done within 3 h of symptom onset, which confirmed the same findings. Mechanical thrombectomy was done, using direct contact

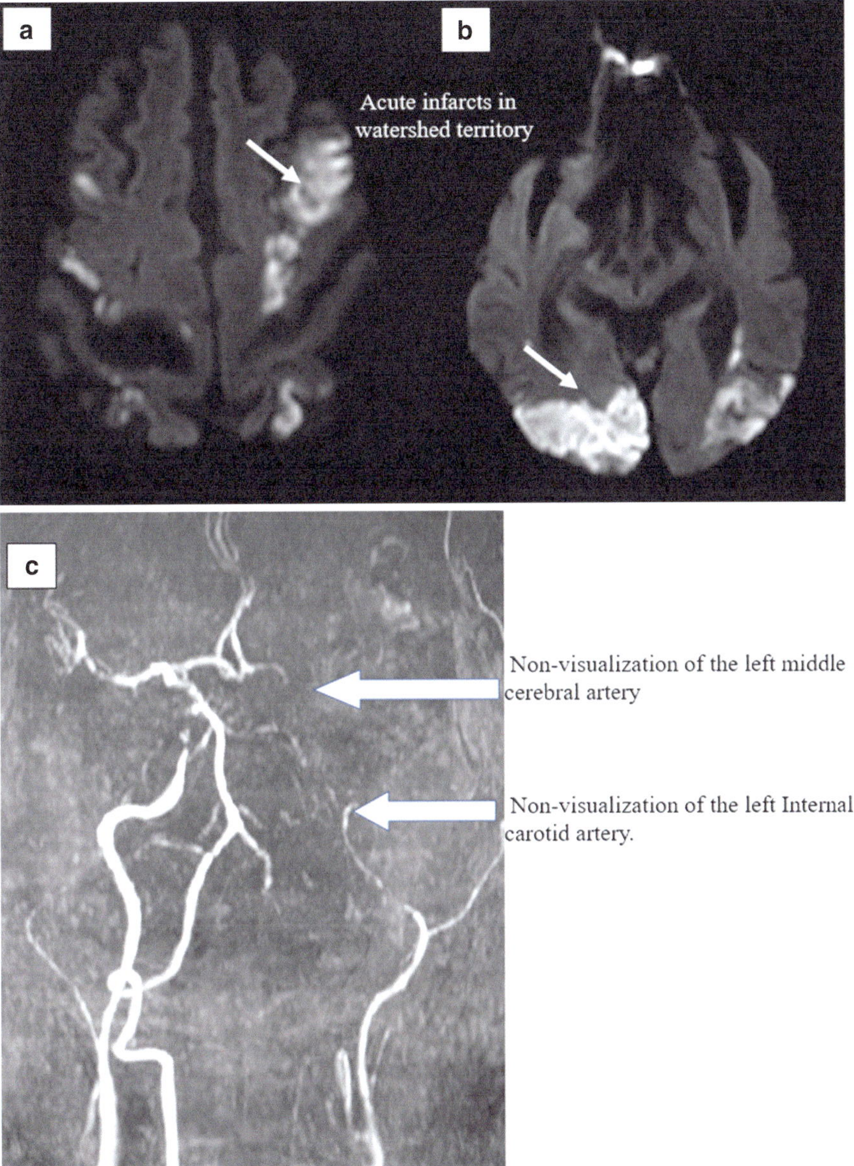

Fig. 7.2 Diffusion-weighted MR image of the brain (**a**, **b**), (**c**) 3D time-of-flight angiography of the circle of Willis

aspiration technique, following which the DSA showed normal opacification of the basilar artery (Fig. 7.3d). This was followed by improvement in the neurological status [2].

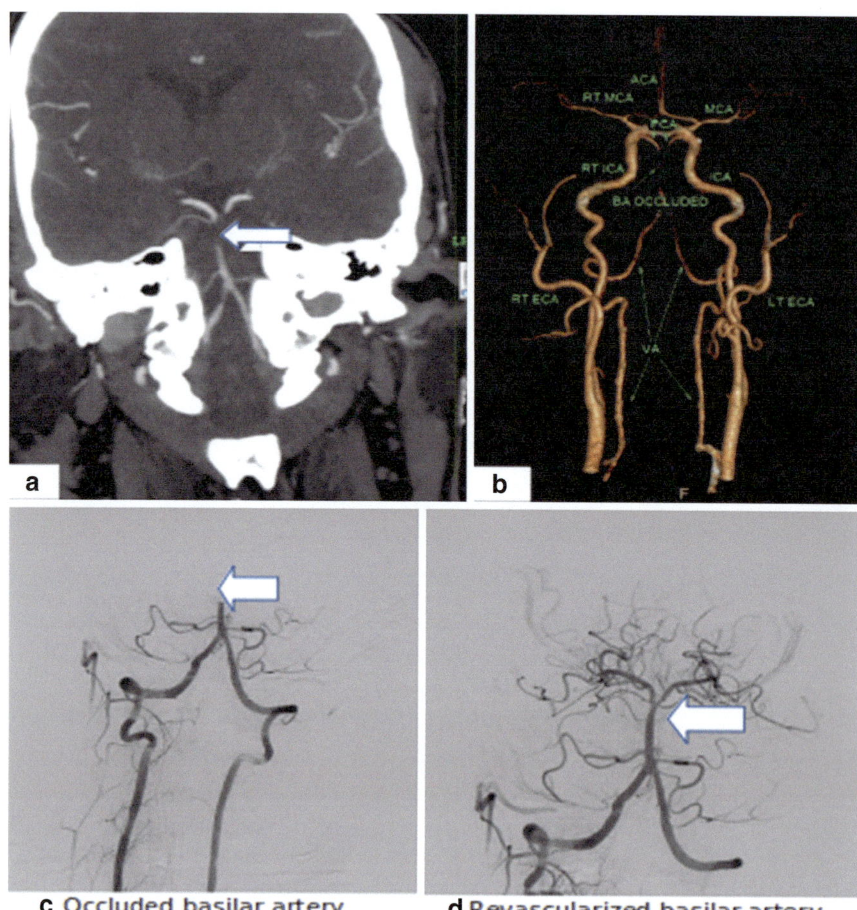

Fig. 7.3 (**a**) Coronal reformatted image of CT angiography of the cerebral vessels, (**b**) 3D volumetric reconstruction of the neck and intracranial arteries showing occluded basilar artery, and (**c**) digital subtraction angiography (DSA) of vertebrobasilar system before and after thrombolysis (**d**)

An 83-year-old diabetic male presented to the emergency department with a history of weakness and slurred speech. MRI brain showed few punctate nonhemorrhagic infarcts in the left internal watershed territory. CT angiography (sagittal and axial reformats—Fig. 7.4a, b) was done. Near complete occlusion of the left internal carotid artery at the origin was identified.

Patient was initially loaded with dual antiplatelet agents.

After a 2-week gap, DSA was done which confirmed the findings (Fig. 7.4c), the patient underwent balloon angioplasty and stenting. Post procedurally, the DSA showed normal flow across the stent and the left internal carotid artery (Fig. 7.4d). The patient showed improvement in his weakness and slurring of speech.

A 75-year-old obese diabetic, DKD stage IIIb with hypertension, has breast cancer and extensive metastasis in the spine, kidneys, and liver. She is being given

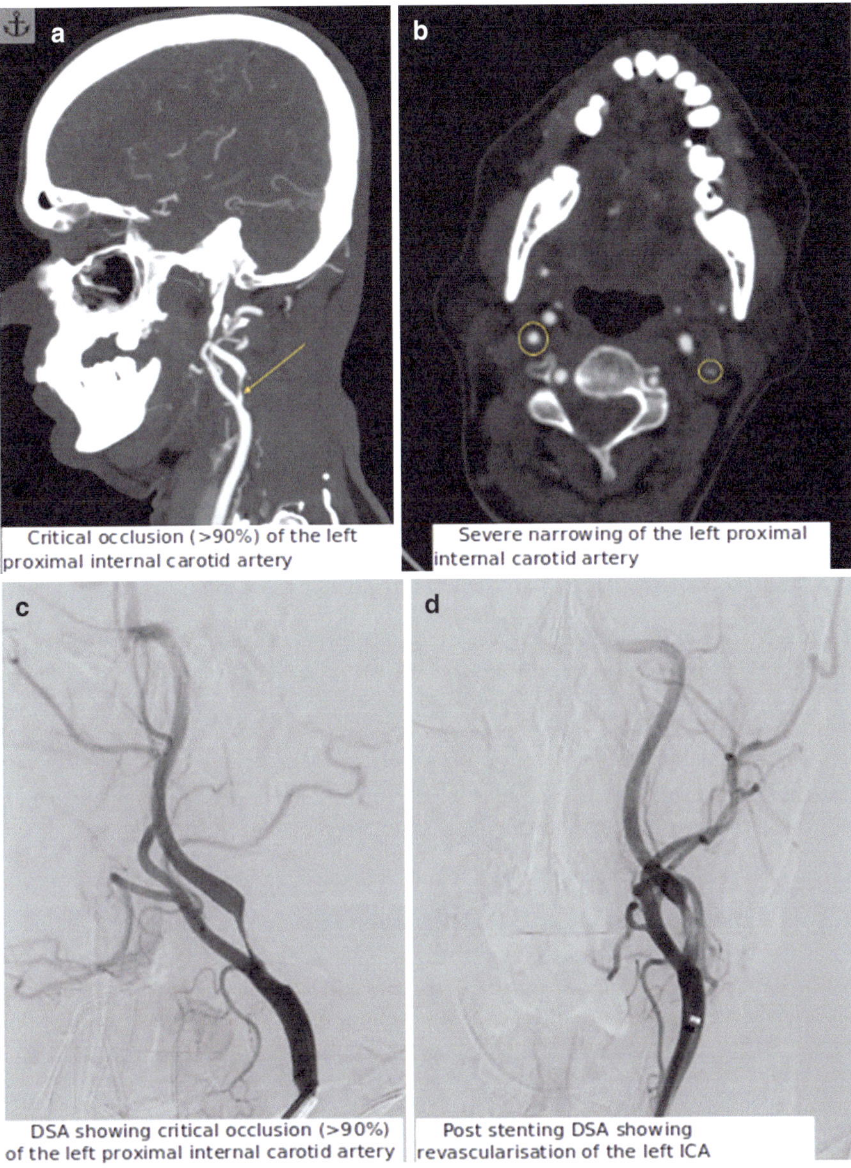

Fig. 7.4 (**a**, **b**) Sagittal and axial reformatted images of CT neck and cerebral vessel angiogram, (**c**) digital subtraction angiogram before, and (**d**) after angioplasty and stenting

chemotherapy which produced tumor lysis syndrome with worsening of kidney function, requiring hemodialysis. She developed a sudden onset of decreased sensorium (Fig. 7.5).

Her hemoglobin was 9.5 mg/dL and platelet count was 55,000/mm^3. CT of the brain showed a large acute intraparenchymal hemorrhage with fluid-fluid level

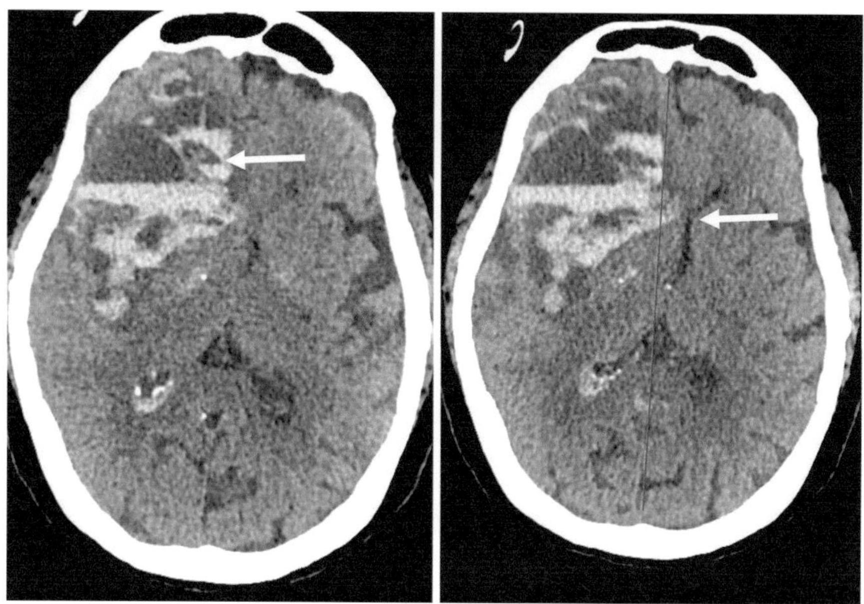

Fig. 7.5 Axial NCCT brain showing hyperacute intraparenchymal bleed in the right frontotemporal region with midline shift and intraventricular extension

(hematocrit sign) in the right frontotemporal and gangliocapsular region. Acute intraventricular hemorrhage and midline shift of 8 mm toward the left side was present [3].

Management consists of decompression with removal of the hematoma.

7.3 Cardiovascular and Respiratory System

A 70-year-old male with more than 20 years of T2DM and chronic kidney disease on home peritoneal dialysis presented with rusty sputum and shortness of breath for 5 days, along with uncontrolled hyperglycemia (blood sugar—380 mg to 420 mg/dL). His SpO_2 at room air was 80% and he was tachypneic.

On CT imaging, the arch of aorta (Fig. 7.6a) and the coronary arteries (Fig. 7.6b) show eccentric calcific plaques indicating atheromatous coronary and aortic disease. He also had multiple patchy areas of consolidation involving the left upper and lower lobes (Fig. 7.6c), indicating infective pneumonia.

Bronchoscopy with BAL showed thickly purulent sputum, growing Gram-negative organism.

A publication by Hariharan et al. from India showed that out of the 50 subjects studied, 39 were hypertensive (78%), 32 were diabetic (64.4%), 20 were on hemodialysis, and 13 were on continuous ambulatory peritoneal dialysis. The mean CACS was 388.6. Twenty-nine patients had high iPTH levels and 92.9% of them

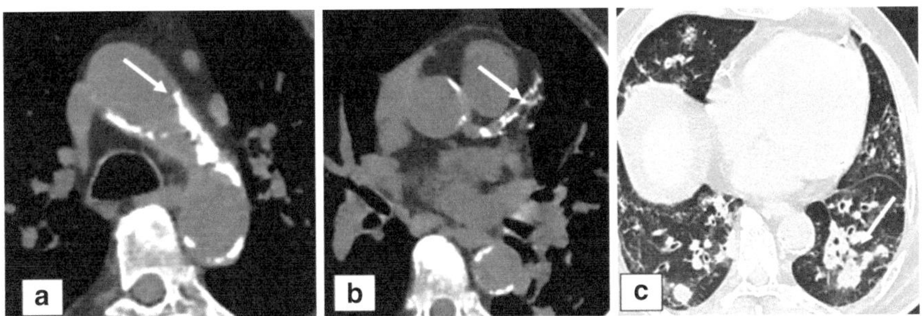

Fig. 7.6 Axial CT chest in mediastinal (**a**, **b**) and lung window (**c**) showing atheromatous calcific plaques and patchy consolidation

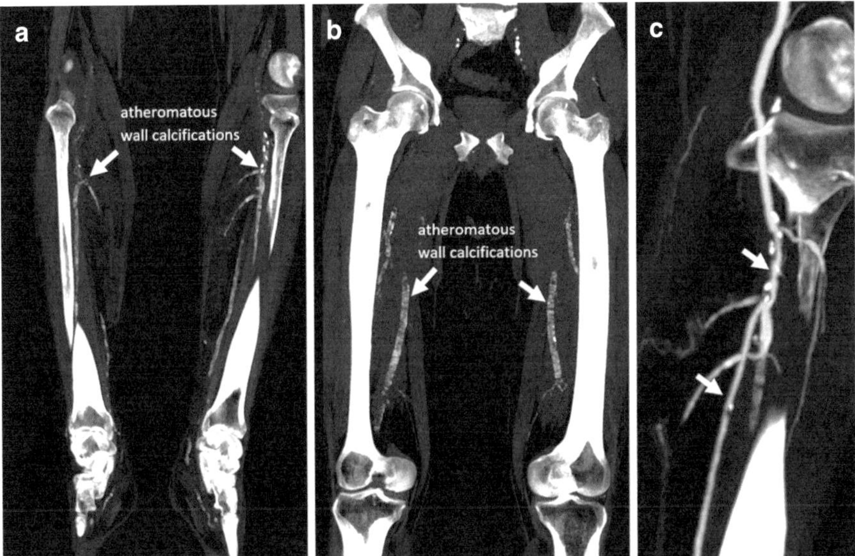

Fig. 7.7 (**a**, **b**, **c**) Coronal reformatted images of CT peripheral angiogram showing diffuse atherosclerotic calcific plaques

had calcium score > 400 (P = 0.013). Twenty-eight patients had high hCRP and 85.7% of these patients had calcium score > 400 (P = 0.048). Patients on dialysis for more than 2 years had higher calcium score > 400 (P = 0.035). 43% of diabetics had calcium score > 400 (P = 0.008). All the six patients who died had calcium score > 400 (P = 0) [4].

A 70-year-old diabetic male, on maintenance hemodialysis (MHD), presented with ischemic ulcers of the left foot with neuropathic symptoms. CT peripheral angiography showed diffuse atheromatous calcifications with multifocal areas of stenosis. Areas of critical narrowing were treated with angioplasty and the ulcers healed. This is a typical example of large vessel disease of the lower limb (Fig. 7.7).

7.4 Genitourinary System

A 63-year-old diabetic woman presented with right loin pain and weight loss. Her serum creatinine level was 2.94 mg/dL, and a urine examination showed plenty of WBCs, 2–4 RBC/hpf, and 2+ proteinuria. Her glycemic control was poor. Blood culture grew multidrug-resistant Klebsiella pneumoniae. CT scan of the abdomen showed a thick-walled exophytic hypodense lesion in the upper pole of right kidney measuring 6.6 × 6 cm. On PET CT, the lesion showed peripheral hypermetabolism (SUVmax—18.7) with focal infiltration of the right hemidiaphragm. She underwent laparatomy and right radical nephrectomy. However, histopathology showed evidence of Xanthogranulomatous pyelonephritis [5].

A 48-year-old female diabetic with left loin pain and fever. CT abdomen showed multiple air pockets within the left kidney, suggestive of emphysematous pyelonephritis. No evidence of renal/ureteric calculi (Fig. 7.8).

A 45-year-old diabetic lady presented with fever and right loin pain. She was diagnosed to have leptospirosis. Her renal functions were abnormal with stage II AKI (acute kidney injury) (Fig. 7.9).

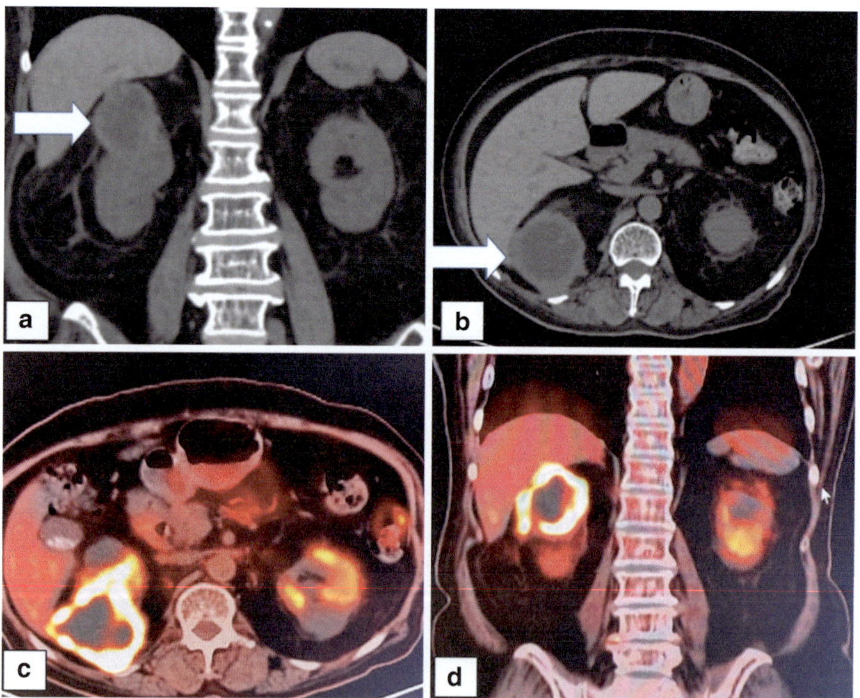

Fig. 7.8 (**a**, **b**) Showing hypodense lesion in the upper pole of right kidney. (**c**, **d**) Axial and coronal sections of PET-CT showing marked peripheral FDG uptake in the wall of the right renal lesion

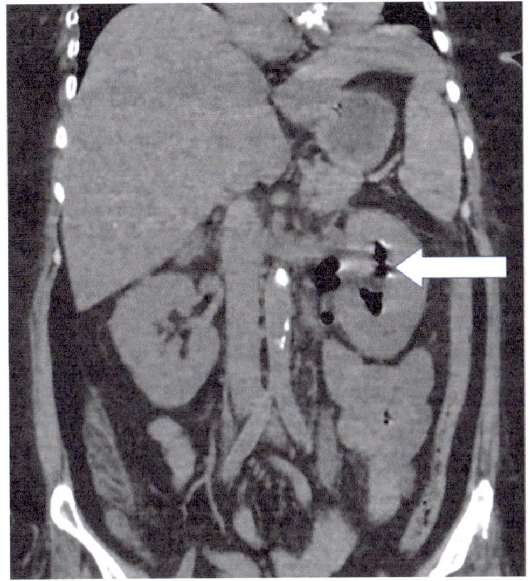

Multiple air pockets seen within the left pelvicalyceal system and the proximal left ureter.

Fig. 7.9 Coronal reformatted image of plain CT abdomen

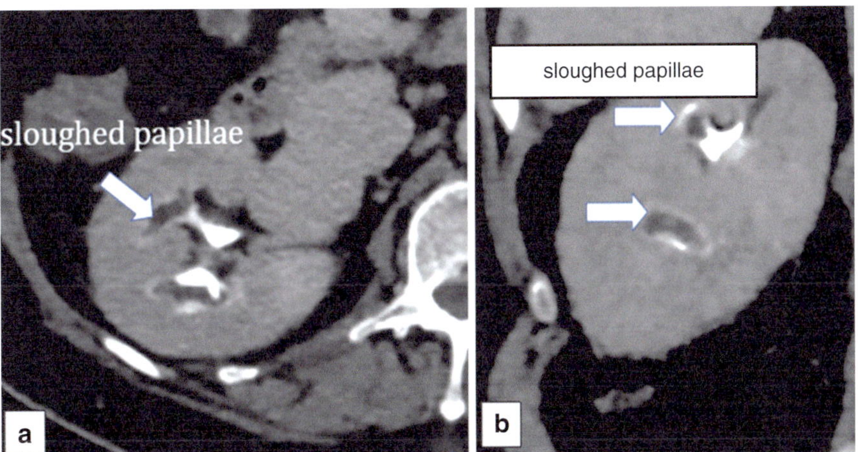

Fig. 7.10 CT urogram in the excretory phase showing filling defects in the kidney suggestive of sloughed papillae shown in white arrows

CT urogram (axial and coronal) in the delayed phase shows multiple hypodense nonenhancing filling defects in the calyceal system suggestive of sloughed papillae (Fig. 7.10). The papillae were recovered from the urine. With the treatment of leptospirosis, her kidney functions improved [6].

7.5 Isotope Studies in Diabetics

A 71-year-old female diabetic with poorly functioning right kidney for 50 years. She is also hypothyroid, on thyroxine supplementation, and has controlled hypertension.

HIDA scan confirmed that there was no leak of bile from the liver/biliary system in a diabetic patient who underwent cholecystectomy (Fig. 7.11).

A 60-year-old female diabetic kidney disease with exit site infection (ESI). Catheter tunnel ultrasound shows a hypoechoic collection in the catheter tunnel, suggestive of tunnel infection (TI). She was treated with appropriate antibiotics, diabetic control, and catheter care (Fig. 7.12).

DKD stage II lady presented with right loin pain and fever with rigor and chills. There was albumin 1+ and many WBCs in the urine. Physical examination showed right renal angle tenderness. On imaging, CT showed an infected cyst with few air pockets, in the posterior subcapsular region of right kidney, displacing the kidney anteriorly. There was no obstruction to the flow of urine in the right kidney. Ultrasound-guided pigtail insertion was done, nearly 1–1.5 L of pus was aspirated, which grew Klebsiella pneumoniae. DJ stenting, appropriate antibiotics, and blood sugar control was also done. Posttreatment repeat CT showed thin rim of residual collection (Fig. 7.13).

A 71-year-old male patient presented with abdominal pain. CT showed the presence of staghorn calculus causing mild hydronephrosis. A staghorn calculus is a nidus for recurrent urinary tract infection including pyelonephritis. An isotope

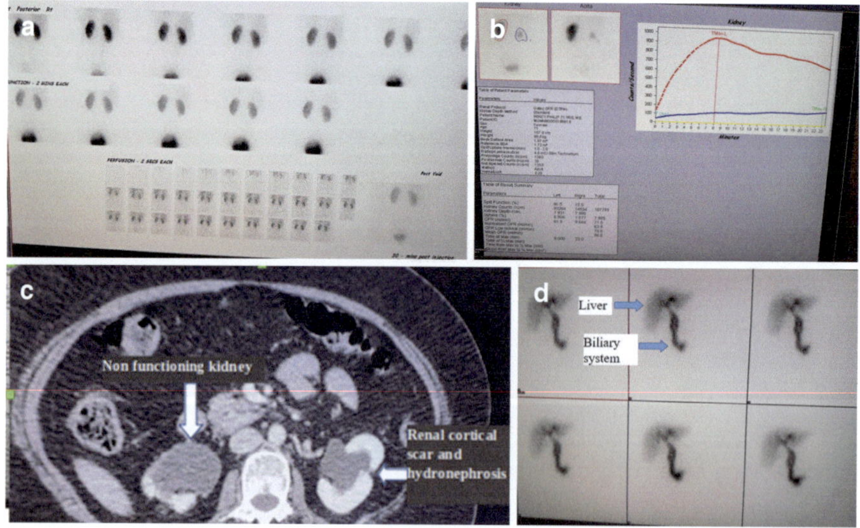

Fig. 7.11 (**a**) Normal isotope renogram, showing uptake and excretion in both kidneys. (**b**, **c**) CT image confirms the diagnosis of right nonfunctioning kidney and left-sided hydronephrosis diagnosed on renogram. (**d**) Serial hepatobiliary iminodiacetic acid (HIDA)

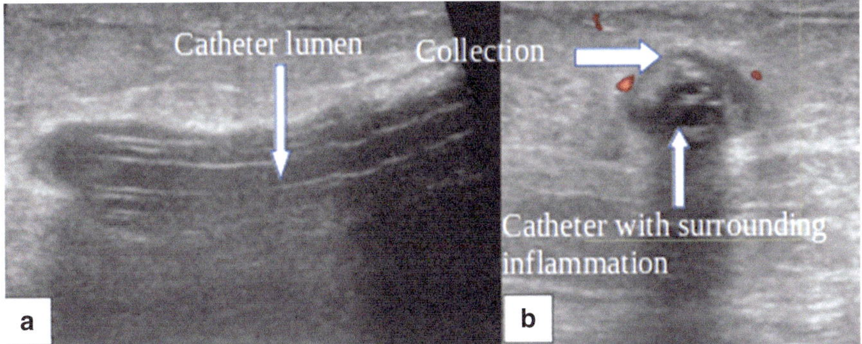

Fig. 7.12 Ultrasound images of the peritoneal dialysis catheter in the abdomen wall showing normal (**a**) and surrounding inflammation (**b**)

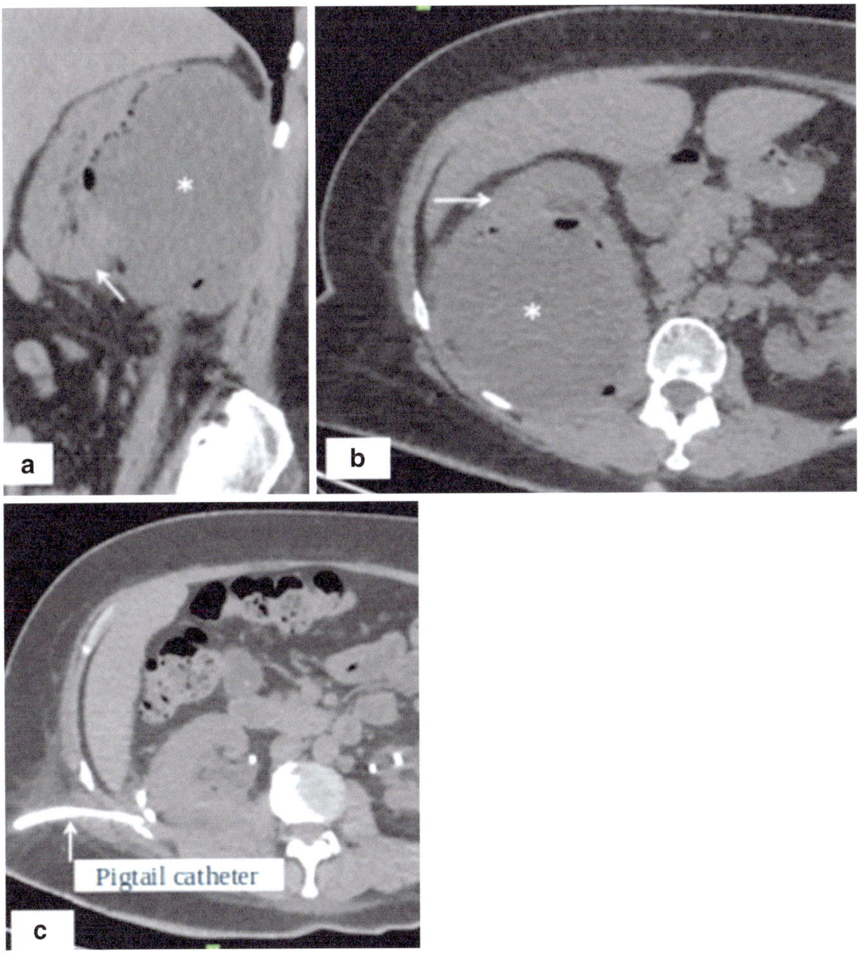

Fig. 7.13 Sagittal, axial sections of CT abdomen done before (**a**, **b**) and after pigtail insertion into the right kidney with subcapsular infected cyst (**c**)

renogram will enable us to see the split functions of the kidney. Removal by extracorporeal shock wave lithotripsy (ESWL) with DJ stenting and antibiotic therapy with glucose control is the treatment of choice. While retrieving the stone, a chemical analysis is required (Fig. 7.14).

Rare neuroendocrine tumor (NET) in a diabetic kidney transplant recipient. A 62-year-old woman, with 22 years of live kidney transplant, presented with intermittent diarrhea and weight loss for 3 months. She is a posttransplant, new onset diabetic (NODAT) taking oral hypoglycemic agents (Fig. 7.15).

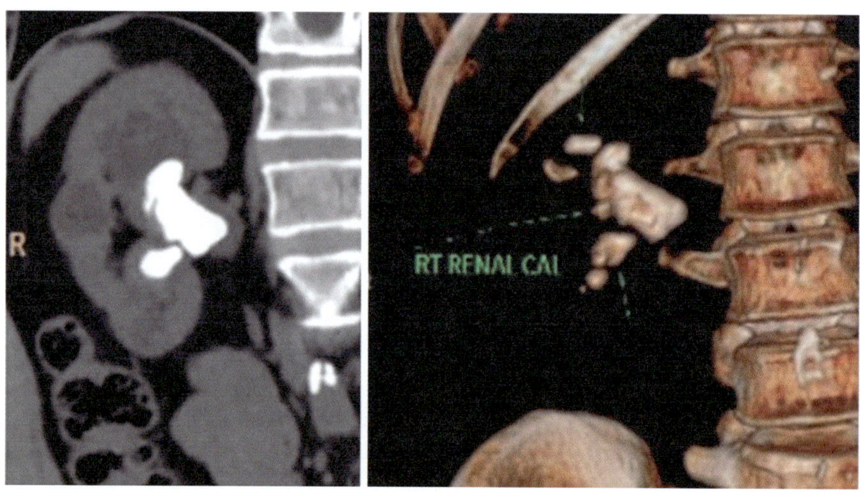

Fig. 7.14 Coronal CT abdomen and 3D volumetric reconstruction images

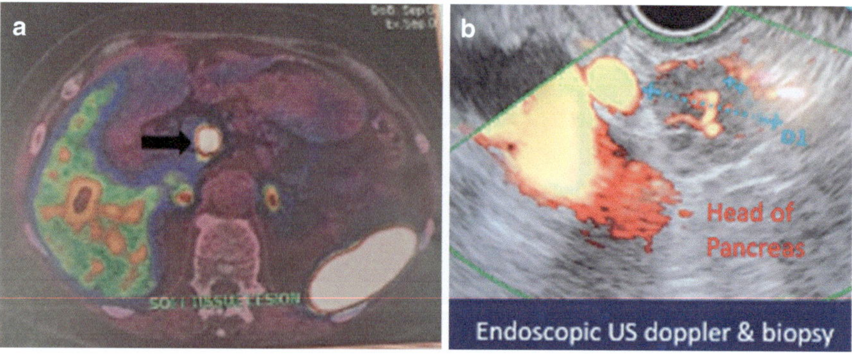

Fig. 7.15 DOTANOC PET CT (**a**) showing increased uptake in the region of head of the pancreas. (**b**) shows a hypoechoic lesion in the head of pancreas from which biopsy was taken

References

1. Mosenzon O, Cheng AY, Rabinstein AA, Sacco S. Diabetes and stroke: what are the connections? J Stroke. 2023;25(1):26–38. https://doi.org/10.5853/jos.2022.02306. Epub 2023 Jan 3. PMID: 36592968; PMCID: PMC9911852.
2. Bradley SA, Spring KJ, Beran RG, Chatzis D, Killingsworth MC, Bhaskar SM. Role of diabetes in stroke: recent advances in pathophysiology and clinical management. Diabetes Metab Res Rev. 2022;38(2):e3495.
3. Hesami O, Kasmaei HD, Matini F, Assarzadegan F, Mansouri B, Jabbehdari S. Relationship between intracerebral hemorrhage and diabetes mellitus: a case-control study. J Clin Diagn Res. 2015;9(4):OC08–10. https://doi.org/10.7860/JCDR/2015/12226.3741. Epub 2015 Apr 1. PMID: 26023579; PMCID: PMC4437093.
4. Iyer H, Abraham G, Reddy YN, et al. Risk factors of chronic kidney disease influencing cardiac calcification. Saudi J Kidney Dis Transpl. 2013;24(6):1189–94. https://doi.org/10.4103/1319-2442.121279.
5. Jaik NP, Sajuitha K, Mathew M, et al. Renal abscess. J Assoc Physicians India. 2006;54:241–3.
6. Thanka J, Kuruvilla S, Abraham G, Shroff S, Kumar BA, Ranjitham M. Bilateral renal papillary necrosis due to Candida infection in a diabetic patient presenting as anuria. J Assoc Physicians India. 2003;51:919–20.

Comprehensive Rehabilitation Program for Diabetes Management and Care

8

A. J. Rajendran and N. Vijayashree

8.1 Introduction

Diabetes mellitus, characterized by chronic hyperglycemia, has evolved into a pervasive global public health crisis, transcending geographical and demographic boundaries. India, in particular, bears the weight of being the second-highest contributor to this crisis globally, with an estimated 77 million diagnosed cases and a concerning number of undiagnosed instances.

Addressing this burgeoning epidemic necessitates a comprehensive, evidence-based approach to diabetes management and care.

Indian Context:

- India hosts the largest population of diabetics [1] outside China, with a prevalence of 7.7% among adults (age 20–79 years) and an estimated prediabetes prevalence of 10.9%.
- The rising burden of diabetes in India is linked to rapid urbanisation, dietary shifts toward processed foods, and sedentary lifestyles.
- Challenges in diabetes care in India encompass limited access to healthcare facilities, a shortage of trained professionals, low awareness, and socioeconomic barriers to medication and treatment.

A. J. Rajendran (✉)
Department of Rehabilitation Medicine, MGM Healthcare, Chennai, Tamil Nadu, India

N. Vijayashree
Department of Dietetics and Nutrition, MGM Healthcare, Chennai, Tamil Nadu, India

G. Abraham et al. (eds.), *Management of Diabetic Complications*,
https://doi.org/10.1007/978-981-97-6406-8_8

8.2 The DREAM Approach

Diabetes, as a chronic metabolic disorder featuring hyperglycemia, significantly impacts global health. While pharmacological interventions are crucial, lifestyle modifications, particularly diet [2–5] and exercise, constitute the cornerstone of successful diabetes management. Diabetes rehabilitation programs present a comprehensive approach to empower patients, optimize glycemic control [6], and prevent complications, ultimately enhancing the quality of life and reducing mortality [6, 7].

The multifaceted nature of diabetes mellitus demands a nuanced management approach, extending beyond medication adherence. The DREAM (diet, relaxation, exercise, attitude, and motivation) program emerges as a comprehensive rehabilitation strategy [7], addressing the biopsychosocial aspects of diabetes and empowering individuals to thrive.

The management of diabetes goes beyond pharmaceutical interventions and extends to comprehensive lifestyle modifications. This chapter explores the cumulative and exponential benefits of diabetes rehabilitation, emphasizing the integration of key components of diet, exercise, relaxation techniques, behavior/lifestyle changes, meditation, and motivation.

The integration of diet, exercise, relaxation, behavior/lifestyle changes, meditation, and motivation in diabetes rehabilitation, the DREAM components, offers cumulative and exponential benefits. Evidence from various studies supports the notion that the long-term commitment to these components significantly improves glycemic control [6], reduces cardiovascular risk factors, and enhances the overall quality of life for individuals with diabetes. Health professionals should emphasize the importance of a comprehensive approach to diabetes management, tailored to individual needs, to achieve optimal and sustainable outcomes.

8.3 Rehabilitation Approach

8.3.1 Diet [4] (D): Tailored Nutrition for Metabolic Balance

- *Evidence:* Personalized dietary plans demonstrably improve glycemic control and reduce chronic disease risk.
- *Approach:* Focus on portion control, balanced macronutrients, and nutrient-dense whole foods.

Implementation

- Collaboration with registered dietitians for individualized meal plans considering participant preferences, health parameters, and lifestyle.

Benefits

- Consistent adherence to a well-balanced, nutrient-dense diet is crucial in diabetes management.
- Gradual reduction of refined sugars and saturated fats contributes to better glycemic control over time.
- Cumulative improvements in insulin sensitivity and weight management lead to reduced cardiovascular risk.
- Studies show that a diet rich in fiber, whole grains, and antioxidants can have a positive impact on blood glucose levels.
- The Dietary Approaches to Stop Hypertension (DASH) and diets, with emphasis on plant-based foods, have demonstrated long-term benefits for individuals with diabetes.

8.3.2 Relaxation (R) [8–13]: Calming the Mind for Metabolic Harmony

- *Evidence:* Stress management techniques effectively reduce cortisol levels, contributing to improved insulin sensitivity and glycemic control.
- *Approach:* Integration of mindfulness meditation, yoga [14–17], and deep breathing [8–10] exercises.
- *Implementation:* Personalized relaxation plans based on individual stress triggers and preferred calming techniques.

Benefits

- Stress management techniques, such as deep breathing [8–10] and progressive muscle relaxation [18, 19] contribute to reduced cortisol levels.
- Consistent relaxation practices mitigate the negative impact of stress on blood glucose levels.
- Long-term stress reduction has been associated with improved insulin sensitivity and enhanced overall well-being.
- Mind–body interventions like yoga [14–16, 20] and meditation [11–13] have shown sustained benefits in glycemic control.

8.3.3 Exercise (E) [21–34]: Moving Toward Metabolic Flexibility

- *Evidence:* Regular physical activity enhances insulin sensitivity and glucose uptake, leading to improved glycemic control.
- *Approach:* Customized exercise routines incorporating aerobic [33, 34] and resistance training [32, 33].
- *Implementation:* Regular monitoring of physical activity through wearable devices or exercise logs.

Benefits

- Regular physical activity contributes to improved insulin sensitivity, facilitating glucose uptake by cells.
- Gradual weight loss and maintenance aid in glycemic control, reducing the risk of diabetes-related complications.
- Cumulative reduction in cardiovascular risk factors, including hypertension and dyslipidemia.
- Evidence suggests that both aerobic and resistance training provide unique benefits in managing diabetes.
- Incremental increases in exercise intensity and duration lead to sustained improvements in insulin sensitivity.

8.3.4 Attitude (A): Cultivating Resilience for Metabolic Empowerment

- *Evidence:* Cognitive-behavioral therapy (CBT) fosters a positive mindset and promotes self-management skills.
- *Approach:* Psychosocial support through group sessions and individual counseling.
- *Implementation:* Collaboration with mental health professionals to provide tailored support.

Benefits

- Gradual adoption of healthy behaviors, such as regular sleep patterns and smoking cessation, contributes to overall diabetes management.
- Consistent adherence to medication regimens and regular monitoring foster better long-term outcomes.
- Studies indicate that sustained positive lifestyle changes lead to improved glycemic control and reduced diabetes-related complications.
- Behavioral interventions, such as cognitive-behavioral therapy, have been effective in promoting lasting lifestyle modifications.

8.3.5 Motivation (M): Fueling the Journey to Metabolic Success

- *Evidence:* Goal-setting and motivational incentives enhance program engagement and adherence.
- *Approach:* Collaborative goal-setting and regular progress tracking.

8.4 Health Parameters Focus of DREAM

The DREAM program emphasizes regular monitoring of key health indicators for optimized diabetes management:

- Height, weight, and BMI.
- Waist-to-hip ratio.
- Blood pressure.
- Blood sugar and lipid levels.

Individualized and Collaborative Care Approach The DREAM program thrives on its tailored approach, considering lifestyle, health parameters, and personal preferences. A multidisciplinary team of healthcare professionals, including diabetes rehabilitation specialists, registered dietitians, and mental health professionals, collaborates to provide holistic care, addressing the physical, emotional, and social aspects of diabetes.

The DREAM holistic rehabilitation program marks a paradigm shift in diabetes management. By addressing diverse needs with a comprehensive, individualized approach, it empowers individuals to proactively manage their health, striving for improved metabolic control and overall well-being. This novel approach holds immense promise for enhancing energy levels, optimizing metabolic function, and promoting a better quality of life for individuals living with diabetes.

8.5 Diet in Diabetes Management

Diet plays a pivotal role in the effective management of diabetes. While medications and other interventions are essential, dietary modifications remain fundamental for achieving and maintaining optimal blood sugar levels, preventing complications, and improving overall health. This chapter explores practical aspects of dietary management, focusing on individualized meal plans, educational strategies, and self-management techniques to empower individuals in successfully navigating their diabetes journey.

Individualized Meal Plans Successful dietary management relies on personalized meal plans tailored to individual needs and preferences. Considerations include

- **Blood glucose monitoring data:** Regular monitoring provides insights into individual responses to different foods, enabling the creation of plans that optimize postprandial glycemic control.
- **Specific dietary needs:** Addressing needs related to carbohydrate counting, portion control, or dietary restrictions ensures an effective and sustainable meal plan.

- **Glycemic index (GI) and glycemic load (GL):** Prioritizing low-GI and low-GL foods helps minimize blood sugar spikes.
- **Nutrient-rich food choices:** Ensure adequate intake of essential nutrients for overall health.

Educational Sessions Effective dietary management extends beyond providing a meal plan. Comprehensive education is crucial to empower individuals with the knowledge and skills to make informed food choices and manage their diabetes effectively. Key areas of focus include

- **Connection between diet and blood sugar control:** Explain how different foods impact blood sugar levels, emphasizing the importance of carbohydrate counting and portion control.
- **Diabetes-specific food choices:** Provide guidance on identifying low-GI and low-GL foods, understanding food labels, and making healthy substitutions.
- **Meal planning tips:** Offer strategies for planning balanced meals and snacks, incorporating cultural preferences, and addressing common challenges.

Monitoring and Self-Management Active self-management is essential for achieving and maintaining glycemic control. Empower individuals with tools and knowledge for active participation in their diabetes care through

- **Regular blood sugar monitoring:** Encourage consistent monitoring to track progress and adjust the dietary plan as needed.
- **Healthy weight management:** Promote a combination of dietary modifications and regular physical activity for maintaining a healthy weight.

8.6 Nutritional Guidelines

Establishing and maintaining a healthy diet and lifestyle are paramount in diabetes rehabilitation program. A heart-healthy diet is not crucial for those seeking to minimize the risk of diabetes-related complications in the future but also healthy eating is a fundamental aspect of overall well-being, emphasizing the importance of sustained positive choices.

8.6.1 Carbohydrates

Carbohydrates consist of sugars and starches and are an important energy source for the body and brain. However, with diabetes, it is important to choose the right carbohydrates that help control blood glucose levels.

The following foods are sources of carbohydrates:

- Starchy carbohydrates
  - Cereals like rice, wheat, millets, noodles.
  - Potatoes, yam, plantain, colacasia, sweet potatoes.
- Simple carbohydrates.
- Sugary/processed foods such as cakes, chocolate, biscuits, jams, marmalades, bread and crackers, nondiet fizzy drinks, etc.
- Naturally occurring sugars.
  - Fruits, pulses (peas, beans, lentils).
  - Dairy food (milk, yogurt).

Starchy foods should form part of each meal. Choose smaller-sized portions of carbohydrate at each main meal and eat more vegetables with carbohydrates as this can help to control your blood glucose levels along with the fiber content of your diet, for example, wholegrain cereals, wholewheat, and brown rice. Adequate fiber in the diet ensures healthy bowel functioning and better sugar control.

- Recommended foods.
- Make your calories count with these nutritious foods:
  - Healthy carbohydrates.
  - During digestion, sugars (simple carbohydrates) and starches (complex carbohydrates) break down into blood glucose. Focus on the healthiest carbohydrates, such as fruits, vegetables, whole grains, legumes (beans, peas, and lentils), and low-fat dairy products.
  - Low glycemic index.

The glycemic index (GI) indicates a number as shown below:

55 or less is considered as low (good).
56–69 is considered as medium.
70 or higher is considered as high (bad).

Smaller the number, lesser will be the impact of that food on your blood sugar. Lower the index, slower the digestion takes place, therefore, the blood sugar levels will increase slowly and steadily. The food with glycemic index:

- Fiber-rich foods

  Dietary fiber includes all parts of plant foods that your body cannot digest or absorb. Fiber moderates how your body digests and helps control blood sugar levels. Foods high in fiber include vegetables, fruits, nuts, legumes (beans, peas, and lentils), whole-wheat flour, and wheat bran.

8.7 Relaxation Techniques in Diabetes Management

Chronic stress plays a pivotal role in the management of diabetes, significantly contributing to hyperglycemia, impaired glycemic control, and an increased risk of complications associated with diabetes. Employing relaxation techniques becomes crucial in diabetes rehabilitation as these techniques alleviate stress, promote psychological well-being, and ultimately enhance glycemic control.

8.7.1 Recommended Relaxation Techniques

1. Deep breathing.
2. Meditation.
3. Progressive muscle relaxation (PMR).

8.7.2 Additional Techniques

- **Visualization:** Shown to lower blood pressure and improve self-management behaviors.
- **Yoga:** Combining physical postures, breathing exercises, and meditation, yoga reduces stress, improves mood, and promotes glycemic control.

8.7.3 Implementation and Benefits

Relaxation techniques, whether in individual or group sessions, can be seamlessly integrated into diabetes rehabilitation programs. By teaching patients self-practice skills, they can incorporate these techniques into daily routines, fostering long-term stress management and potentially improving glycemic control.

Here is a guided meditation exercise for stress reduction:

1. Find a comfortable position: Sit or lie down in a quiet space where you would not be disturbed. Close your eyes or soften your gaze.
2. Body scan: Focus your attention on your body, scanning for areas of tension. Gently release any tightness you find through deep, slow breaths.
3. Mantra repetition: Choose a single word, phrase, or sound that resonates with you, such as "calm," "peace," or "om." silently repeat your chosen mantra as you inhale and exhale, letting its presence occupy your mind.
4. Nonjudgmental observation: When thoughts intrude, acknowledge them without judgment and gently redirect your focus back to your mantra. This is a natural process; persistence is key.
5. Gradual return: After 15–20 min, slowly open your eyes and take a few moments to reorient yourself. Notice the feeling of inner peace and relaxation.

Benefits of meditation for diabetes management

- Reduces stress hormones like cortisol, which can elevate blood sugar levels.
- Improves glucose control through enhanced self-awareness and emotional regulation.
- Promotes healthy sleep patterns, crucial for diabetes management.
- Enhances positive coping mechanisms, increasing resilience against stress-induced setbacks.

Progressive muscle relaxation (PMR)

Here is a guided PMR exercise for general relaxation:

1. Get comfortable: Lie down or sit in a supported position, close your eyes, and take a few deep breaths.
2. Muscle group focus: Select a muscle group, such as your hands and forearms. Clench your fists tightly for a few seconds, focusing on the sensation of tension.
3. Release and refocus: Slowly release the tension and observe the feeling of relaxation that washes over the muscles. Breathe deeply and hold this relaxed state for a few moments.
4. Repeat and progress: Repeat this tensing and releasing process with all major muscle groups, progressing from your hands and arms to your face, neck, shoulders, torso, legs, and feet.
5. Enjoy the relaxation: After completing the cycle, lie quietly for several minutes, savoring the feeling of peace and relaxation throughout your body.

Integrating meditation and PMR into diabetes rehabilitation

Both meditation and PMR are easily incorporated into a comprehensive diabetes rehabilitation program which includes education/learning, provide guided practice, use of audio resources.

8.8 Exercise in Diabetes Rehabilitation Program

Exercise is a crucial component of the diabetes rehabilitation education.

8.8.1 Types of Exercise and Supporting Evidence

- **Breathing Exercises**
  - *Pursed lip breathing technique:* Benefits include reducing anxiety, improving lung function, and promoting relaxation.
- **Range of Motion Exercises**
  - Maintaining full joint mobility promotes joint health, flexibility, and pain prevention.

- **Stretching Exercises**
  - Enhances flexibility, reduces pain, and prevents injuries, particularly in older adults.
- **Strengthening Exercises**
  - *Thera-band exercises:* Progressive resistance exercises using elastic bands improve muscle strength and stability.
- **Aerobic Exercises**
  - Activities like cycling, swimming, and walking improve cardiovascular health, glycemic control, and mood.
- **FITT Principle (Frequency, Intensity, Time, and Type)**
  - Guides exercise prescription for optimal results, emphasizing individualization based on fitness level and health status.
- **Home Exercises**
  - Simple exercises like sit-to-stand improve balance, strengthen leg muscles, and prevent falls.

The FITT Principle and Its Importance in Diabetes Rehabilitation Programs

The FITT principle stands for frequency, intensity, time, and type, and it serves as a framework for designing effective exercise programs. In diabetes rehabilitation, incorporating the FITT principle allows tailoring exercise plans to optimize blood sugar control, improve physical fitness, and enhance overall well-being.

Here is a breakdown of each element and its relevance to diabetes rehabilitation:

Frequency:

- Aim for at least 3–5 days per week of moderate-intensity exercise or a combination of moderate-intensity and vigorous-intensity activity. Consistency is key to reaping the benefits.

Intensity:

- Moderate intensity for people with diabetes generally translates to a perceived exertion level of 5–6 on the Borg rating of perceived exertion scale (somewhat hard).
- Individualizing intensity based on fitness level and health conditions is crucial.

Time:

- Accumulate at least 150 min of moderate-intensity aerobic activity or 75 min of vigorous-intensity exercise per week.
- Shorter sessions spread throughout the week can be equally effective.

Type:

- Choose a variety of activities you enjoy, aerobic exercises like brisk walking, swimming, or cycling, and strength training to build muscle mass. Flexibility and balance exercises are also important for overall fitness.

Why is the FITT principle important in diabetes rehabilitation?

- Improves blood sugar control: Regular exercise increases insulin sensitivity, helping the body use insulin more effectively to lower blood sugar levels.
- Reduces risk of complications: Exercise prevents or delays the onset of diabetes-related complications like heart disease, neuropathy, and retinopathy.

Tailoring the FITT principle:

- Consulting a healthcare professional and certified exercise specialist is crucial for creating a safe and effective exercise plan specific to individual needs and limitations.
- Starting slowly and gradually increasing duration, intensity, and frequency as tolerated is vital to prevent injuries and maintain motivation.
- Monitoring blood sugar levels before, during, and after exercise is essential for managing hypoglycemia risk.

Managing Vulnerability: Shoulder and Foot Care in Diabetes

Diabetes poses unique challenges to individuals, and attention to specific areas of vulnerability, such as the shoulders and feet.

Shoulder Care

1. Regular range of motion exercises: Diabetic individuals should perform regular shoulder exercises to maintain flexibility and prevent stiffness. These exercises, guided by healthcare professionals, can help minimize the risk of frozen shoulder, a common complication in diabetes.
2. Blood sugar control: Maintaining optimal blood sugar levels is essential for preventing complications like adhesive capsulitis (frozen shoulder). Consistent glucose control supports joint health and reduces the likelihood of shoulder-related issues.

Foot Care

1. Daily inspection and hygiene: Inspect their feet daily for any cuts, blisters, or signs of infection. Keeping feet clean, dry, and moisturized is vital to prevent complications such as infections and neuropathy.
2. Proper footwear: Wearing comfortable, well-fitting shoes is imperative to prevent foot ulcers and pressure points. Diabetics should avoid going barefoot and choose footwear that provides support and protection.
3. Regular podiatric check-ups: Routine visits to a podiatrist are essential for monitoring foot health, identifying potential issues early, and receiving professional advice on proper foot care practices.
4. Circulation management: Diabetes can affect blood circulation to the extremities. Maintaining good circulation through regular exercise and avoiding tobacco products is critical for preventing complications like peripheral arterial disease.

Enhancing Well-Being Through Medical Approaches
Section 1: Respiratory wellness
Subsection 1.1: Deep breathing exercise

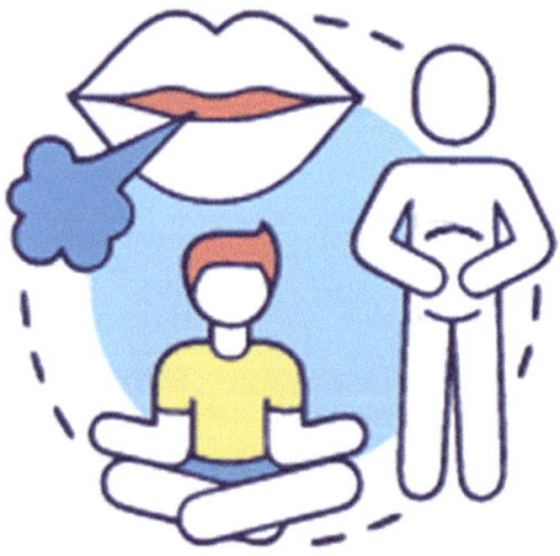

Utilization of breath

A single breath carries a profound responsibility for vital living, influencing emotions and thoughts. Ancient practices, such as yoga and Patanjali, suggest that controlling one's breath can lead to emotional control, a proposition substantiated by recent scientific studies. Shallow and rapid breathing can be indicative of anxiety and stress, while focused and intentional breathing has been found to have powerful effects on stress reduction, combating depression, improving sleep, and overall well-being.

Positive coping technique I: Deep breathing exercise

Steps

1. Find a comfortable position, either sitting upright or lying down, and loosen constricting clothing.
2. Close your eyes and place hands on the abdomen and chest.
3. Inhale through the nose, counting slowly to four, pause for two counts, then exhale through the mouth for a count of six (or eight, if comfortable).
4. Focus on the movement of the lower hand, encouraging abdominal expansion during inhalation and contraction during exhalation.
5. After several minutes, transition to normal breathing and open your eyes, maintaining a state of quietude.

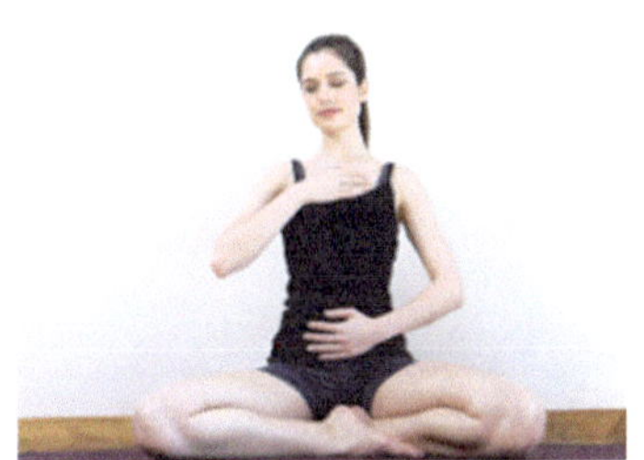

This technique is especially helpful for emotional calming

Section 2: Mindful relaxation

Subsection 2.1: Meditation

A fundamental aspect of meditation is accepting the natural occurrence of thoughts without attempting to suppress them. The basics involve starting with short sessions, gradually increasing duration, and observing the resulting conditions post-meditation.

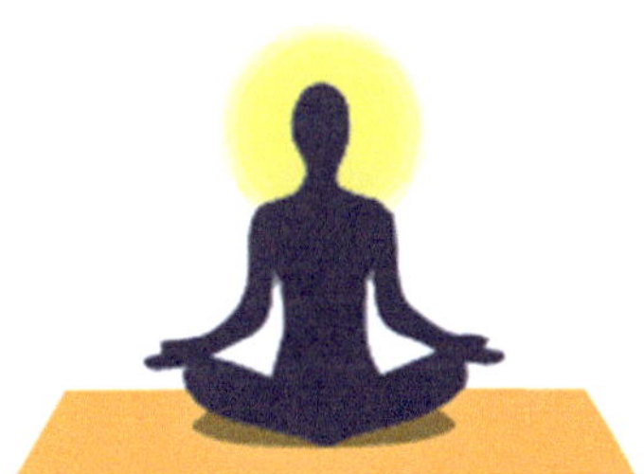

Positive coping technique II: Meditation

Steps:

1. Sit comfortably, close your eyes, and scan your body for tension.
2. Breathe slowly from the abdomen.
3. Focus on a chosen word, phrase, or sound, repeating it rhythmically.
4. Adopt a passive attitude, redirecting your focus when intrusive thoughts occur.
5. After 15–20 min, slowly open your eyes, feeling refreshed and energized.

Subsection 2.2: Progressive muscle relaxation (PMR)

PMR is a widely used strategy for stress relief, involving sequential tensing and relaxing of muscles. This mind–body technique aims to reduce tension, lower perceived stress, and induce overall relaxation.

Benefits of PMR

- Slows heart rate and lowers blood pressure.
- Reduces stress hormone activity and muscle tension.
- Improves concentration, mood, and sleep quality.

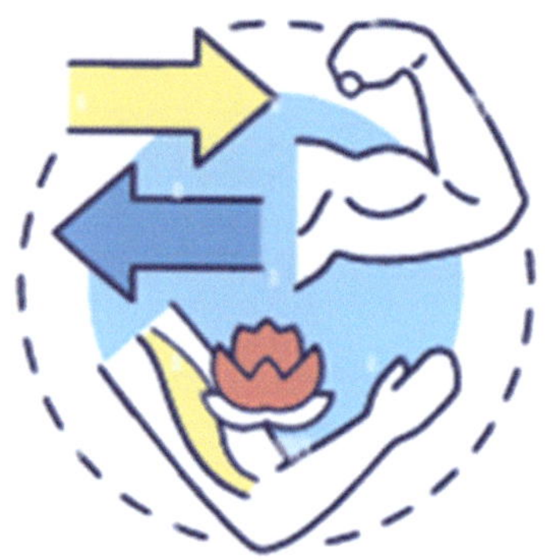

Positive coping technique III: Progressive muscle relaxation

Steps

1. Get into a comfortable position with support for your head and neck.
2. Close your eyes and sequentially tense and release different muscle groups.
3. Focus on the contrast between tight and relaxed muscles.
4. Sit quietly after completion, relishing the sensation of a relaxed body.

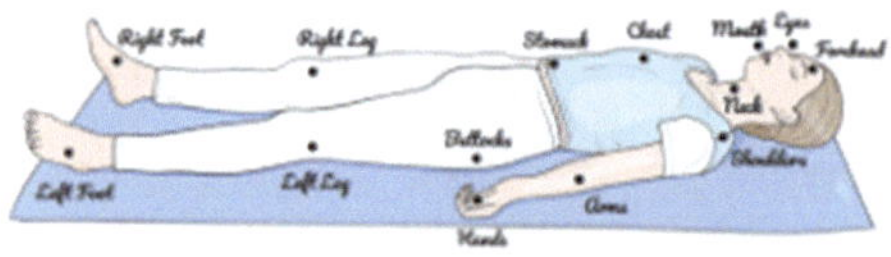

This technique is especially helpful for relaxing the body.

Section 3: Integrating exercise for diabetes

Exercise program recommendations

- Warm up before exercising.
- Cool down after exercising.

Warm up
helps your muscles get ready for exercise
helps make your heart stronger & ready for activity
helps reduce your risk of injury

Cool down
helps bring your heart rate back to normal
helps improve your flexibility
helps your muscles feel less sore

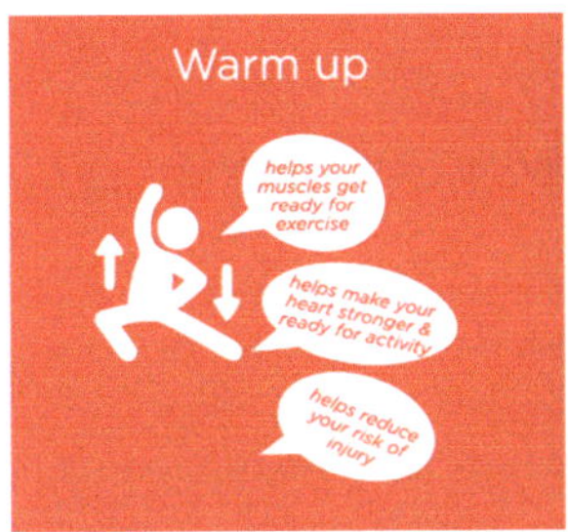

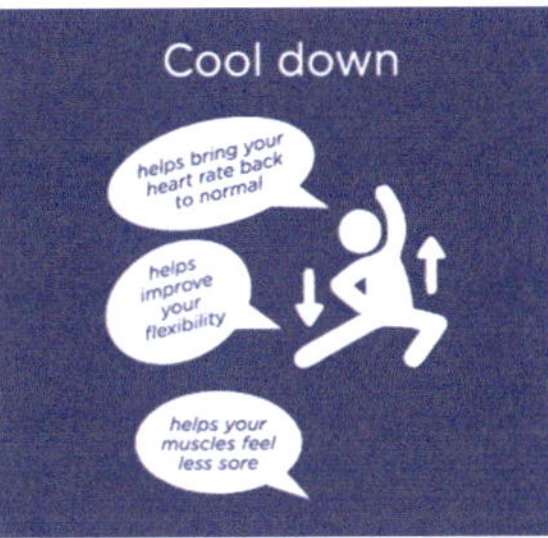

By incorporating these medical approaches into daily life, individuals can foster a holistic approach to well-being, addressing both physical and mental aspects for a healthier lifestyle.

8.9 Attitude in Diabetes Management

The "Attitude" component of the DREAM program highlights the crucial link between one's inner world and health in diabetes management. Addressing negative behaviors rooted in attitudes like stress, anxiety, and negative coping mechanisms empowers individuals with diabetes to take control of their well-being.

8.9.1 Strategies for Attitude Management

1. Smoking cessation [35, 36]
   (a) Cognitive-behavioral therapy (CBT) effective in the COMMIT trial.
   (b) Mindfulness-based interventions boost smoking cessation rates.
2. Alcohol rethink [37]
   (a) Recent research suggests a nuanced approach to alcohol consumption, emphasizing personalized assessments and potential abstinence.
3. Stress busters.
   (a) Yoga, known for stress reduction, significantly improves glycemic control and quality of life.
4. Beyond the anger
   (a) Internet-based CBT [17] designed for anger management reduces anger expression and improves emotional well-being.
5. Worry warriors [38]
   (a) Mindfulness-based cognitive therapy [38] (MBCT) effectively reduces worry and improves emotional regulation.

   By addressing underlying attitudes through research-backed strategies, the DREAM program transforms diabetes management, promoting not only blood sugar control but also inner peace and well-being.

Smoking

- Increased insulin resistance.
- Greater risk of complications such as end organ damage.
- Reduced circulation.
- Impaired lung function.

Substance use

- Chewing ghutka and tobacco can interfere with the body's ability to regulate blood sugar, increased risk of infections, and mental health challenges.

Excessive alcohol consumption [37]

- Can lead to hypoglycemia, if ingesting hypoglycemic agents, and weight gain from empty calories. May function as a diuretic leading to dehydration and threat of pancreatitis.

Additionally, healthcare professionals should routinely screen their patients with diabetes for smoking, substance use, and alcohol abuse and offer appropriate interventions and support to help them manage these challenges and improve their overall health outcomes.

The Role of Cognitive Behavioral Therapy (CBT) [17] in Diabetes Rehabilitation

In diabetes rehabilitation programs, addressing both physical and mental Well-being is crucial. Cognitive behavioral therapy (CBT) has emerged as a valuable tool in enhancing psychological resilience and improving outcomes for individuals with diabetes.

Key components of CBT in diabetes care: **Cognitive restructuring, behavioral activation, stress management techniques, and emotional regulation.** The benefits include **improved glycemic control, enhanced quality of life,** and **long-term behavioral change.**

8.10 Motivation in DREAM's Diabetes Rehabilitation Program

DREAM recognizes the importance of nurturing motivation to actively engage individuals in their care.

8.10.1 Strategies for Enhancing Motivation

1. *Clinical research*
   (a) Motivational interviewing coupled with diabetes education improves medication adherence and self-efficacy.

2. *Goal setting*
   (a) Individualized, achievable goals foster a sense of purpose and progress.
3. *Self-determination theory*
   (a) Intrinsic motivation driven by autonomy, competence, and relatedness leads to sustained behavior change.
4. *Cognitive behavioral therapy (CBT)*
   (a) Techniques like identifying self-defeating thoughts can help individuals overcome negativity and boost confidence.
5. *Positive psychology*
   (a) Practices like gratitude and visualizing success cultivate a positive mindset.

8.10.2 DREAM Motivation Tool

Incorporating the DREAM Motivation Tool into clinical practice empowers individuals with diabetes, fostering patient engagement and contributing to an enhanced quality of life.

While diabetes is commonly associated with regulating blood sugar, it also affects other bodily systems, including the respiratory system. Individuals with diabetes have an increased risk of respiratory infections, such as pneumonia. Additionally, diabetes can lead to a condition called diabetic lung, which causes structural and functional changes in the lungs, impacting lung function. Understanding this connection is crucial for a holistic approach to health.

8.11 The Role of Respiratory Health in Diabetes Management

"Diabetes mellitus can have a significant impact on respiratory health, leading to decreased lung function and an increased risk of respiratory infections. It is crucial for individuals with diabetes to prioritize their respiratory well-being through regular monitoring and management of blood sugar levels, engaging in physical activity, and adopting a healthy lifestyle overall," says *endocrinologist* Bob Kagan.

Healthy lungs play a crucial role in maintaining optimal blood sugar control. They enable efficient delivery of oxygen to the bloodstream, which helps the body effectively utilize glucose. Individuals with well-functioning lungs are more likely to engage in physical activities that regulate blood sugar levels. On the other hand, impaired lung function can hinder physical activity and negatively affect diabetes management. Therefore, addressing respiratory health is vital for individuals with diabetes.

8.12 Practical Tips for Diabetes Management and Respiratory Health

Control your blood sugar levels: Maintaining good blood sugar levels is vital to both diabetes and respiratory health. Monitor your glucose levels regularly, take medication as prescribed, and follow a healthy diet.

8.12.1 Get Vaccinated

People with diabetes are more susceptible to respiratory infections like flu and pneumonia. Stay up-to-date with vaccinations, including COVID-19 pneumococcal infection and seasonal flu.

Here are a few types of breathing exercises that experts often recommend:

Diaphragmatic breathing

Also known as belly breathing, diaphragmatic breathing involves deep breaths that engage the diaphragm and expand the belly. This technique helps to increase oxygen intake and promote relaxation.

Pursed lip breathing

Pursed lip breathing involves inhaling through the nose and exhaling slowly through pursed lips as if blowing out a candle. This technique promotes better control of breathing, increases lung airflow, and can help reduce shortness of breath.

Alternate nostril breathing

Also known as Nadi Shodhana, this technique involves closing one nostril with a finger while inhaling through the other nostril, then switching sides and exhaling through the opposite nostril. Alternate nostril breathing can help balance the body and calm the mind.

Kapalbhati pranayama

This yoga breathing technique involves forceful exhalation through the nose using quick abdominal contractions, followed by passive inhalation. Kapalbhati breathing stimulates the pancreas and improves digestion, which can be helpful for individuals with diabetes.

It is important to note that before starting any new exercise or breathing technique, it is advisable to consult with a healthcare professional or a certified yoga instructor, especially if you have any underlying health conditions or concerns.

8.13 Uniting Diabetes and Respiratory Well-Being

In summary, it is crucial to understand the impact of diabetes on your breathing and the significance of addressing both your diabetes and respiratory health. By attending to both aspects, you can markedly enhance your overall well-being and relish a healthier, more satisfying life characterized by vitality and an improved quality of life.

8.13.1 Positive Adaptation to Change

Internal control	External control
I want to	I have to…because if I do not, I pay a terrible price
I choose to	

8.13.2 Health Achievement Plan

Six essentials for an active and healthy life

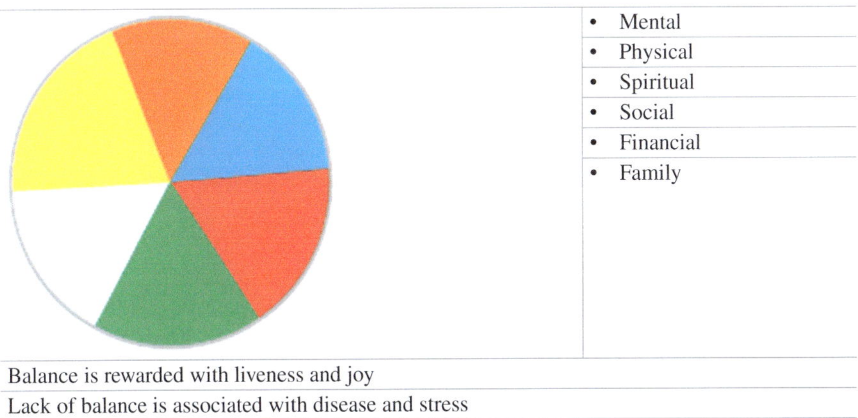	• Mental • Physical • Spiritual • Social • Financial • Family
Balance is rewarded with liveness and joy	
Lack of balance is associated with disease and stress	

8.13.3 Pain Management Techniques

- The rehabilitation team conducts a thorough assessment to identify pain sources.
- Utilize advanced electrotherapy modalities for optimal pain relief:
  - Interferential therapy.
  - Transcutaneous electrical nerve stimulation (TENS).
  - Ultrasound therapy.
  - Shockwave therapy.
  - Laser therapy.
  - Segmental mechanical traction for neck and back pain.
  - Cryotherapy.
  - Heat therapy.

These medical guidelines aim to enhance overall well-being by addressing both psychological and physical aspects, promoting a comprehensive and sustainable approach to health.

EXERCISE INTENSITY

Rating of Perceived Exertion - Borg RPE Sacle		
6 7 8 9 10 11	 Extremely Light Very Light Fairly light	How you feel when lying in bed or sitting in a chair, relaxed Little or no effort
12 13 14 15 16	 Somewhat hard Hard 	Target Range How you should feel with exercise or activity
17 18 19 20	Very hard Extremely Hard Maximum exertion	How you felt with the hardest work you have every done Don't work this hard!

References

1. https://www.ncbi.nlm.nih.gov/pmc/articles/PMC8725109/
2. American Diabetes Association. Standards of medical care in diabetes-2023. Diabetes Care. 2023;46(Supplement 1):S1–S154. https://doi.org/10.7332/dc-23-S001.
3. American Dietetic Association. Dietary guidelines for Americans, 2020–2025. Washington, DC: U.S. Department of Agriculture and U.S. Department of Health and Human Services; 2020.
4. https://www.nin.res.in/downloads/DietaryGuidelinesforNINwebsite.pdf
5. https://www.ncbi.nlm.nih.gov/books/NBK279012/
6. https://www.health.harvard.edu/diseases-and-conditions/the-lowdown-on-glycemic-index-and-glycemic-load
7. https://ph.health.mil/topics/healthyliving/Pages/default.aspx
8. American Diabetes Association (ADA) Standards of Medical Care in Diabetes—2023: recommends deep breathing exercises as a non-pharmacological approach for stress management and glycemic control.
9. Study showing deep breathing effectively reduces anxiety and lowers blood pressure. J Clin Endocrinol Metab. 2000;85(6):2090–7.
10. Study showing deep breathing improves heart rate variability in individuals with diabetes. Diabetes Care. 2003;26(10):1601–6.
11. Study highlighting the benefits of mindfulness-based meditation for stress management and overall well-being in individuals with diabetes. Diabetes Care. 2017;40(10):1236–43.
12. Study supporting the effectiveness of meditation in reducing anxiety and depressive symptoms. J Consult Clin Psychol. 2014;82(4):504–12.
13. ADA Standards of Medical Care in Diabetes—2023: acknowledges the potential benefits of meditation and emphasizes the need for further research on its specific role in diabetes management.
14. Study highlighting yoga's benefits for reducing stress, improving mood, and promoting glycemic control in individuals with diabetes. Diabetes Care. 2017;40(10):1236–43.

15. Study demonstrating yoga's effectiveness in improving physical and mental health outcomes in individuals with diabetes. J Diabetes Complications. 2012;26(4):236–42.
16. EASD/ADA 2023 Clinical Practice Guidelines on Cardiovascular Disease and Diabetes: recommends yoga as a lifestyle intervention for improving cardiovascular health in individuals with diabetes.
17. Davis, et al. Yoga Power: A 2022 Diabetes Care study found yoga led to significant improvements in glycemic control and quality of life for individuals with type 2 diabetes. 2022.
18. Study demonstrating PMR's effectiveness in reducing anxiety and muscle tension in individuals with diabetes. Diabetes Care. 2009;32(9):1590–5.
19. Study showing PMR's effectiveness in reducing pain in individuals with chronic conditions not explicitly recommended by major diabetes guidelines, but can be considered as a complementary technique. J Psychosom Res. 2004;56(5):407–12.
20. ADA Standards of Medical Care in Diabetes—2023: acknowledges the potential benefits of yoga for individuals with diabetes.
21. Chen Y, Yang Z, Xu M, Wang W. Effects of pursed-lip breathing with an expiratory resistor on anxiety and respiratory function in healthy adults. Respir Care. 2010;55(4):458–64.
22. Purssell E, Byrne N, Singh B. Breathing retraining reduces dyspnea in chronic obstructive pulmonary disease patients: a randomized controlled trial. Respir Physiol Neurobiol. 2013;192(1):87–92.
23. Wilson R, Elkins RK, Alton DG. Airway clearance techniques for bronchiectasis and chronic bronchitis. Chest. 2004;125(2):555–62.
24. Rochester CL, Grant BB, Welte KA. Chest physiotherapy techniques for acute and chronic pulmonary disease. Respir Care. 2006;51(8):1035–46.
25. Incentive spirometry for preventing pulmonary complications after surgery. Cochrane Database Syst Rev. 2013. https://doi.org/10.1002/14651858.CD004134.pub3.
26. O'Donnell DE, Barnes HW, Rogers RM. Incentive spirometry for postoperative pulmonary complications: a meta-analysis. Respir Care. 2011;56(10):1421–35.
27. American College of Sports Medicine. Clinical practice guidelines for exercise and physical activity testing: American College of Sports Medicine. Am J Med. 2009;122(5):S1–S14.
28. Bennell KL, Bryant CR, Holloway GJ. Exercise interventions for improving physical function and gait in older adults with knee osteoarthritis: a systematic review. Clin Gerontol. 2010;29(3–4):189–207.
29. Viana RF, Pereira AS, Cardoso VT, Tessaro PH, Oliveira GC. The effect of a static stretching program on range of motion and balance in healthy older adults: a randomized controlled trial. J Gerontol Ser A Biol Sci Med Sci. 2017;72(2):283–90.
30. Bahr R, Gleim GW. The effects of stretching on performance and injury in sports: a systematic review. Int J Sports Med. 2016;37(7):560–71.
31. Villareal DT, Borod M, Snelling K, Unverdorben MT. Resistance training improves functional performance and gait in frail older adults: a meta-analysis. J Gerontol Ser A Biol Sci Med Sci. 2009;64(8):1204–12.
32. Alves BB, Oliveira SL, Fernandes VG, Teixeira LC. Effectiveness of Thera-band resistance training on functional mobility in patients with chronic hip and knee osteoarthritis: a randomized controlled trial. Physiother Res Int. 2010;15(4):239–50.
33. American Diabetes Association. Standards of medical care in diabetes—2023. Diabetes Care. 2023;46(Supplement 1):S114–32.
34. American College of Sport Medicine. American College of Sport Medicine Guideline on Exercise Testing and Prescription, Tenth Edition. Medicine & Science in Sports & Exercise. 2023;55(Supplement 8):S1–S67.
35. Taylor, et al. Landmark Study: COMMIT trial (Cold Turkey or Gradual Smoking Reduction to Quit? A Trial to Help Smokers Quit) demonstrated the effectiveness of CBT in smoking cessation for diabetics. 2001.
36. Tang, et al. Mindfulness Approach: A 2023 study in Nicotine & Tobacco Research found mindfulness-based interventions significantly boosted smoking cessation rates among diabetics. 2023.

37. Berr, et al. New Perspective: A 2023 Lancet Diabetes & Endocrinology study suggests even moderate alcohol intake can adversely affect blood sugar control and increase complication risk in some diabetics. 2023.
38. Yang X, Li Z, Sun J. Effects of Cognitive behavioural therapy- based Intervention on Improving Glyceamic, Psychological, and Physiological outcomes in Adult patients with Diabetes Mellitus: A Meta analysis pf Randomized Controlled trials. Front Psychiatry. 2020;11:711. https://doi.org/10.3389/fpsyt.2020.00711.

9 The Management of Overweight and Obese Diabetic Patient

N. Vijayashree, Deepak Subramanian, and Megha Mariam George

9.1 Introduction

Obesity and type 2 diabetes mellitus (T2DM) are closely linked and are increasing in prevalence worldwide. Both chronic conditions have multisystem impact and are associated with increased cardiovascular risk and mortality [1].

Obesity is a key modifiable risk factor for the development of T2DM, with 90% of adults classified as overweight or obese. There is an estimated threefold increase in the development of diabetes associated with being overweight and a sevenfold increase in those with obesity.

According to the ADA guidelines, there is a strong and consistent evidence base to support that vigilant obesity management can delay the progression from prediabetes to T2DM and improve glycemic control as well as reduce the need for glucose-lowering therapies in patients with established T2D. Therefore, weight management forms the core of the treatment plan in patients with diabetes. However, weight reduction remains a significant challenge owing to multiple factors such as glucose-lowering therapies, insufficient lifestyle modifications, and socioeconomic status. Before deciding on a goal for a given patient, it is critical to be aware of the patient's perspective on his or her weight, cultural or economic barriers, and correct BMI classification. BMI cut points may differ based on ethnicity (e.g., Asian and Asian American populations define obesity at a lower cut point owing to differences and cardiovascular risk) as well as on whether the individual is highly muscular or frail [2].

N. Vijayashree (✉)
MGM Healthcare, Chennai, Tamil Nadu, India

D. Subramanian · M. M. George
Kings College, London, UK

G. Abraham et al. (eds.), *Management of Diabetic Complications*,
https://doi.org/10.1007/978-981-97-6406-8_9

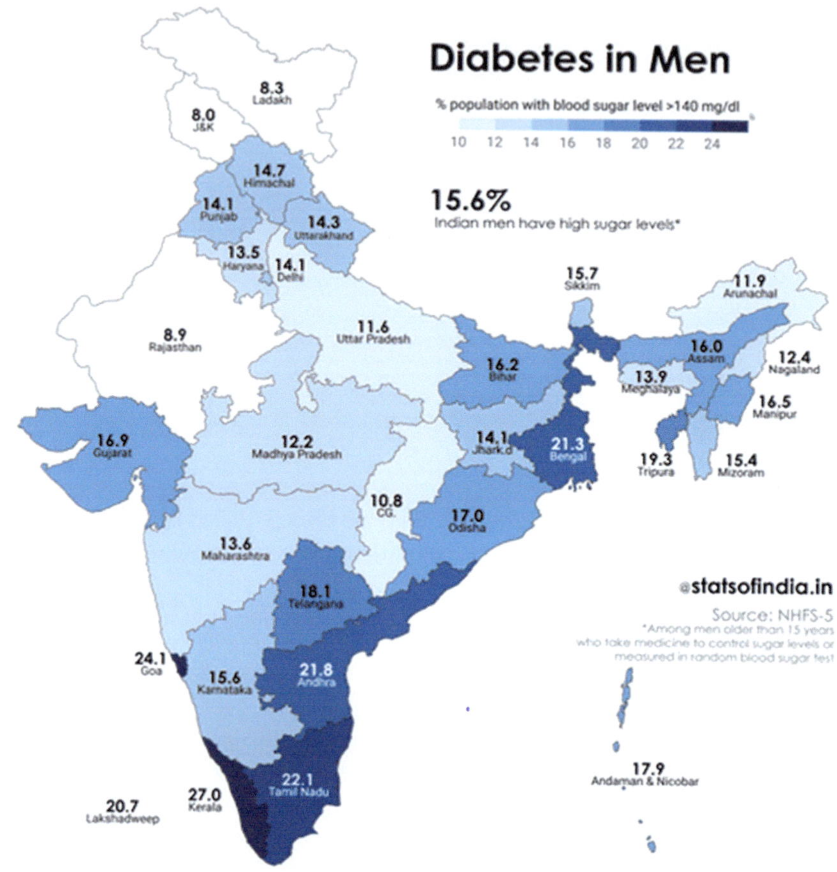

Fig. 9.1 Prevalence of diabetes in Indian men

The prevalence of T2DM in Indian men is given in Fig. 9.1. A study of the prevalence of diabetes mellitus and obesity is shown in Figs. 9.2 and 9.3 [3].

9.2 Classification of Obesity

WHO recognizes two distinct classifications of obesity:

1. Generalized obesity, which is defined as having a body mass index (BMI) of 30 or higher,
2. Central/abdominal obesity, which is assessed using waist circumference and/or waist-to-hip ratio (WHR) [4, 5].

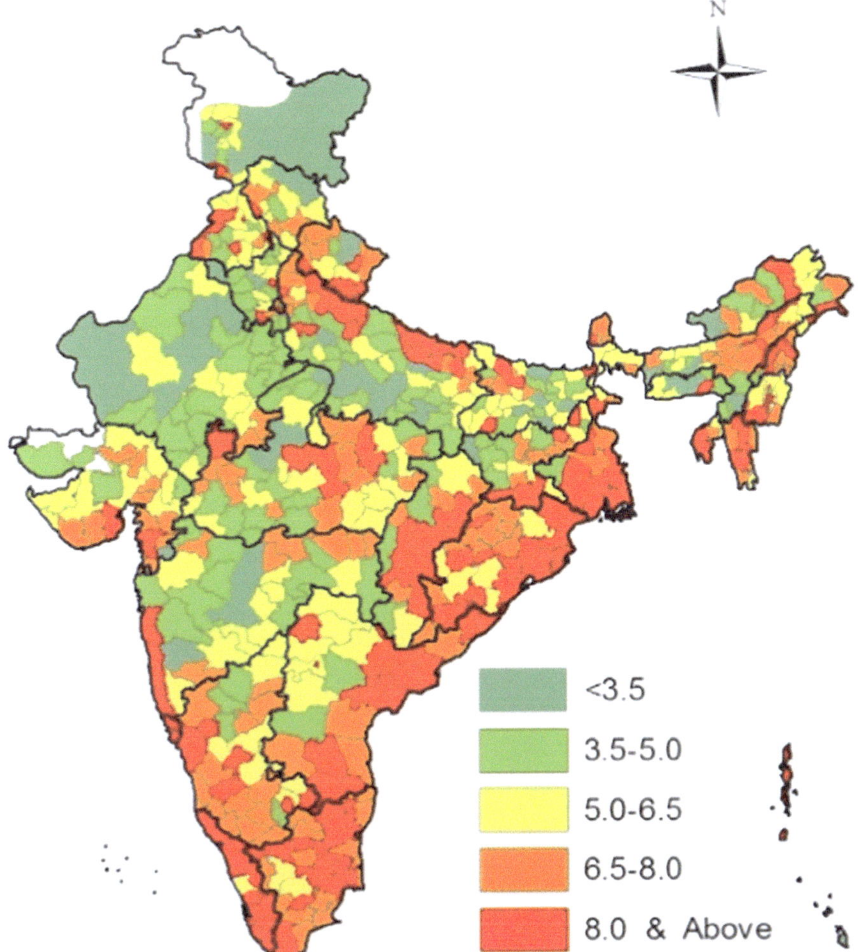

Fig. 9.2 Prevalence of diabetes mellitus in India

Abdominal obesity, specifically, has emerged as a major public health concern globally. Hindsight emphasizes the profound impact of abdominal obesity on both the development of diabetes mellitus and its detrimental effects on overall health [6].

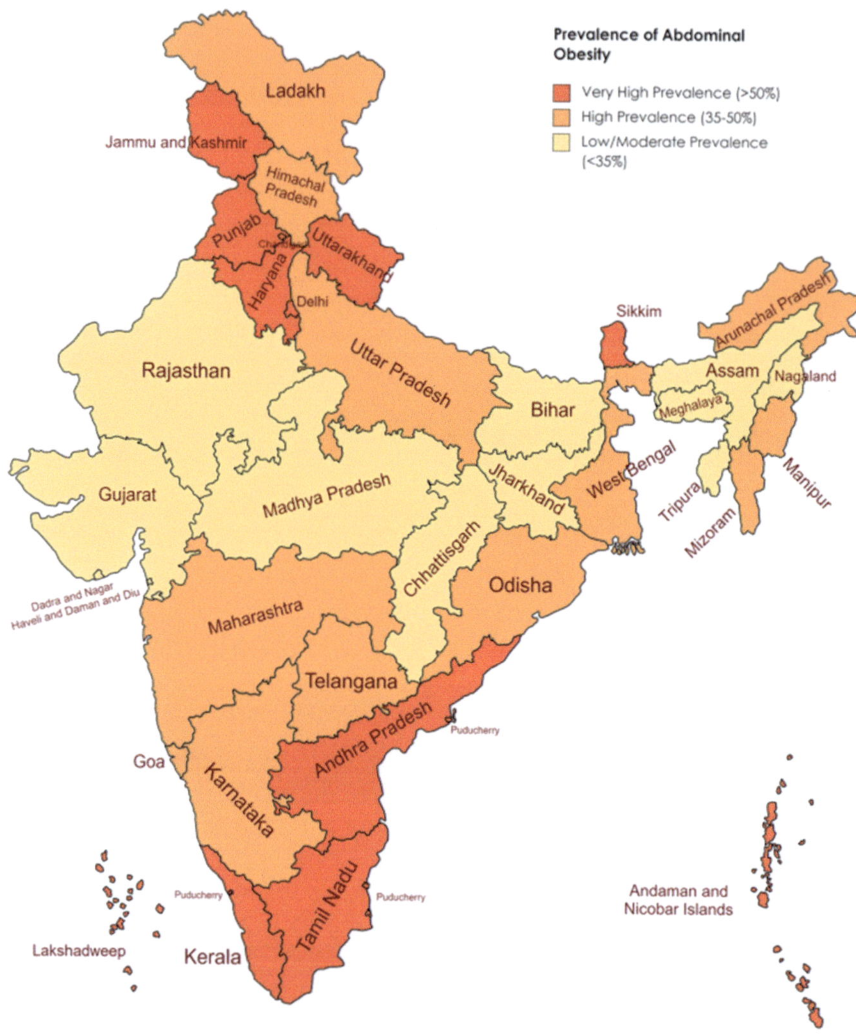

Fig. 9.3 Prevalence of abdominal obesity in Indian states

9.3 Pathophysiology of Obesity and T2DM

The mechanisms linking obesity and T2DM are complex and still being understood, but likely involve a combination of

- Adipose tissue release of excess circulating fatty acids, glycerol, hormones and pro-inflammatory cytokines, impairing cellular insulin signalling and increasing insulin resistance.
- Chronically raised lipid levels leading to impaired islet beta-cell function and lower levels of insulin production [6].

9.4 Assessment and Diagnosing Obesity

Detailed history taking and evaluation are described elsewhere. Aspects to consider include:

- Age at onset of excess weight, onset in early childhood, suggestive of genetic syndromes.
- Family history of obesity and its pattern, especially if severe obesity is dichotomously present with normal weight.
- Pattern of weight gain, noting periods of acceleration or weight loss and their relation to health or life events.
- Intake of alcohol or other highly calorific liquids.
- Success and failure of previous attempts at losing weight.

National Institute for Health and Care Excellence (NICE) guidelines (CG189) also provide further advice on the assessment of obesity. During examination of a person with diabetes and obesity, aspects to consider include cardiovascular risk, secondary obesity (including genetic causes and endocrinopathies such as Cushing's syndrome), and sequelae (e.g., osteoarthritis and obstructive sleep apnea). A thorough assessment, combined with a sensitive approach which considers context, provides the foundation to discuss intervention [7].

9.5 Anthropometry

In general, measurements of body weight and body dimensions (anthropometry) are used to reflect body fat in large studies or in clinical settings, as they provide a rapid and cheap way to estimate body fatness and fat distribution. A new wearable device from Inbioz, as well as densitometry and imaging techniques, are used in smaller-scale studies such as clinical trials.

Obesity is traditionally defined as a percentage body fat of >25% in men and >32% in women. Asians, and Indians in particular, have a greater amount of fat and less muscle mass than whites for the same weight and BMI [8].

Asian Indians have more abdominal (visceral) fat deposition than Europids. For the same BMI, percentage of body fat is 7%–8% points higher for Asian Indians compared to Europids. Conversely, for the same percentage body fat, BMI is 3–6 units lower for Asian Indians compared to Europids. The exact opposite occurs in Pacific Islanders and blacks who have 4% points lower percentage of body fat than whites for the same BMI [8, 9]. WHO criteria for diagnosing obesity based on BMI for Asians is given in Table 9.1.

The BMI interpretation for Asians [10] are given below:

There is ample evidence to indicate that having excess fat in the abdominal area is a significant risk factor for T2DM and cardiovascular disease. However, the most commonly employed method for determining obesity in medical and research settings is BMI although there is ongoing debate about its diagnostic accuracy [11].

Table 9.1 Obesity classification according to WHO and Asia-Pacific guidelines

	WHO (BMI kg/m^2))	Asia-Pacific (BMI kg/m^2)
Underweight	<18.5	<18.5
Normal	18.5–24.9	18.5–22.9
Overweight	25–29.9	23–24.9
Obese	≥30	≥25
BMI in the general population (kg/m^2)	BMI in certain ethnic groups (kg/m^2)[a]	
Overweight	25–29.9	23–27.4
Obesity Class 1	30–34.9	27.5–32.4
Obesity Class 2	35–39.9	32.5–37.4
Obesity Class 3	>40	>37.5

BMI body mass index

[a]South Asian, Chinese, other Asian, Middle Eastern, Black African, and African-Caribbean

9.6 Waist Circumference

Evidence supports a strong correlation between increasing waist circumference and the dangerous central, or visceral, fat that sits in and around central organs (as distinct from subcutaneous fat) that increases cardiometabolic risk [12]. Apart from BMI, other measures can be used. Waist circumference (WC) measured with a tape around the waist midway between the bottom of the ribs and top of the pelvis (Fig. 9.4) is a good measure of central adiposity [13].

For Indian-Asian men, a waist circumference below 94 cm (37 in.) is “low risk,” 94–102 cm (37–40 in.) is “high risk,” and more than 102 cm (40 in.) is “very high.” For women, below 80 cm (31.5 in.) is low risk, 80–88 cm (31.5–34.6 in.) is high risk, and more than 88 cm (34.6 in.) is very high.

Waist-to-height ratio (WHtR) is calculated by dividing the WC by the height in the same units [14].

Increased health risks are associated with a WHR of 0.5 to 0.59, and further increased risk if the ratio is >0.6. The target range is a ratio of <0.5, that is, the weight should be less than half the height. Although there are many indicators using WC to help assess central adiposity, WHtR appears to be a preferable indicator for the assessment of cardiovascular disease [15]. The remainder of the examination should be focused on the effects of obesity, secondary causes, complications, and multiple health conditions of obesity.

9.7 An Approach to the Patient with Obesity and Diabetes

The treatment of obesity is always intimately linked to the reduction of body weight. This can be achieved by different weight loss strategies, including lifestyle interventions, diet and exercise, pharmaceutical interventions, or bariatric surgery. There is strong and consistent evidence that obesity management can delay the progression from prediabetes to T2DM. In patients with T2DM who are also overweight or obese,

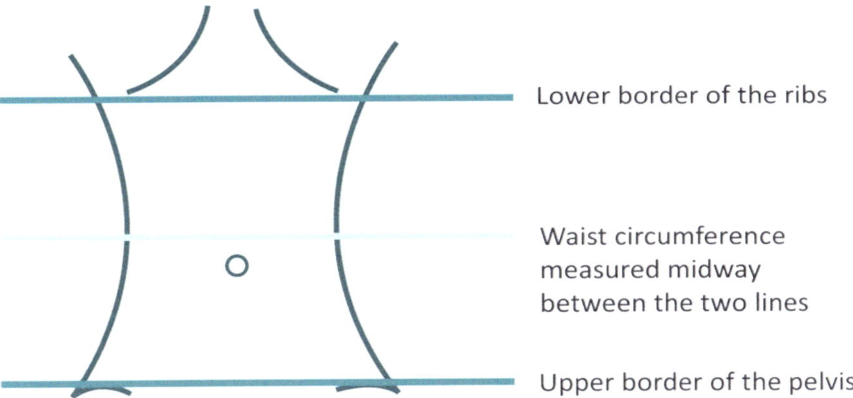

Fig. 9.4 Point at which waist circumference is measured

modest and sustained weight loss has been shown to improve glycemic control and reduce the need for glucose-lowering medications [6]. Several studies have demonstrated that in patients with type 2 diabetes and obesity, more intensive dietary energy restriction with very-low-calorie diets can substantially reduce fasting blood glucose and HbA1C, and promote sustained diabetes remission through at least 2 years [10].

9.8 Weight Loss Strategies: Lifestyle Management

Individualized advice on diet and physical activity, combined with a personalized diabetes care plan, underpins all approaches. The Look AHEAD Trial compared a 4-year intensive program (including lifestyle counsellor, dietary interventions, portion-controlled meal plans, physical activity, and behavioral modification techniques) with a diabetes support/education (DSE) group and usual medical care [16]. The intensive intervention group showed mean weight loss at 1 year of −8.6% versus −0.7% in the DSE group. This was sustained over 4 years with a mean weight loss of −6.15% and −0.88% in the intervention and DSE groups, respectively. In a separate study, an intensive diet intervention soon after diagnosis was shown to improve glycaemic control [17]. Unfortunately, weight maintenance has been reported to be a challenge following lifestyle-induced weight loss [18].

9.8.1 Low-Calorie Diet

Very-low-calorie diets (VLCDs, often referred to as very-low-energy diets [VLEDs]), which reflect a calorie intake of less than 1,000 kcal/day), are an option for some overweight and obese people, but in the author's opinion, should be used under supervision if the individual is on medication or has a medical condition, such as T2DM. The short-term use of a VLCD is very effective in rapidly improving glycemic control and promoting substantial weight loss in obese people with

T2DM. T2DM has often been described as a chronic and progressive condition. The landmark Diabetes Remission Clinical Trial (DiRECT) demonstrated, however, that diabetes remission was possible through a low-calorie total diet replacement program [19]. In South Asian countries, especially in India, the dietary pattern is diverse, as shown in Fig. 9.5. Therefore, trained nutritionists should play a major

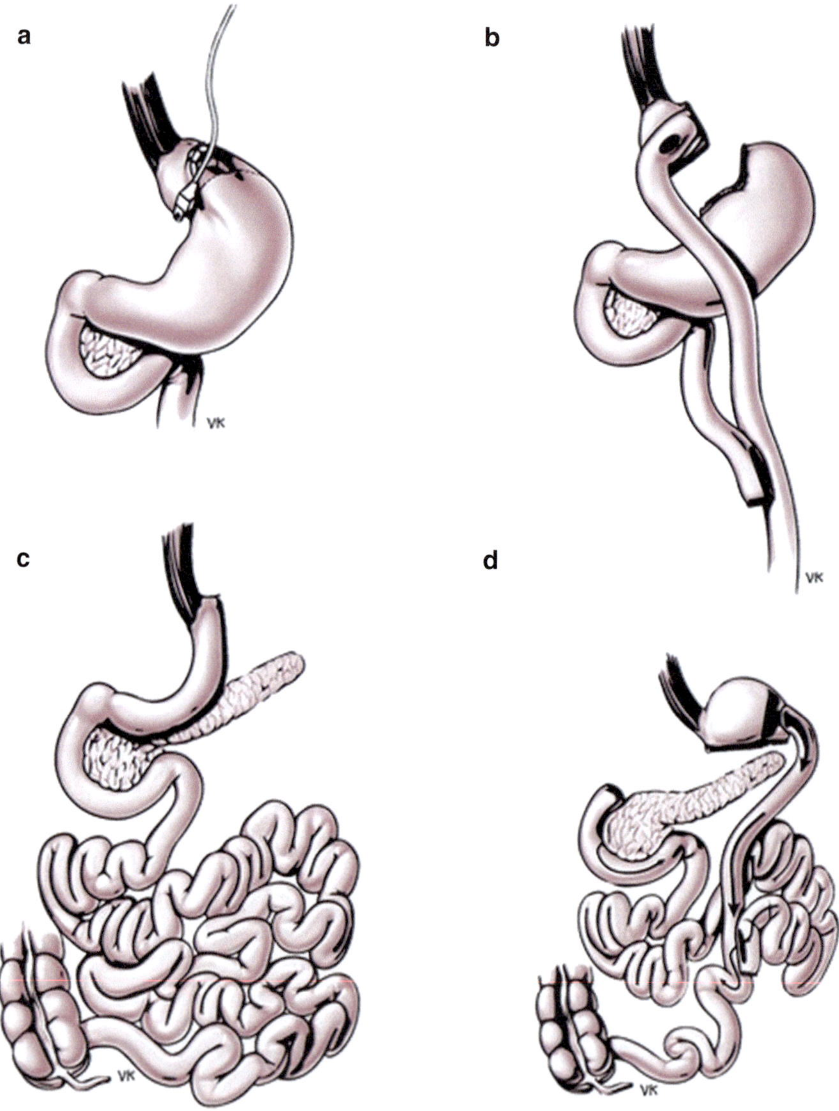

Fig. 9.5 Metabolic surgery for weight loss. (**a**) Laparoscopic adjustable gastric band. (**b**) Laparoscopic Roux en Y gastric bypass. (**c**) Laparoscopic sleeve gastrectomy. (**d**) Laparoscopic biliopancreatic diversion

role in prescribing diet as per the socioeconomic and cultural beliefs. The practical implementation of literature regarding diet of Caucasians, Africans, Chinese, Japanese, and Middle East are not applicable for nonvegetarian, ova-vegetarians, and vegans in South Asian population. This requires interplay of patients, physicians, and nutritionists coming together to encourage patients to follow medical nutrition therapy suitable for each individual.

9.8.2 Low-Carbohydrate Diet (LCD)

There is no universal consensus over what is considered to be low-carbohydrate diet; however, general recommendations are summarised in Table 9.2 [20]. Carbohydrates heighten the postprandial glycemic response along with insulin resistance, and it is suggested that increased carbohydrate intake is associated with higher levels of insulin secretion, which leads to weight gain through mechanism of increase in adipose tissue [21]. LCDs have shown improvements in HbA1c in individuals with T2DM in the first 12 months of intervention. A positive correlation has been observed between the carbohydrate restriction and lower HbA1c.

9.8.3 Diabetic Remission

T2DM has long been regarded as a chronic, irreversible illness, requiring a continuous titration of add-on pharmacotherapy, and which inexorably progresses in over 50% of patients to insulin dependence within 9–10 years [9]. The World Health Organization and Diabetes UK acknowledge that diabetes mellitus is metabolically reversible—at least for a period of time. Four approaches are detailed on the Diabetes UK website: low carbohydrate diets, very-low-calorie diets, exercise, and bariatric surgery. As a result of the debate around and interest in diabetes remission, a joint consensus statement has emerged around the definition of diabetes remission from the American Diabetes Association (ADA), the Endocrine Society, the European Association for the Study of Diabetes (EASD), and Diabetes UK. The consensus position now defines remission as being a return to below the World Health Organization (WHO)/American Diabetes Association (ADA) original diagnostic thresholds for diabetes mellitus and this return should be maintained for 3 months without any glucose-lowering pharmacotherapy (see Table 9.3) [22].

Table 9.2 Carbohydrate content of named diets

Diet	Carbohydrate (g) per day	Percentage of total calories (%)
Very-low-carbohydrate ketogenic diet (VLCKD)	20–50 g	10
Low carbohydrate	<130	26
Moderate carbohydrate	130–230	26–45
High carbohydrate	>230	>45

Table 9.3 Published criteria for T2DM in remission

	Criteria for remission	Confirmation
ADA, Endocrine Society, EASD, and Diabetes UK joint consensus statement on the definition of T2DM remission	Complete remission (no longer having prediabetes): HbA1c < 6.5% (<48 mmol/mol) or fasting blood glucose <7 mmol/L, or estimated HbA1c less than 6.5% calculated from continuous glucose monitoring values; maintained without antidiabetes drugs for at least 3 months. Testing of HbA1c to document a remission should be performed just prior to an intervention and no sooner than 3 months after initiation of the intervention or withdrawal of any glucose-lowering pharmacotherapy	Reviewed annually as a minimum

Measurement of either HbA1c or blood glucose can be used to confirm remission. Patients in remission should thereafter be kept under regular review with annual testing. It is important to note that the term "cure" has not been applied to T2DM, as weight regain is always a risk factor for its recurrence. Although the terms "reversal" and "remission" are used interchangeably, recent consensus supports the use of "remission" in the context of T2DM. Furthermore, a distinction could be made between mere reversal (return to normoglycaemia) and true remission (normoglycamia maintained for at least 3 months in the absence of glucose-lowering drugs) [23].

9.9 Pharmacotherapy

Clinicians should consider altering the diabetes medication regimen and using weight loss agents for these patients.

Clinicians should consider using the following glucose-lowering medications that are weight neutral or may promote weight loss: metformin, pramlintide, glucagon-like peptide 1 (GLP-1) receptor agonists, dipeptidyl peptidase 4 (DPP-4) inhibitors, and sodium–glucose cotransporter 2 (SGLT2) inhibitors. Metformin has been associated with a 3-kg weight loss. In addition to being associated with a 3.7-kg weight loss, pramlintide can also lower daily insulin requirements in patients with diabetes on insulin therapy. GLP-1 receptor agonists have been associated with a 5.3-kg weight loss. DPP-4 inhibitors are generally weight neutral. Finally, SGLT2 inhibitors can promote a 2.4-kg weight loss and lower insulin requirements. Of note, there is generally no benefit to using DPP-4 inhibitors and GLP-1 receptor agonists simultaneously because they work on the same pathway. Further discussion on pharmacotherapy for obesity in patients with diabetes is covered elsewhere in this issue.

The AACE/ACE guidelines recommend that patients with diabetes and a BMI ≥27 kg/m^2 be prescribed weight loss medications. Treatment of obesity through pharmacotherapy, in conjunction with a healthy lifestyle, directly improves glycemic control. Five medications are now approved by the U.S. Food and Drug Administration (FDA) for long-term use for weight loss. Table 9.4 [24] provides an overview of their weight loss and A1C outcomes and their side effects . Additionally,

Table 9.4 Medications approved by the FDA for long-term use for weight management

Medication (trade names)	Mechanism of action	Five most common side effects	Possible safety concerns[a]	Mean 1-year weight loss compared to placebo (dose)	A1C change in patients with diabetes (%)
Decreases absorption of food					
Orlistat (Alli, Xenical)	Lipase inhibitor	Abdominal pain, flatulence, fecal urgency, back pain, and headache	Fat-soluble vitamin deficiencies, altered absorption of medications, cholelithiasis, nephrolithiasis	3.4 kg, 4.0% (120 mg TID)	−0.7
Suppresses appetite					
Lorcaserin (Belviq)	Serotonin receptor agonist	Headache, nausea, dizziness, fatigue, and nasopharyngitis	Serotonin syndrome, hypertension, and edema are potential side effects. Avoid use in patients with liver and renal failure	3.3 kg, 3.6% (10 mg BID)	−1.1[b]
Phentermine/ topiramate (Qsymia)	Norepinephrine release, GABA receptor modulation	Constipation, paresthesia, insomnia, nasopharyngitis, and xerostomia	Birth defects, cognitive impairment, acute angle-closure glaucoma, lactic acidosis with metformin, avoid in renal failure	6.7 kg, 6.6% (7.5/46 mg daily) 8.9 kg, 9.0% (15/92 mg daily)	−0.4
Naltrexone/bupropion (Contrave)	Opiate antagonist, decreased re-uptake of norepinephrine	Constipation, nausea, headache, xerostomia, and insomnia	Depression, anxiety, acute angle-closure glaucoma, avoid in patients with uncontrolled hypertension and renal failure	4.1 kg, 5.2% (16/80 mg BID)	−0.6
Liraglutide (Saxenda)	GLP-1 receptor agonist	Hypoglycemia, constipation, nausea, headache, and indigestion	Gastroparesis, suicidal ideation, increased heart rate, caution in pancreatitis and cholelithiasis	4.5 kg, 5.6% (3 mg daily)	−0.6 to −1.8

BID twice daily, *GABA* gamma-aminobutyric acid, *TID* three times daily
[a]A comprehensive list of safety concerns can be found in each medication's package insert, which is available from the manufacturing pharmaceutical company
[b]HbA1C change has only been assessed in patients with prediabetes

sympathomimetic appetite suppressant medications are approved for short-term use (up to 12 weeks). To avoid weight regain, the ADA recommends long-term use of weight loss medication for patients who successfully lose weight on the medication. Therefore, this article will focus only on medications approved for long-term use. For patients whose weight loss is <5% of initial body weight after the initial treatment period on a given medication (various medications have different initial treatment periods), the medication should be discontinued and an alternative medication or approach should be tried. The AACE/ACE guidelines recommend monitoring patients who are on insulin or sulfonylureas for hypoglycemia after starting any weight loss medication. When considering these medications, clinicians should discuss typical weight loss results, side effects, and medication costs with their patients [25].

9.9.1 Surgical Therapy

Bariatric surgery has shown to be beneficial in the resolution of T2DM. But there seems to be limited data on its impact on diabetic-related complications especially, DKD and ESKD (R). Obesity or overweight reduction following bariatric surgery has a beneficial effect in reducing albuminuria and slowing the progression of DKD. The weight loss obtained reduce the requirement for insulin and OHAs. Here, we describe the different bariatric surgery procedures and selection criteria for diabetes with overweight and obesity [26].

9.9.1.1 Effect of Bariatric Surgery on Diabetes Mellitus: Mechanisms

These surgeries involve gastrointestinal manipulations with the objective of resolution of T2DM. The mechanisms involved are effects on insulin sensitivity, Beta-cell function and incretin responses. The incremental effects include bile acid composition and flow which plays a significant role for weight loss and its metabolic side effects. The altered gut microbiota and its negative influence (dysbiosis), is negated by bariatric surgery (symbiosis). The increased metabolic activity of brown adipose tissue and Intestinal glucose metabolism has a direct effect on the glucose homeostasis and resolution of diabetes mellitus [27].

Further bariatric surgery/metabolic surgery produces significant weight loss through a variety of mechanisms such as decreased calorie intake, modulation of energy balance, appetite regulation, and gut brain signaling pathways. The caloric restriction leads to an increased incretin effect which also is sustained for a longer duration by patients. This caloric restriction that most patients have has proven to have a direct effect on hepatic insulin sensitivity. The weight loss that occurs in all bariatric surgery patients leads to increasing skeletal muscle insulin sensitivity patterns [28].

9.9.1.2 The Foregut and Hindgut Hypothesis

The hindgut hypothesis states that the surgical rerouting of nutrients to the distal part of the small intestine results in increased secretion of GLP 1 and lowering blood glucose. GLP 1 is produced in the mucosal endocrine M cells from the epithelium of the intestinal tract with maximum concentration in the ileum. GLP 1 has very strong insulinotropic properties and has shown to help in all steps of insulin biosynthesis. GLP 1 stimulates beta-cell proliferation, inhibits glucagon secretion, and reduces appetite and GI motility. The passage of the nutrients directly to the distal small bowel after metabolic surgeries has all these beneficial effects [29].

The foregut hypothesis was introduced by Rubino and his colleagues Hickey and his colleagues proposed that type 2 DM is due to the excessive production of diabetogenic signal generated in the proximal part of the small intestine. Pories et al. elaborated this hypothesis and proposed that bariatric procedures that include a bypass of the duodenum and proximal jejunum would prevent the nutrients from eliciting this diabetogenic signal and help in resolution of diabetes mellitus [27].

9.9.2 Common Bariatric Procedures Done

A. Laparoscopic Adjustable Gastric Band

Laparoscopic adjustable gastric band involves encircling the upper part of the stomach with a silicone adjustable band with an inflatable balloon at the inner surface connected with a port placed subcutaneously, through which pressure on the vagal endings can be adjusted by adding and removing fluid.

B. Laparoscopic Roux en Y Gastric Bypass (RYGB)

RYGB is a mixed technique where there is a restrictive and a malabsorptive effect. It includes creation of a gastric pouch with a volume of 20–30 mL. The pouch is isolated from its gastric remnant and anastamosed to the jejunum leaving a alimentary limb of 100–150 cm. Jejeuno-jejunostomy is also done to ensure continuity of the bowel which is performed 150 cm from the gastro-jejunostomy.

C. Sleeve gastrectomy is based on the resection of main part of the fundus and body of the stomach, starting 4 cm from the pylorus. This procedure which was initially used as first step of a staged procedure for a super obese but now it is one of the commonest procedures performed. Significant weight loss and metabolic improvement was seen after sleeve gastrectomy.

D. Biliopancreatic diversion with or without duodenal switch creates caloric malabsorption. This consists of a horizontal gastrectomy and an anastomosis between the remaining remnant and the small intestine about 250 cm away. The bypassed duodenum, jejunum, and proximal ileum, which carries the bile and pancreatic secretions are connected to the alimentary limb very close to the IC valve thereby making the hindgut hypothesis very effective [30].

9.10 Conclusion

A range of options are available for the treatment of diabetes mellitus and obesity, with significant advances made in recent years. In order to provide the most effective treatment plan, it is important to assess the benefits and risks and communicate the overweight individual in a lucid and comprehensive way. Patients should understand that glycemic improvement and diabetes remission are realistic goals. They should be empowered to seek out such options through multidisciplinary approach.

References

1. Hossain P, Kawar B, El Nahas M. Obesity and diabetes in the developing world—a growing challenge. N Engl J Med. 2007;356:213–5.
2. American Diabetes Association. 8. Obesity management for the treatment of type 2 diabetes: Standards of Medical Care in Diabetes—2021. Diabetes Care. 2021;44(suppl 1):S100–10.
3. Chaudhary M, Sharma P. Abdominal obesity in India: analysis of the National Family Health Survey-5 (2019–2021) data. Lancet Reg Health Southeast Asia. 2023;12:100208.
4. World Health Organization. Diabetes. In: Diabetes [Internet]; 2023. Accessed 27 May 2023.
5. Liu YK, Ling S, Lui LMW, Ceban F, Vinberg M, Kessing LV, et al. Prevalence of type 2 diabetes mellitus, impaired fasting glucose, general obesity, and abdominal obesity in patients with bipolar disorder: a systematic review and meta-analysis. J Affect Disord. 2022;300:449–61.
6. Meeks KAC, Freitas-Da-Silva D, Adeyemo A, Beune EJAJ, Modesti PA, Stronks K, et al. Disparities in type 2 diabetes prevalence among ethnic minority groups resident in Europe: a systematic review and meta-analysis. Intern Emerg Med. 2016;11:327–40.
7. Crane JD, Mcgowan BM. Clinical assessment of the patient with overweight or obesity. In: Sbraccia P, Finer N, editors. Obesity. Endocrinology. Berlin: Springer; 2017.
8. National Institute for Health and Care Excellence. Obesity: identification, assessment and management: clinical guideline [CG189]. London: NICE; 2014.
9. Rush E, Plank L, Chandu V, et al. Body size, body composition, and fat distribution: a comparison of young New Zealand men of European, Pacific Island, and Asian Indian ethnicities. N Z Med J. 2004;117(1207):U1203.
10. Jackson AS, Ellis KJ, McFarlin BK, Sailors MH, Bray MS. Body mass index bias in defining obesity of diverse young adults: the training intervention and genetics of exercise response (TIGER) study. Br J Nutr. 2009;102(7):1084–90.
11. Deurenberg-Yap M, Chew SK, Deurenberg P. Elevated body fat percentage and cardiovascular risks at low body mass index levels among Singaporean Chinese, Malays and Indians. Obes Rev. 2002;3(3):209–15.
12. Pischon T, et al. General and abdominal adiposity and risk of death in Europe. N Engl J Med. 2008;359(20):2105–20. https://doi.org/10.1056/NEJMoa0801891.
13. Mallik R, et al. Assessment of obesity. Clin Med. 2023;23:299–303.
14. Yearwood L, Masood W. Behavioral approaches to obesity treatment. Treasure Island, FL: StatPearls; 2022.
15. Xue R, Li Q, Geng Y, et al. Abdominal obesity and risk of CVD: a dose–response meta-analysis of thirty—one prospective studies. Br J Nutr. 2021;126:1420–30.
16. Wing RR, Bolin P, Brancati FL, et al. Cardiovascular effects of intensive lifestyle intervention in type 2 diabetes. N Engl J Med. 2013;369:145–54.
17. Andrews RC, Cooper AR, Montgomery AA, et al. Diet or diet plus physical activity versus usual care in patients with newly diagnosed type 2 diabetes: the early ACTID randomised controlled trial. Lancet. 2011;378:129–39.
18. Mann T, Tomiyama AJ, Westling E, et al. Medicare's search for effective obesity treatments: diets are not the answer. Am Psychol. 2007;62:220–33.
19. Lean MEJ, Leslie WS, Barnes AC, et al. Durability of a primary care-led weight-management intervention for remission of type 2 diabetes: 2-year results of the DiRECT open-label, cluster-randomised trial. Lancet Diabetes Endocrinol. 2019;7:344–55.

20. Snorgaard O, Poulsen GM, Andersen HK, et al. Systematic review and meta-analysis of dietary carbohydrate restriction in patients with type 2 diabetes. BMJ Open Diabetes Res Care. 2017;5:e000354.
21. Noto H, Goto A, Tsujimoto T, et al. Low-carbohydrate diets and all-cause mortality: a systematic review and meta-analysis of observational studies. PLoS One. 2013;8:e55030.
22. Feinman RD, Pogozelski WK, Astrup A, et al. Dietary carbohydrate restriction as the first approach in diabetes management: critical review and evidence base. Nutrition. 2015;31:1–13.
23. Riddle MC, Cefalu WT, Evans PH, et al. Consensus report: definition and interpretation of remission in type 2 diabetes. Diabetes Care. 2021;44(10):2438–44. https://doi.org/10.2337/dci21-0034.
24. Shibib L, et al. Reversal and remission of T2DM—an update for practitioners. Vasc Health Risk Manag. 2022;18:417–43.
25. Bramante CT, et al. Treatment of obesity in patients with diabetes. Diabetes Spectr. 2017;30(4):237–43. https://doi.org/10.2337/ds17-0030.
26. Koliaki C, Liatis S, le Roux CW, Kokkinos A. The role of bariatric surgery to treat diabetes: current challenges and perspectives. BMC Endocr Disord. 2017;17:50.
27. Rubino F, Forgione A, Cummings DE, et al. The mechanism of diabetes control after gastrointestinal bypass surgery reveals a role of the proximal small intestine in the pathophysiology of type 2 diabetes. Ann Surg. 2006;244:741–9.
28. Rubino F, Gagner M. Potential of surgery for curing type 2 diabetes mellitus. Ann Surg. 2002;236:554–9.
29. Hickey MS, Pories WJ, MacDonald KG Jr, et al. A new paradigm for type 2 diabetes mellitus: could it be a disease of the foregut? Ann Surg. 1998;227:637–43.
30. Pories WJ, Albrecht RJ. Etiology of type II diabetes mellitus: role of the foregut. World J Surg. 2001;25:527–31.

10 Ophthalmological Causes of Visual Impairment in Diabetes Mellitus

Meenakshi Mahesh, Harshita Sanjeev, Srinivas K. Rao, and Mahesh P. Shanmugam

10.1 Introduction

Diabetic eye disease is a broad term used for the various eye problems that develop due to diabetes mellitus. Vision loss in diabetics can be due to the short-term fluctuations in blood sugar levels resulting in transient episodes of blurred vision. However, serious complications can result from long-term exposure to high blood sugar levels.

Diabetes is a disease that is strongly associated with both microvascular and macrovascular changes and these are associated with commonly seen ocular complications like diabetic retinopathy. Diabetes is also responsible for other conditions like cataract, glaucoma, ocular infections, and nerve palsies, which are also discussed in this chapter.

Diabetic eye disease is one of the causes of preventable blindness. Early screening and control help in reducing the morbidity of the disease. The development of better screening and awareness programs, along with newer treatment protocols, have contributed toward the same.

Cross section image of the human eye (Fig. 10.1).

M. Mahesh · M. P. Shanmugam
Sankara Eye Hospital, Bangalore, Karnataka, India

H. Sanjeev · S. K. Rao (✉)
Darshan Eye Care and Surgical Centre, Chennai, Tamil Nadu, India

G. Abraham et al. (eds.), *Management of Diabetic Complications*,
https://doi.org/10.1007/978-981-97-6406-8_10

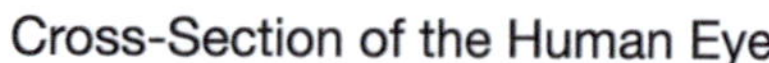

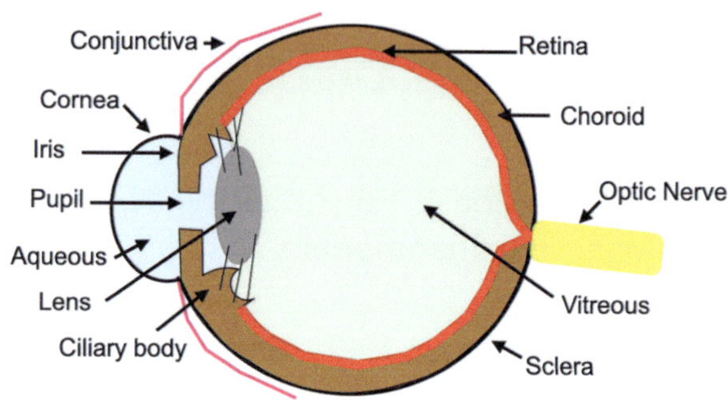

Fig. 10.1 Drawing showing various parts of the human eye

10.1.1 Epidemiology

Globally, diabetic retinopathy (DR) was the fifth most common cause of blindness among people of age 50 years or older in 2020 [1]. Incidence of diabetic retinopathy is significantly associated with a future risk of cerebrovascular disease and myocardial infarction. This risk corresponds directly to the degree of retinopathy [2].

The prevalence of any retinopathy in individuals with type 1 diabetes was 56.0%, and in type 2 diabetes was 30.3% according to the 2015 UK National diabetic retinopathy screening service report [3]. The reduced incidence compared to older reports can be explained by increasing awareness, better screening, and improved treatment options.

The incidence of diabetic retinopathy is higher in type 1 group with an annual incidence of 15.2 ± 2.2% as compared with 8.4 ± 2.2% in type 2 diabetes [4].

10.1.2 For Diabetics: When to Consult an Ophthalmologist?

While the duration of diabetes or exposure to high blood sugar levels is the most common risk factor, type 1 diabetics tend to have a higher incidence of early onset diabetes-related complications. The duration of diabetes is probably the strongest predictor for the development and progression of retinopathy. Among younger patients with diabetes in the Wisconsin epidemiological study of diabetic retinopathy (WESDR), the prevalence of any retinopathy was 8% at 3 years, 25% at 5 years, 60% at 10 years, and 80% at 15 years.

In a study of type 1 diabetes patients from South India, the incidence of diabetic retinopathy changes was 3% in patients with less than 5-year disease duration and 57.8% incidence in patients with 15 years disease duration [5].

Type 2 diabetics are advised to have fundus examination at diagnosis of diabetes mellitus and type 1 diabetics can get screening fundus examination 3–5 years after diagnosis [6].

However, in the Indian scenario, it is preferable to have an earlier fundus screening after the diagnosis of diabetes, and periodic follow-up is mandatory. Follow-up intervals vary widely depending on the duration of disease, glycemic index, and ocular status. Patients with diabetic eye disease need closer follow-up and strict glycemic control. The higher rate of retinopathy seen in type 1 diabetic patients is believed to be a result of the longer diabetes duration, fluctuating blood glucose, and uncontrolled diabetes status.

10.2 Pathophysiology of Diabetic Eye Disease

Even though high blood sugar levels are the main cause for the diabetes-related eye problems different theories have been proposed for different complications. Hyperglycemia leads to the activation of alternative pathways of glucose metabolism such as the polyol pathway, advanced glycation end product formation, protein kinase C activation, hexosamine pathway flux, and poly (ADP-ribose) polymerase activation which are responsible for ocular manifestations [7].

10.2.1 Polyol Pathway

Glucose is converted to sorbitol by aldolase reductase enzymes inside the cells. Normally, sorbitol is converted to fructose by sorbitol dehydrogenase. However, in diabetics, excess intracellular sorbitol accumulation leads to osmotic changes, resulting in hydropic lens fibers, which has a low level of sorbitol dehydrogenase activity. These fibers degenerate, resulting in diabetic cataract.

10.2.2 Advanced Glycation End (AGE) Products

The release of reactive oxygen species (ROS) causes oxidative stress-induced retinal cell damage and pericyte loss leading to the changes seen in diabetic retinopathy. Oxidative stress is an important cause of pericyte loss, mitochondrial dysfunction, and thickening of basement membrane. Pericyte loss or endothelial cell injury leads to break down of the blood retinal barrier and accumulation of fluid in the retinal layers leading to macular edema. A higher expression of AGE products has been reported in the diabetic rat cornea, indicating that this may be implicated in the development of diabetic keratopathy as a result of apoptosis.

10.2.3 Inflammation and Microvasculopathy

Diabetes can be described as a state of chronic low-grade inflammation due to the effects of simultaneous, multiple metabolic pathways like AGE, ROS, and oxidative stress. The end result is vascular endothelial dysfunction resulting in microvasculopathy. Leucocyte adhesion to the vessel walls leads to capillary occlusion resulting in VEGF expression. The end result is new vessel formation (neovascularization), which forms the basis for the pathogenesis of proliferative diabetic retinopathy. Diabetic retinopathy (DR), diabetic kidney disease (DKD), and diabetic peripheral neuropathy are the most prevalent microvascular complications of type 2 diabetes (T2DM).

10.2.4 Neuropathy

Elevated glucose levels increase oxidative metabolism inside the mitochondria and increased transport of electrons leading to the release of reactive oxygen species and super oxides. Super oxides cause a dangerous imbalance in the mitochondrial electron transport chain. Accumulation of super oxides at nerve endings causes mitochondrial stress injury resulting in conduction block and demyelination of axons. This leads to ocular complications like corneal and peripheral neuropathy.

10.2.5 Protein Kinase C Pathway

Elevated intracellular glucose stimulates the synthesis of endogenous protein kinase C (PKC) activator and, diacylglycerol (DAG). Activation of PKC can adversely affect sodium potassium ATPase activity, and other enzymes that are crucial in creating cellular membrane potential, nerve conduction, and nerve regeneration, thus causing diabetic motor neuropathy complications.

PKC is also responsible for cellular apoptosis, which can be seen as pericyte loss and endothelial dysfunction. These factors, along with increased vascular permeability, lead to different stages of diabetic retinopathy [8].

10.3 Clinical Features and Management

10.3.1 Orbit and Adnexal Infection

Diabetes is a state of immune suppression, increasing the risk of intra- and extraocular infections. It has been described as a risk factor in most of the literature for a wide range of infections, varying from mild conjunctivitis to serious complications like mucormycosis and endophthalmitis [9], especially in those with poor control of diabetes. There is also an increased risk of panophthalmitis (Fig. 10.2), which involves infection of all layers of the eye ball and orbital spaces.

Diabetics have a higher chance of developing preseptal infections such as hordeolum, chalazion, and blepharitis, which are treatable with topical and oral antibiotics. However, a spread of infections posterior to the septum can result in orbital cellulitis (Fig. 10.3). which if uncontrolled can lead to cavernous sinus thrombosis and intracranial infections.

Mucor mycosis is an aggressive fungal infection caused by fungi of the phylum mucoromycetes, and is commonly seen in immunocompromised states such as

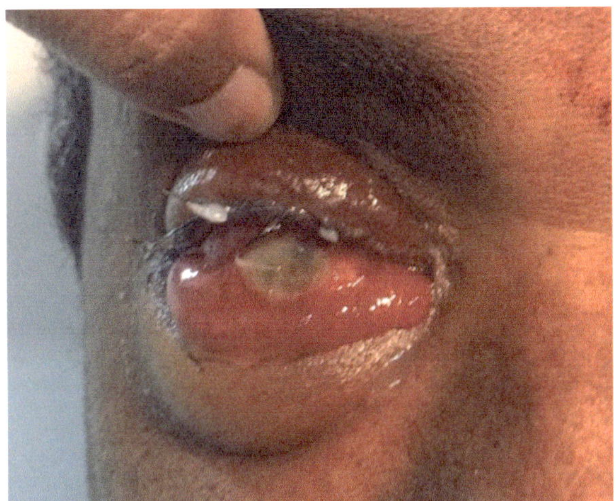

Fig. 10.2 Orbital cellulitis with panophthalmitis

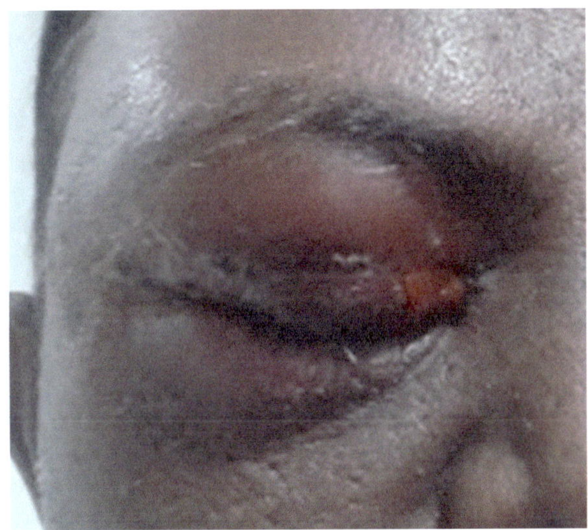

Fig. 10.3 Orbital cellulitis showing increasing redness and swelling of the eyelid with a secondary ptosis and proptosis

diabetes, posttransplantation, patients on immunosuppressants, and associated infections like covid.

It may present as mild sinusitis or occur after dental procedures, with later spread to the eye. Initially, the presentation may resemble preseptal cellulitis, but this can rapidly progress to involve extraocular muscles, cranial nerves, and later spread to the cavernous sinus resulting in involvement of the fellow eye.

Rhizopus oryzae is a subtype of mucoromycetes causing mucormycosis especially in people with diabetic ketoacidosis. These organisms produce the enzyme ketoreductase, which allows them to utilize the patient's ketone bodies, thereby resulting in fulminant and rapid spread [10].

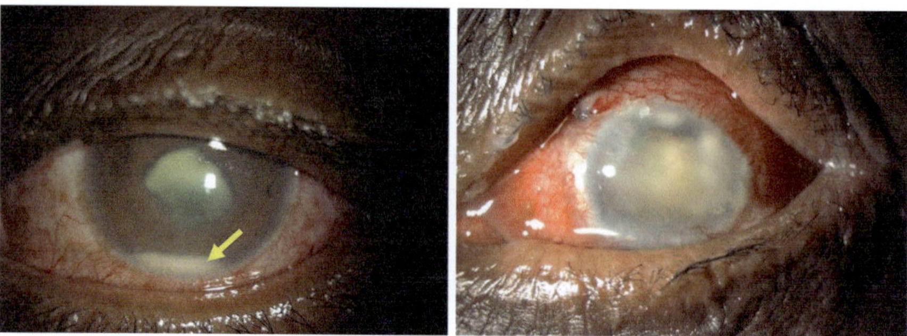

Fig. 10.4 Endophthalmitis—congestion, intense anterior segment inflammation with hypopyon (yellow arrow) with posterior segment inflammation and membranes

Treatment involves aggressive diabetic management and antifungal medications like amphotericin B and posaconazole given intravenously, orally, and in the form of intra-orbital injections. Surgical debridement can help in some patients.

Endophthalmitis (Fig. 10.4) is another serious complication which may lead to complete vision loss. Endophthalmitis can be endogenous or exogenous or can be seen in postoperative cases as well. Any ocular surgery requires strict diabetic control in the pre- and postoperative period, in order to optimize the outcome and prevent inadvertent infection. Fourteen to twenty-one percent of patients who develop postoperative endophthalmitis are diabetic [9]. The most common organism isolated from diabetic patients with acute endophthalmitis is coagulase-negative Staphylococcus [11]. Diabetics tend to have a poorer outcome posttreatment for endophthalmitis.

Endogenous endophthalmitis caused by *Escherichia coli* was reported to be almost exclusively found in diabetic patients [12]. Medical management of endophthalmitis which is an emergency, involves topical steroids, antibiotics, and intravitreal injections. Severe cases may require vitreoretinal surgery. Cases may also require physician monitoring for diabetic control during the course of admission. Severe cases with no light perception may require evisceration of the affected eye in order to prevent intra-orbital or intracranial spread, which may become a life-threatening complication.

10.3.2 Cornea

Corneal neuropathy is a well-described and frequent complication seen in diabetics. Clinically, patients may present with recurrent corneal erosions and neurotrophic corneal ulcers. The tear film, which functions as an important immunological defense for the ocular system, is altered in patients with DM. There is a documented decrease in the breakup time and Schirmer's test values in diabetics, resulting in dry eye [13].

As neuropathy is a frequent complication in diabetes, the densely innervated cornea can be affected, leading to recurrent corneal erosions and nonhealing corneal epithelial defects. Corneal neuropathy changes can be controlled with good glycemic control but cannot be reversed completely.

In diabetes, there is also a reduction in concentration of growth factors, leading to disruption of epithelial integrity (Fig. 10.5), epithelial fragility, thinning of epithelium and reduced epithelial cell density. This results in detrimental changes to the ocular surface.

Approximately 50% of patients with diabetes complain of dry eye disease (Fig. 10.6). Dry eye symptoms and signs show a similar correlation with diabetic retinopathy and peripheral neuropathy (Figs. 10.7 and 10.8). Microvascular damage to the lacrimal gland from hyperglycemia reduces binding sites for androgens and estrogens on the lacrimal gland resulting in reduced tear production [14].

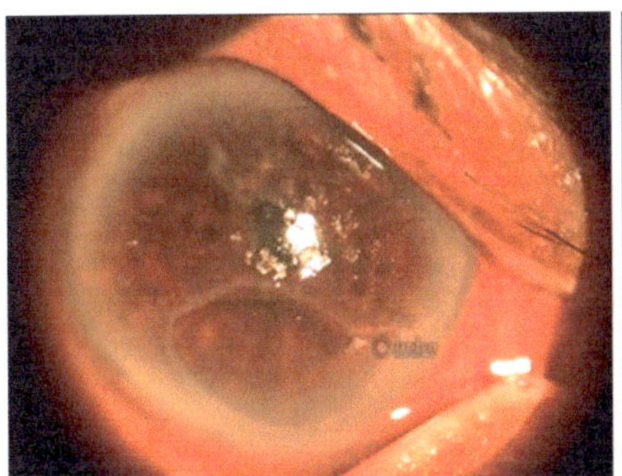
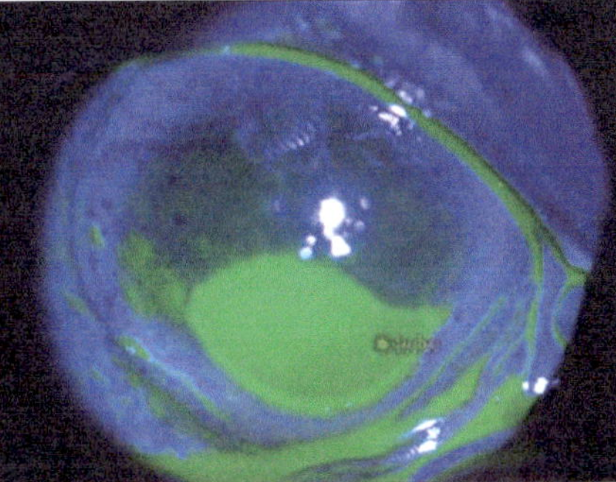

Fig. 10.5 Eye showing an epithelial defect. The defect appears to be in the inferior third of the cornea with corresponding conjunctival congestion. This is typical of exposure keratopathy caused by inadequate lid closure associated with lagophthalmos

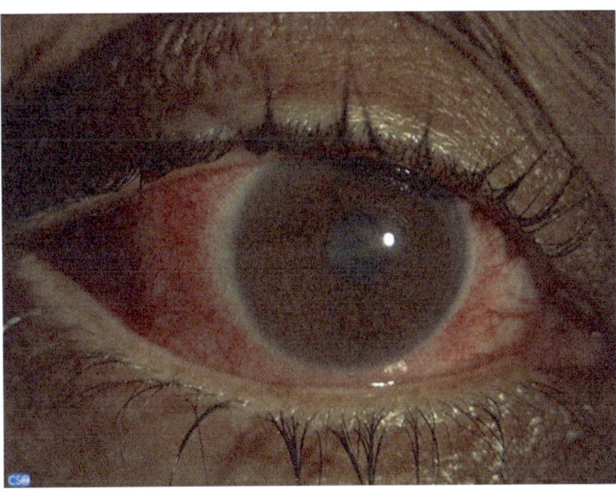

Fig. 10.6 Eye showing diffuse congestion due to decreased tear film production, a case of severe dry eye

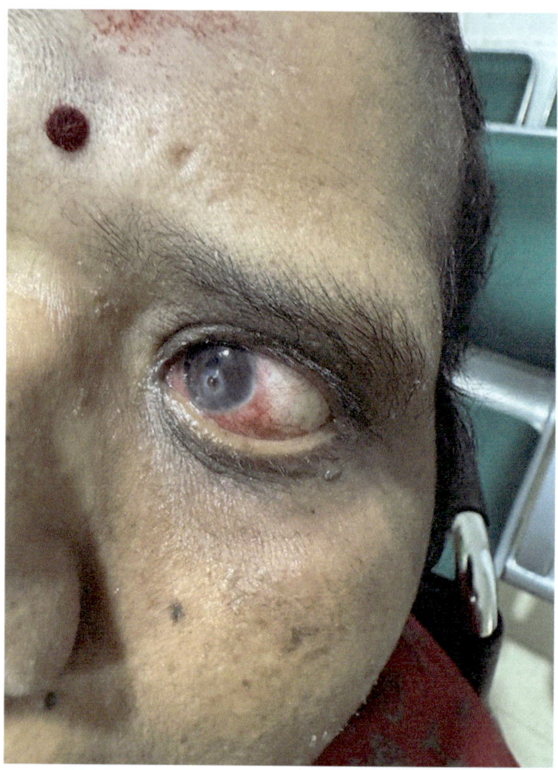

Fig. 10.7 An elderly woman with multiple cranial nerve palsy (III, IV, V, and VII), complete lagophthalmos and corneal perforation with iris tissue prolapse caused by corneal desiccation and melt

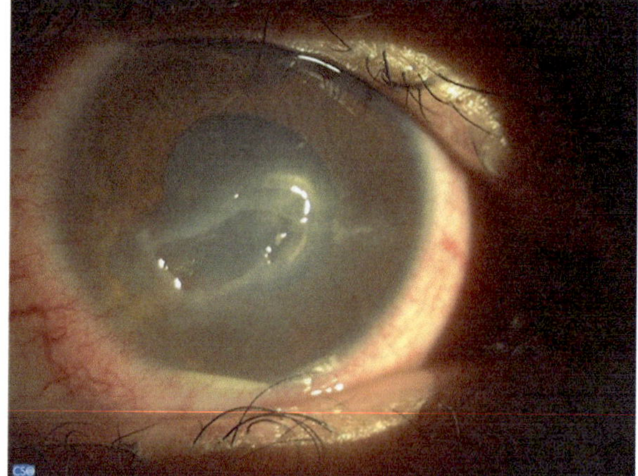

Fig. 10.8 Neurotrophic corneal ulcer which occurs as a result of improper corneal epithelial healing due to loss of corneal innervation

10.3.3 Glaucoma

The association of glaucoma in diabetes has not been unequivocally described. However, many theories exist to support the same. The suggested pathophysiology includes microvascular leakage and vascular dysregulation resulting in compromised optic nerve head perfusion. Other proposed theories talk about trabecular mesh work damage causing disrupted aqueous outflow. Dysregulated glial cell apoptosis and loss of neuroprotective function has also been described as a cause of glaucoma in diabetics.

The glaucoma prevalence is approximately two to three times higher in diabetic populations compared to nondiabetic populations [15]. Primary open-angle glaucoma is more common. Once glaucoma develops, patients require topical antiglaucoma therapy. Refractory cases may need glaucoma surgery.

Neovascular glaucoma occurs in patients with advanced diabetic retinopathy, as a result of significant retinal ischemia. They develop new vessels in the iris or angle of anterior chamber, which can be detected on slit lamp examination or gonioscopy. This is a serious condition in which patients present with symptoms like pain, redness, and reduced vision. The rise in intraocular pressure in these cases is usually refractory. Patients require urgent attention and need to be treated with topical medications and laser photocoagulation to areas of avascular retina to prevent VEGF (vascular endothelial growth factors) that are responsible for new vessels. Coexisting glaucoma may also need to be managed to prevent irreversible blindness.

10.3.4 Cataract

Cataract is the commonest cause of curable blindness in the world and can be caused by multiple factors like age, trauma, and a whole host of systemic conditions. Unregulated polyol production and AGE have been described as important causes in the pathogenesis of cataract in diabetics.

Diabetics have an increased risk of developing cataracts at an early age, and are 2–5 times more at risk for cataract than nondiabetics [5]. A snowflake-like cataract is commonly seen in young diabetics.

Cataract does not have any medical treatment to reduce or cease its progression. Surgical management is the only viable option of treatment. In spite of newer surgical techniques like minimally invasive phacoemulsification and femto-laser-assisted cataract surgery, which have lesser chances of postoperative infection due to better wound integrity and healing, surgical intervention still requires strict perioperative diabetes control.

A thorough fundus examination should be done before surgery to correlate loss of vision with grade of cataract as underlying diabetic retinopathy can be missed in preoperative screening due to the media opacity caused by cataract.

Diabetics have higher chances of developing postoperative infections, dry eye and worsening of existing diabetic retinopathy following surgery, and thereby need a regular follow-up.

Post-operative cystoid macular edema is a common complication seen after cataract surgery. Long duration of diabetes (>5 years), insulin dependency, high HBA1C, long ultrasound time during cataract surgery, and preexisting diabetic retinopathy or diabetic macular edema are the important predisposing factors for developing postoperative cystoid macular edema in diabetics [16]. Initially, treatment in early postoperative period is conservative, with the use of topical NSAID drops and other anti-inflammatory agents. However, refractory macular edema may need intravitreal injections.

10.3.5 Diabetic Retinopathy (DR)

Diabetic retinopathy is one of the leading causes of blindness, across the globe. With the rampant increase in the incidence of diabetes, diabetic retinopathy and its complications are quite prevalent. Retinopathy is seen in 30–50% of the diabetic population and every year 1% are affected by severe forms of the disorder [17]. The risk factors associated with occurrence and progression of the disease include duration of diabetes, uncontrolled blood sugar levels, and arterial hypertension [17]. Some other compounding risk factors include anemia, hyperlipidemia, and renal disease, which need to be ruled out and managed alongside the retinopathy. One study predicted that the total number of people with diabetes would rise from 171 million in 2000 to 366 million by 2030 [18].

10.3.5.1 Pathogenesis of Diabetic Retinopathy

1. Lesions in the vessel walls—thickening of basement membrane, alterations in vessel wall endothelial tight junctions, changes in pericytes, and alterations of the internal blood retinal barrier—cause **edema** and **exudation—diabetic macular edema (DME).**
2. Changes in blood flow—increased viscosity of blood, decreased deformability of erythrocytes, hyper aggregation of erythrocytes, and reduction in fibrinolysis—can cause capillary occlusions, ischemia, and increased vascular endothelial growth factor (VEGF) load, further causing **neovascularization** and glaucoma.
3. Platelet alteration—hyper aggregation and increased adhesiveness—also contributes to capillary occlusion.
4. Growth factors involved in pathogenesis of diabetic retinopathy include
   - VEGF—increased levels have been detected in the vitreous and retina [19].
   - Insulin-like growth factor-1.
   - Platelet-derived growth factor.
   - Pigment epithelium-derived factor.
   - Placental growth factor [20].

Stages of diabetic retinopathy—Nonproliferative diabetic retinopathy (NPDR) and proliferative diabetic retinopathy (DR). Proliferative disease is when fibrovascular proliferation occurs causing retinal detachment.

1. Classification of nonproliferative disease (NPDR) [21]
   - Mild (Fig. 10.9)
   - Moderate (Fig. 10.10)
   - Severe (Fig. 10.11)
   - Very severe

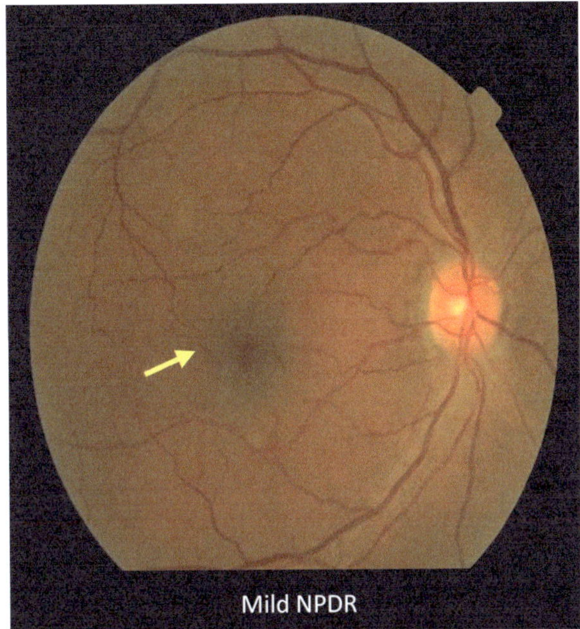

Fig. 10.9 Mild NPDR—at least 1 microaneurysm (yellow arrow) or dot-blot hemorrhage

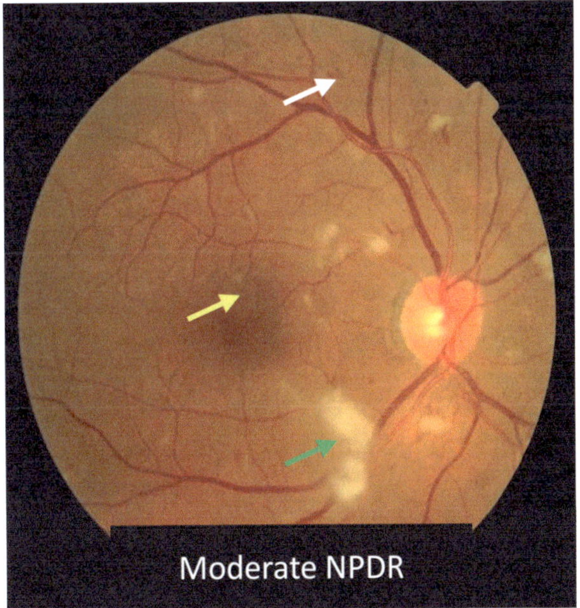

Fig. 10.10 At least 1 microaneurysm (yellow arrow) or dot-blot hemorrhage (white arrow) in 1–3 quadrants with at least 1 of the following: hard exudate, cotton wool spots (green arrow), or venous beading

2. Classification of proliferative DR (PDR) [21]
   - Early (Figs. 10.12 and 10.13)
   - High risk PDR (Fig. 10.14)

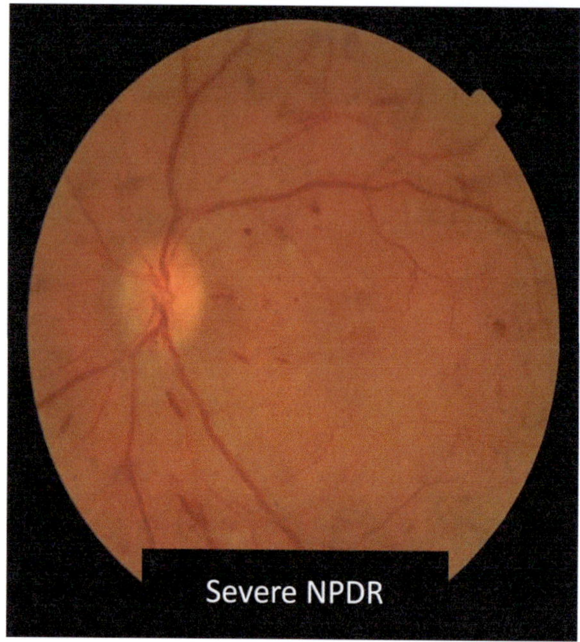

Fig. 10.11 Microaneurysm and dot-blot hemorrhages in all 4 quadrants with at least 2 quadrants of venous beading and 1 or more quadrant of IRMA

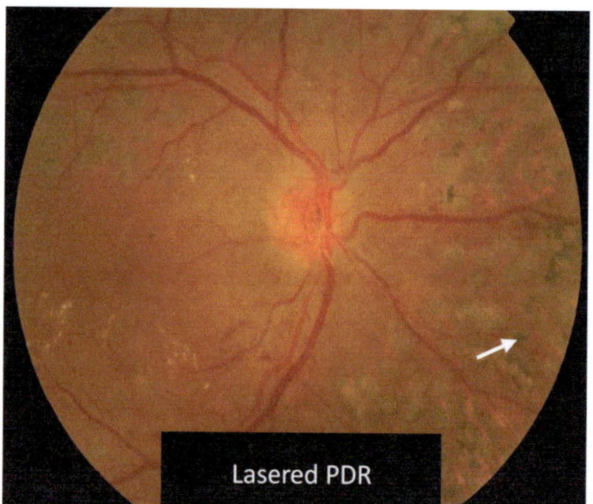

Fig. 10.12 Lasered PDR (white arrow depicts old laser marks)

3. Diabetic macular edema (Fig. 10.15) is accumulation of exuded fluid within and under the macula causing impairment of vision. Clinically significant macular edema (CSME) as defined by the early treatment diabetic retinopathy study (ETDRS) requires one of the following criteria: thickening at or within 500 μm (1/2 DD) of the center of the fovea, hard exudates at or within 500 μm (1/2 DD) of the center of the fovea with associated thickening, and/or 1 DD of thickening that is within 1 DD of the center of the fovea [21].

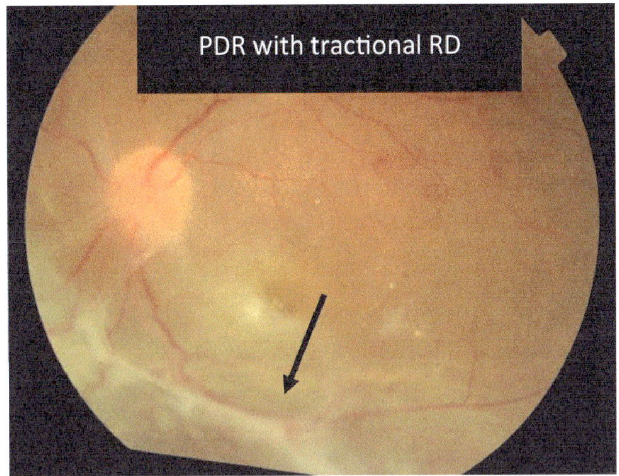

Fig. 10.13 PDR with fibrovascular proliferation and tractional retinal detachment (black arrow)

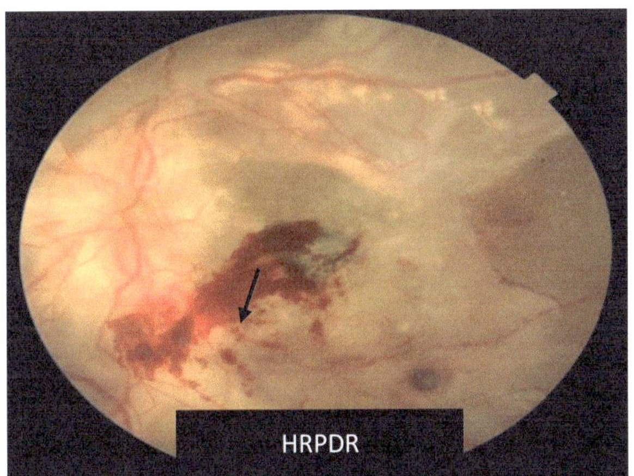

Fig. 10.14 PDR with preretinal hemorrhage (black arrow)

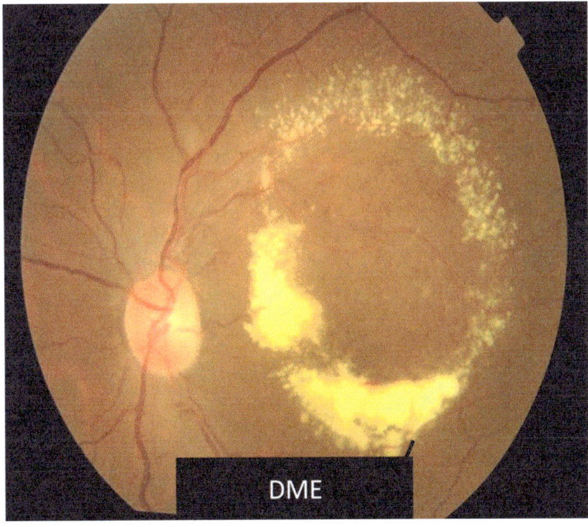

Fig. 10.15 Diabetic macular edema with hard exudates (black arrow)

Diabetic macular edema is one of the main causes of vision loss in diabetic retinopathy. DME can occur in nonproliferative or proliferative stage of the disease.

4. Optical coherence tomography (OCT) classification of DME is based on the involvement of the fovea. Retinal thickening located within the central subfield zone (1 mm in diameter) of the fovea is considered center-involving DME, and retinal thickening outside the central subfield zone of the fovea is considered non-center-involving DME [22].

   As management of each differs, DME is currently classified as center-involving DME and non-center involving DME, with center involving DME causing more vision loss.

10.3.5.2 Classification and Follow-Up

Stage	Fundus findings	Follow-up
Mild NPDR	At least 1 micro-aneurysm (MA) or dot-blot hemorrhage	6–12 months depending on glycemic status
		5% progression to PDR in 1 year
Moderate NPDR	At least 1 MA or dot-blot hemorrhage in 1–3 quadrants with at least 1 of the following: Hard exudate, cotton wool spots, or venous beading	6–8 months, depending on glycemic status
		25% progression to PDR in 1 year
Severe NPDR	4-2-1 rule	2–4 months, depending on glycemic status
	MA and dot-blot hemorrhages in all 4 quadrants with at least 2 quadrants of venous beading and 1 or more quadrant of IRMA	52% progression to PDR in 1 year
Very severe NPDR	2 or more characteristics of NPDR in the absence of neovascularization	2–3 months, depending on glycemic status
		75% progression to PDR in 1 year
Early PDR	Neovascularization of disk (NVD) or elsewhere (NVE)	75% progress to high risk PDR in 5 years
	NVD <1/3 disk diameters with no vitreous hemorrhage	
High—Risk PDR	• NVD ≥ 1/3 to 1/2 disc diameters • Any NVD associated with preretinal or vitreous hemorrhage • NVE ≥ 1/2-disk diameters with vitreous/preretinal heme	
Advanced diabetic eye disease	Pre-retinal hemorrhage, tractional retinal detachment, or rubeosis iridis	

10.3.5.3 Diagnosis of Diabetic Retinopathy and DME

1. Systemic evaluation

   Fasting and postprandial blood sugars, HbA1c levels, renal function test, lipid profile, hemoglobin, and blood pressure.
2. Ophthalmic evaluation—The most important diagnostic modality is the dilated fundus examination, using direct and indirect ophthalmoscope, along with visual acuity, intraocular pressure, gonioscopy, and slit lamp evaluation.
3. Fundus photography is useful in documentation and documentation.
4. Imaging methods like optical coherence tomography (OCT) (Fig. 10.16) and OCT-angiography aid in diagnosis and staging of diabetic retinopathy and macular edema.
5. In select situations, a dye-based angiography test called fluorescein angiography may be performed to identify new blood vessels in PDR and microaneurysms and areas of leakage associated with DME. FFA also identifies degree of retinal capillary non perfusion.

10.3.5.4 Treatment Modalities

Diabetic retinopathy needs treatment when DME affects vision and also when proliferative diabetic retinopathy causes vision loss due to vitreous hemorrhage or retinal detachment.

Earlier stages of NPDR do not need treatment but periodic follow-up along with systemic control of blood sugar, hypertension, hyperlipidemia, coexisting renal disease, and anemia.

Diabetic macular edema may be asymptomatic in its early stages, and proliferative diabetic retinopathy can also be asymptomatic until new vessels cause hemorrhage. However, PDR can be treated effectively with laser photocoagulation at this

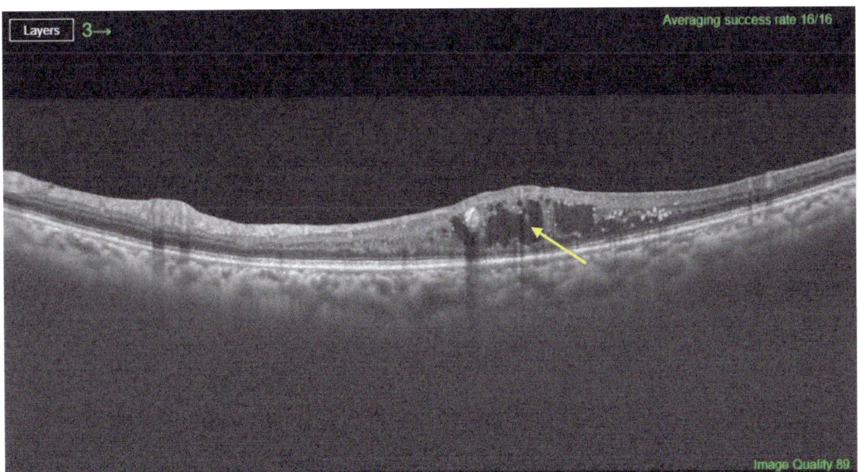

Fig. 10.16 Optical coherence tomography of diabetic macular edema showing intraretinal cystic spaces (yellow arrow) with hyper-reflective foci

stage—when the patient is asymptomatic and has no hemorrhage. This can arrest progression of the disease and help maintain vision. Similarly, prompt treatment of DME can prevent vision loss and help patient maintain good vision. Restoration of vision in late, established stages of DME will need prolonged treatment and may often not restore vision completely.

This underlines the need for prompt diagnosis of diabetic retinopathy and appropriate treatment. This can be possible only with regular fundus exam or screening. Recent evidence also suggests that presence of retinopathy is often an indicator of other target organ damage and helps the physician screen for the same and treat appropriately. For all these, reasons, it is essential that a diabetic patient is referred for a fundus screening at diagnosis and at periodic intervals as suggested by the ophthalmologist.

1. Strict glycemic control and lifestyle modifications—regular exercise, a diabetic diet, and appropriate medical therapy.
2. Associated systemic diseases such as hypertension, renal disease, hyperlipidemia, and anemia need to be corrected.

   Glitazones have been known to cause macular edema and hence they have to be replaced with other drugs in the presence of DME.
3. Very mild NPDR follow-up every year.
4. Mild-to-moderate NPDR follow-up 6–12 monthly.
5. Severe to very severe NPDR close follow-up within 2–3 months.
6. Diabetic macular edema - if center involving - anti-VEGF injections, intravitreal steroids or intravitreal steroid implants. The intravitreal injections would need to be repeated on a periodic basis, depending on patient's response to treatment.
7. DME-non-center involving - focal/grid laser photocoagulation.
8. Tractional DME—due to vitreomacular traction (VMT) or ERM (epiretinal membrane)—should consider vitrectomy.
9. Refractory DME—The definition of refractory or persistent DME varies, including macular edema not responding to multiple injections of anti-VEGF and, at least one sitting of laser, and suboptimal response (central macular thickness on OCT of more than 250 μm with associated visual loss) to 6 consecutive monthly injections of anti-VEGF agents [23, 24]. These patients need evaluation of systemic diabetic control, higher dosing, or frequency of anti-VEGF medications or use of steroid implants [25, 26].
10. PDR-laser pan retinal photocoagulation. Pan retinal photocoagulation destroys ischemic retina, thereby decreasing secretion of factors promoting neovascularization, such as VEGF, thereby arresting the progression of the proliferative disease.
11. PDR with DME-combined anti-VEGF injection along with PRP.
12. Advanced diabetic eye disease—Indications of vitrectomy include
    - Non-clearing vitreous/sub-hyaloid hemorrhage
    - Tractional retinal detachment
    - Combined retinal detachment
    - Anterior segment neovascularization with no view of the posterior segment

- Ghost cell glaucoma
- Thick epiretinal membrane
- Vitreomacular traction
- Vitrectomy is microsurgery, wherein the vitreous gel along with blood or abnormal fibrovascular tissue causing vision loss or retinal detachment is removed to clear the media and also allow retinal reattachment, thereby allowing the patient to see once again. This is usually combined with pan-retinal photocoagulation or injection of anti-VEGF agent.

10.3.6 Neurology and the Eye

Factors like oxidative stress, reactive oxygen species, polyol pathways, and microvascular changes causing nerve microinfarctions are responsible for the mononeuropathies commonly seen in diabetics. Patients with diabetes have a ten-fold increase in the incidence of cranial nerve palsies, with an incidence of 1% among diabetics compared with an incidence of 0.1% for the nondiabetic population [27].

Cranial nerves III, IV, VI, and VII are commonly affected in diabetes and can present either as individual mononeuropathies or as multiple nerve palsies. Third cranial nerve palsy is the most common of these [28]. Common symptoms include diplopia (double vision) and ptosis. Other cranial nerve palsies like IV and VI produce diplopia which is gaze specific, occurring in the direction of gaze involving the affected extraocular muscle.

No specific treatment strategy is available for nerve palsies. Strict metabolic control is required, and in most the cases, the nerve palsies are transient and recover with very minimal residual symptoms. Rare instances produce residual permanent nerve damage. These cases are treated with prism glasses or surgery on the affected muscles to overcome diplopia.

Facial nerve palsy leads to weakness of one side of the face and inability to close the eyelid. This may further lead to complications like exposure keratopathy, which needs symptomatic treatment like lid closure tapes, lubricants, or surgical tarsorrhaphy.

All nerve palsies should be examined in detail and other causes should be ruled out. Although not mandatory, neuroimaging is advisable for all cases in order to rule out other serious intra cranial causes.

10.3.6.1 Diabetic Papillopathy (Fig. 10.17)

Diabetic papillopathy is an uncommon ocular manifestation of unilateral or bilateral disk edema seen in patients with diabetes. The prevalence of papillopathy in both types of DM is about 0.5%, regardless of glycemic control and seriousness of diabetic retinopathy [29].

The disk edema is usually self-limiting and reverses on control of diabetes with the probable pathophysiology being compromise to the peripapillary vasculature.

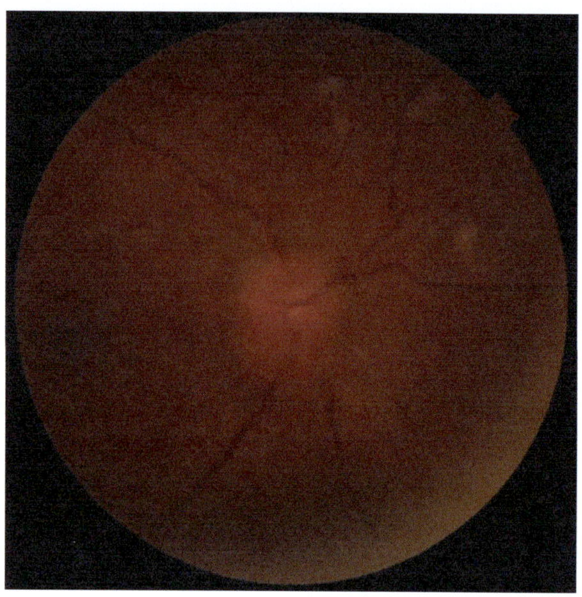

Fig. 10.17 Diabetic papillopathy

Despite its benign nature, it is always prudent to rule out other causes of disk edema. Long-standing disk edema may lead to disk pallor leading to permanent impairment or complete loss of vision.

10.4 Diabetes and the Eye: Outreach and Community

In many low-middle income countries, tertiary centers alone may not be sufficient to cater to the large population of diabetics. Many local population-based screening and awareness programs have been conducted across the countries through camps, and outreach programs. The major activities in community outreach programs are screening, diagnosis, providing advice to people with early DR regarding glycemic control, life style modification, and regular follow-up (systemic management) and referring those requiring ocular management to secondary and tertiary eye care centers [30].

Some of the successful outreach programmes for diabetic eye disease include

1. Screening in healthcare services such as optical shops, pharmacies, etc.
2. Risk-based screening
3. Tele-ophthalmology-based screening model
4. Fundus photography technique
5. Mobile screening modalities

Methods of screening for DR include direct and indirect ophthalmoscopy, stereoscopic seven field fundus photography, and nonmydriatic, or mydriatic digital retinal color fundus photography [31].

10.5 Diabetes and the Eye: Future Treatment Pathways and Artificial Intelligence (AI)

The American Academy of Ophthalmology recommends that individuals with type 1 diabetes should undergo annual eye examinations 5 years after the onset of diabetes. Individuals with type 2 diabetes should undergo annual eye examinations at the time of diagnosis [32].

Screening the eye for diabetic eye disease can be done by a clinical examination or by tele-screening wherein a photograph of the fundus is obtained and digitally transmitted to a specialist to diagnose presence of DR and also stage the same.

Current interest is in using artificial intelligence (AI) to diagnose DR from fundus photographs. Using AI frees precious human resource such as the medical professionals from the screening process and filters only those requiring human intervention to be routed to the treating physician.

In the field of ophthalmology, AI assists in the diagnosis of DR, glaucoma, age-related macular degeneration, and retinopathy of prematurity.

In 2018, the Food and Drug Administration approved the first AI software for DR (IDx-DR). IDx-DR captures fundus images, and the technician uploads the images to the cloud server. The software provides results according to the images: if the image quality is high enough, and mild or severe DR is detected, the physician will then be prompted to refer the patient to an ophthalmologist; if the severity is not higher than mild DR, it will prompt the patient to retest in 12 months [33].

Some of the other AI-based screening systems include

- EyeArt (Eyenuk Inc., Los Angeles, USA) was approved by the Food and Drug Administration in August 2020 [34].
- Retmarker DR (Retmarker, Coimbra, Portugal) has been certified as a Class IIa medical device in Europe [35].
- In China, AI-based screening software for DR by Shenzhen SiBionics Co. Ltd. (Shenzhen, China) and the AI-based analysis software for DR by Airdoc (Beijing, China) were also approved in August 2020 [36].
- With the advent of AI-based screening tools, early detection and management of diabetic eye disease is more feasible in countries with a large population of diabetics, with inaccessible healthcare systems for all.
- Currently, some of the fundus camera systems used to obtain the retinal image have in-built AI to aid prompt diagnosis and referral.

10.6 Conclusion

Diabetes has multiple manifestations in the eye, and can cause complications in all ocular structures, if not identified early and treated appropriately. Hence, awareness and regular examination by the ophthalmologist can prevent the progression of these conditions in the eye.

References

1. GBD 2019 Blindness and Vision Impairment Collaborators; Vision Loss Expert Group of the Global Burden of Disease Study. Causes of blindness and vision impairment in 2020 and trends over 30 years, and prevalence of avoidable blindness in relation to VISION 2020: the Right to Sight: an analysis for the Global Burden of Disease Study. Lancet Glob Health. 2021;9(2):e144–60. https://doi.org/10.1016/S2214-109X(20)30489-7. Epub 2020 Dec 1. Erratum in: Lancet Glob Health. 2021 Apr;9(4):e408. PMID: 33275949; PMCID: PMC7820391.
2. Modjtahedi BS, Wu J, Luong TQ, Gandhi NK, Fong DS, Chen W. Severity of diabetic retinopathy and the risk of future cerebrovascular disease, cardiovascular disease, and all-cause mortality. Ophthalmology. 2021;128(8):1169–79. https://doi.org/10.1016/j.ophtha.2020.12.019. Epub 2020 Dec 25. PMID: 33359888.
3. Thomas RL, Dunstan FD, Luzio SD, Chowdhury SR, North RV, Hale SL, et al. Prevalence of diabetic retinopathy within a national diabetic retinopathy screening service. Br J Ophthalmol. 2015;99:64–8.
4. Romero-Aroca P, Navarro-Gil R, Valls-Mateu A, Sagarra-Alamo R, Moreno-Ribas A, Soler N. Differences in incidence of diabetic retinopathy between type 1 and 2 diabetes mellitus: a nine-year follow-up study. Br J Ophthalmol. 2017;101(10):1346–51. https://doi.org/10.1136/bjophthalmol-2016-310063. Epub 2017 Mar 7. PMID: 28270484; PMCID: PMC5629951.
5. Ramachandran A, Snehalatha C, Sasikala R, Satyavani K, Vijay V. Vascular complications in young Asian Indian patients with type 1 diabetes mellitus. Diabetes Res Clin Pract. 2000;48(1):51–6. https://doi.org/10.1016/s0168-8227(99)00134-5.
6. Flaxel CJ, Adelman RA, Bailey ST, Fawzi A, Lim JI, Vemulakonda GA, Ying GS. Diabetic retinopathy preferred practice pattern®. Ophthalmology. 2020;127(1):P66–145. https://doi.org/10.1016/j.ophtha.2019.09.025. Epub 2019 Sep 25. Erratum in: Ophthalmology. 2020 Sep;127(9):1279.PMID: 31757498.
7. Srikanth KK, Orrick JA. Biochemistry, polyol or sorbitol pathways. [Updated 2022 Nov 14]. In: StatPearls. Treasure Island, FL: StatPearls Publishing; 2023.
8. Pan D, Xu L, Guo M. The role of protein kinase C in diabetic microvascular complications. Front Endocrinol (Lausanne). 2022;13:973058. https://doi.org/10.3389/fendo.2022.973058. PMID: 36060954; PMCID: PMC9433088.
9. Doft BH, Wisniewski SR, Kelsey SF, Fitzgerald SG, The Endophthalmitis Vitrectomy Study Group. Diabetes and postoperative endophthalmitis in the endophthalmitis vitrectomy study. Arch Ophthalmol. 2001;119(5):650–6. https://doi.org/10.1001/archopht.119.5.650.
10. Marx RE, Stern D. Inflammatory, reactive and infectious diseases in oral and maxillofacial pathology. Carol Stream, IL: Quintessence Publishing; 2003. p. 104–6.
11. Dev S, Pulido JS, Tessler HH, et al. Progression of diabetic retinopathy after endophthalmitis. Ophthalmology. 1999;106(4):774–81.
12. Walmsley RS, David DB, Allan RN, Kirkby GR. Bilateral endogenous *Escherichia coli* endophthalmitis: a devastating complication in an insulin-dependent diabetic. Postgrad Med J. 1996;72:361–3.
13. Bilen H, Ates O, Astam N, Uslu H, Akcay G, Baykal O. Conjunctival flora in patients with type 1 or type 2 diabetes mellitus. Adv Ther. 2007;24(5):1028–35.
14. Lv H, Li A, Zhang X, Xu M, Qiao Y, Zhang J, et al. Meta-analysis and review on the changes of tear function and corneal sensitivity in diabetic patients. Acta Ophthalmol. 2014;92:e96–104.
15. Song BJ, Aiello LP, Pasquale LR. Presence and risk factors for glaucoma in patients with diabetes. Curr Diab Rep. 2016;16(12):124. https://doi.org/10.1007/s11892-016-0815-6. PMID: 27766584; PMCID: PMC5310929.
16. Yang J, Cai L, Sun Z, Ye H, Fan Q, Zhang K, Lu W, Lu Y. Risk factors for and diagnosis of pseudophakic cystoid macular edema after cataract surgery in diabetic patients. J Cataract Refract Surg. 2017;43(2):207–14. https://doi.org/10.1016/j.jcrs.2016.11.047. Erratum in: J Cataract Refract Surg. 2017 Aug;43(8):1126. PMID: 28366368.

17. Diabetic retinopathy, 1st edn. 2015. ISBN 978-93-5152-898-2.
18. Wild S, Roglic G, Green A, et al. Global prevalence of diabetes: estimates for the year 2000 and projections for 2030. Diabetes Care. 2004;27(5):1047–53.
19. Williams B. Vascular permeability/vascular endothelial growth factors: a potential role in the pathogenesis and treatment of vascular diseases. Vasc Med. 1996;1:251–8.
20. Cai J, Boulton M. The pathogenesis of diabetic retinopathy: old concepts and new questions. Eye. 2002;16:242–60.
21. Grading diabetic retinopathy from stereoscopic color fundus photographs—an extension of the modified Airlie House classification. ETDRS report number 10. Early Treatment Diabetic Retinopathy Study Research Group. Ophthalmology. 1991;98(5 Suppl):786–806. https://doi.org/10.1016/S0161-6420(13)38012-9.
22. Diabetic Eye Care. International Council of Ophthalmology. www.icoph.org/enhancing_eyecare/diabetic_eyecare.html. Accessed 15 Oct 2021.
23. Hussain RM, Ciulla TA. Treatment strategies for refractory diabetic macular edema: switching anti-VEGF treatments, adopting corticosteroid-based treatments, and combination therapy. Expert Opin Biol Ther. 2016;16(3):365–74.
24. Shah SU, Maturi RK. Therapeutic options in refractory diabetic macular oedema. Drugs. 2017;77(5):481–92.
25. Jiang AC, Srivastava SK, Hu M, Figueiredo N, Babiuch A, Boss JD, Reese JL, Ehlers JP. Quantitative ultra-widefield angiographic features and associations with diabetic macular edema. Ophthalmol Retina. 2020;4(1):49–56.
26. Khan Z, Kuriakose RK, Khan M, Chin EK, Almeida DR. Efficacy of the intravitreal sustained-release dexamethasone implant for diabetic macular edema refractory to anti-vascular endothelial growth factor therapy: meta-analysis and clinical implications. Ophthalmic Surg Lasers Imaging Retina. 2017;48(2):160–6.
27. Watanabe K, Hagura R, Akanuma Y, et al. Characteristics of cranial nerve palsies in diabetic patients. Diabetes Res Clin Pract. 1990;10:19–27.
28. Greco D, Gambina F, Pisciotta M, Abrignani M, Maggio F. Clinical characteristics and associated comorbidities in diabetic patients with cranial nerve palsies. J Endocrinol Investig. 2012;35(2):146–9. https://doi.org/10.3275/7574. Epub 2011 Mar 7. PMID: 21399393.
29. Sayin N, Kara N, Pekel G. Ocular complications of diabetes mellitus. World J Diabetes. 2015;6(1):92–108. https://doi.org/10.4239/wjd.v6.i1.92. PMID: 25685281; PMCID: PMC4317321.
30. Wadhwani M, Vashist P, Singh SS, Gupta N, Malhotra S, Gupta A, et al. Diabetic retinopathy screening programme utilising non-mydriatic fundus imaging in slum populations of New Delhi, India. Trop Med Int Health. 2018;23:405–14.
31. Wong TY, Sun J, Kawasaki R, Ruamviboonsuk P, Gupta N, Lansingh VC, et al. Guidelines on diabetic eye care: the International Council of Ophthalmology recommendations for screening, follow-up, referral, and treatment based on resource settings. Ophthalmology. 2018;125:1608–22.
32. Preferred practice pattern® guidelines. San Francisco: American Academy of Ophthalmology Preferred Practice Patterns Committee; 2019.
33. DA permits marketing of artificial intelligence-based device to detect certain diabetes-related eye problems. U.S. Food and Drug Administration; 2018.
34. August 2020 510(K) clearances. U.S. Food and Drug Administration; 2020.
35. Roy R, Lobo A, Pal BP, Oliveira CM, Raman R, Sharma T. Automated diabetic retinopathy imaging in Indian eyes: a pilot study. Indian J Ophthalmol. 2014;62:1121–4. https://doi.org/10.4103/0301-4738.149129.
36. Announcement of the State Food and Drug Administration on approval of registration of 96 medical devices (August 2020) (No. 98 of 2020). National Medical Products Administration; 2020.

Diabetes and Dermatology 11

Deepika Lunawat and Georgi Abraham

11.1 Introduction

Diabetes mellitus is a debilitating disease that affects skin amongst various other organs. In total, 30–70% of patients with DM, both type 1 and type 2, will present with a cutaneous complication at some point during their lifetime [1]. Individuals with type 2 diabetes are more likely to develop cutaneous manifestations than type 1. These dermatologic changes can range from being benign, aesthetically concerning to deforming and life-threatening. Such changes can aid in diagnosis of diabetes as sometimes cutaneous disease can appear as the first sign of DM. It can often offer an insight into a patient's glycemic control. Management of these conditions is important in improving the quality of life and in avoiding serious adverse effects.

11.1.1 Diabetes and Skin

There are many proposed pathological mechanisms for skin involvement in DM, which include abnormal carbohydrate metabolism, production of advanced glycation end products (AGEs), other altered metabolic pathways, atherosclerosis, microangiopathy, neuron degeneration, and impaired host mechanism [2].

Skin manifestations of DM may be classified as

1. Skin manifestations strongly associated with DM
2. Nonspecific dermatologic signs and symptoms

D. Lunawat (✉)
Mahi Skin Hair and Laser Clinic, Chennai, Tamil Nadu, India

G. Abraham
Department of Nephrology, MGM Healthcare, Chennai, Tamil Nadu, India

G. Abraham et al. (eds.), *Management of Diabetic Complications*,
https://doi.org/10.1007/978-981-97-6406-8_11

3. Dermatologic diseases associated with DM
4. Infections
5. Cutaneous changes associated with diabetes medications

11.1.2 Skin Manifestations Strongly Associated with DM

11.1.2.1 Acanthosis Nigricans

Acanthosis nigricans (AN), a classic dermatologic manifestation of diabetes, is more common in type 2 diabetes mellitus [3] and affects both sexes equally. AN may be associated with various endocrinopathies that involve insulin resistance such as acromegaly, Cushing syndrome, obesity, and polycystic ovarian syndrome. AN can also be associated with malignancies such as gastric adenocarcinomas and other carcinomas.

AN presents as asymptomatic hyperpigmented velvety to verrucous plaques (Fig. 11.1a–c). It is symmetrically present in intertriginous or flexural surfaces such as the back of the neck, axilla, elbows, palmer hands (also known as "tripe palms"), inframammary creases, umbilicus, or groin. Facial AN is also seen commonly and is a cutaneous indicator of Metabolic syndrome [4]. AN can be associated with skin tags (acrochordons). Microscopy shows hyperkeratosis and epidermal papillomatosis with acanthosis. The presence of AN should prompt evaluation for diabetes mellitus and other signs of insulin resistance. Burke et al. have proposed a scoring system for AN based on the degree of severity and number of affected sites.

The pathogenesis of AN is not completely understood. The predominant theory is that a hyperinsulin state activates insulin growth factor receptors, IGF-1, on keratinocytes and fibroblasts, provoking cell proliferation.

AN is best managed with lifestyle changes such as dietary modifications, increased physical activity, and weight reduction. In patients with diabetes, pharmacologic adjuvants, such as metformin, help. However, in those with thickened or macerated areas of skin, oral retinoids or topical agents such as ammonium lactate, retinoic acid, vitamin D analogs-calcipotriene, urea, and salicylic acid can be used. Chemical peels also help.

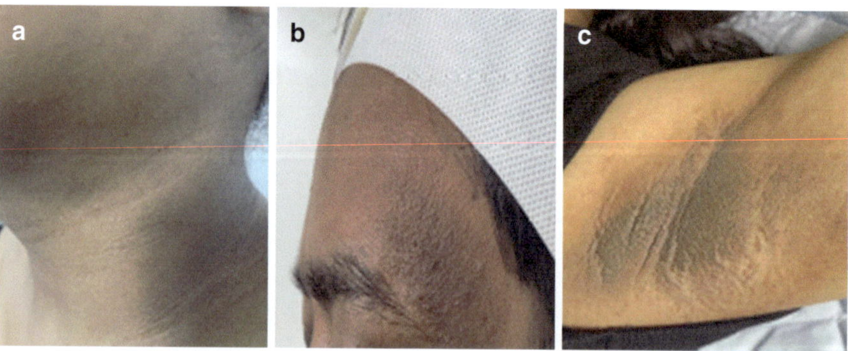

Fig. 11.1 (a–c) Acanthosis nigricans of *neck, face and axilla*

11.1.2.2 Diabetic Dermopathy

Dermopathy (DD), also known as pigmented pretibial patches or diabetic shin spots, is the most common dermatologic manifestation of diabetes, presenting in as many as one-half of those with diabetes [5] (Fig. 11.2). Some studies consider it to be pathognomonic for diabetes. DD has a strong predilection for older men. DD may be associated with diabetics having microvascular complications, nephropathy, neuropathy, retinopathy, and cardiovascular issues.

DD presents with round red papules that become well-circumscribed, atrophic, scaly brown macules. As the lesions progress, they leave behind an area of concavity and hyperpigmentation. At any time, different lesions can present at different stages of evolution. The lesions are bilaterally symmetrical over bony prominences like the pretibial area (most common), other bony prominences such as the forearms, lateral malleoli, or thighs may also be involved. This predilection for shin is due to sluggish blood flow, increased vascular fragility, increased plasma viscosity, and lower skin temperature [6].

Histologically, DD is rather nonspecific; it is characterized by lymphocytic infiltrates surrounding vasculature, engorged blood vessels in the papillary dermis, and dispersed hemosiderin deposits.

The origin of DD remains unclear, though mild trauma, hemosiderin and melanin deposition, microangiopathic changes, and destruction of subcutaneous nerves have been suggested.

Treatment is avoided as the disease per se is asymptomatic and self-resolving.

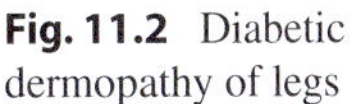

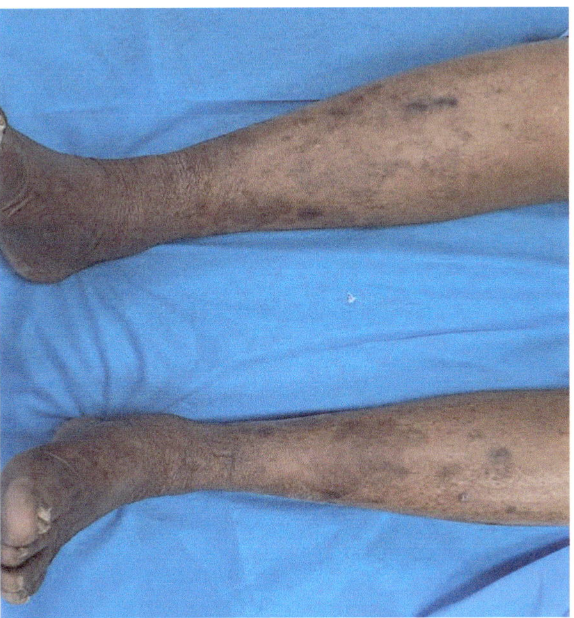

Fig. 11.2 Diabetic dermopathy of legs

11.1.2.3 Diabetic Foot Syndrome

Diabetic foot syndrome (DFS) encompasses the neurovascular complications that develop in the feet of patients with diabetes. Although preventable, DFS is a significant cause of morbidity, mortality, hospitalization, and reduction in quality of life of patients with diabetes (Fig. 11.3).

In the early stages, it presents with callosities and dry skin. Chronic ulcers which may be neuropathic, ischemic, or mixed and a variety of other malformations of the feet develop in the later stages. Neuropathic ulcers are painless resulting from peripheral neuropathy. Ulcers associated with peripheral vascular ischemia are painful. Ulcers tend to occur in areas prone to trauma, classically presenting at the site of calluses or over bony prominences like the toes, forefoot, and ankles. Secondary infection of ulcers can lead to gangrenous necrosis, osteomyelitis, and may even require lower extremity amputation. Another complication, diabetic neuro-osteoarthropathy (also known as Charcot's foot), is an irreversible debilitating and deforming condition involving progressive destruction of weight-bearing bones and joints. It can result in collapse of the midfoot, referred to as "rocker-bottom foot." Clawing deformity of the toes is also seen. Erythromelalgia presents with redness, warmth, and a burning pain involving the lower extremities, most often the feet.

The pathogenesis of DFS involves a combination of neuropathy [7], atherosclerosis [7], and impaired wound healing [8]. Due to long-standing hyperglycemia, there is an increase in advanced glycosylation end products, proinflammatory factors, and oxidative stress which results in the demyelination of nerves and

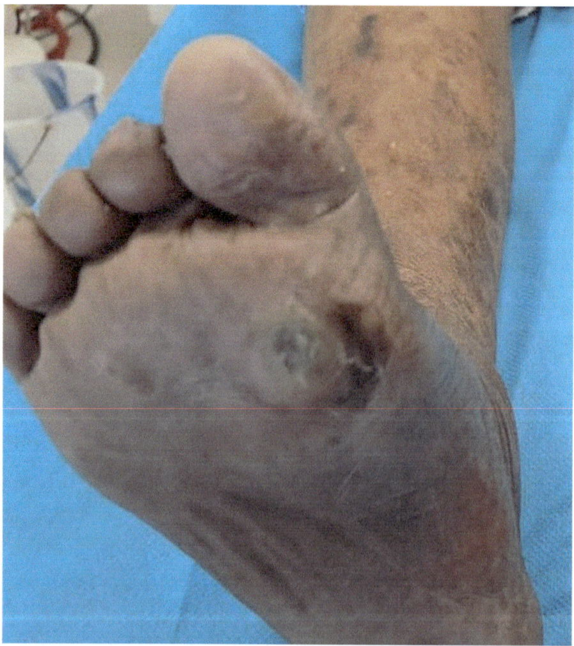

Fig. 11.3 Callosity over the plantar aspect of forefoot

subsequent neuropathy. This in turn can blunt the perception of adverse stimuli and produce an altered gait, increasing the likelihood of developing callosities, foot ulcers, and malformations. In addition, damage to autonomic nerve fibers causes a reduction in sweating making it prone to fissures and secondary infection [9]. In addition to neuropathy, accelerated arterial atherosclerosis can lead to peripheral ischemia and ulceration. Finally, hyperglycemia impairs macrophage function, prolongs the inflammatory response, and slows the healing of ulcers (Fig. 11.4).

Prevention encompasses daily surveillance, appropriate foot hygiene, and proper footwear to prevent infection, promote healing, and reduce amputation risk. Treatment involves offloading with therapeutic shoes, braces, and casts to reduce pressure. Oral antibiotics targeted at the growth help. Surgical intervention involves removing infected tissue, draining abscess, and reconstructing the foot. Adjuvant treatment in the form of Granulocyte colony-stimulating factor (G-CSF), Negative pressure wound therapy (NPWT), hyperbaric oxygen therapy, topical growth factors, and biofabricated skin grafts are available.

11.1.2.4 Diabetic Thick Skin

Skin thickening in diabetics can appear as thickened, waxy, or edematous skin. It is often asymptomatic but can present as a reduction in sensation and pain. The hands and feet are most frequently involved. Ultrasound evaluation of the skin can be

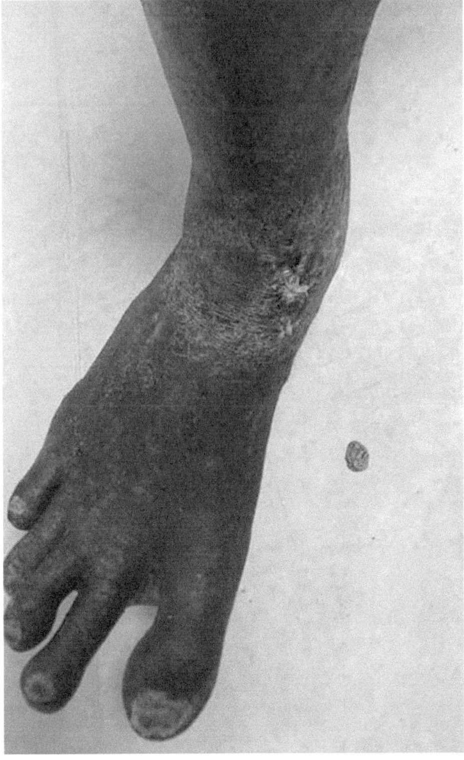

Fig. 11.4 Diabetic ulcer over the right ankle joint on the medial side

diagnostic and exhibit thickened skin. Histology shows thickened and disorganized collagen bundles. Subclinical generalized skin thickening is the most common type of skin thickening. Diabetic thick skin can present as scleroderma-like skin changes or limited joint mobility.

11.1.2.5 Scleroderma-Like Skin Changes

Scleroderma-like skin changes occur more commonly in those with type 1 diabetes and in those with longstanding disease. This presents as bilaterally symmetric painless, indurated, waxy appearing, thickened skin in acral areas. It involves the dorsum of the fingers (sclerodactyly), proximal interphalangeal, and metacarpophalangeal joints. Severe disease may extend centrally from the hands to the arms or back. The risk of developing nephropathy and retinopathy is increased in those with scleroderma-like skin changes who also have type 1 diabetes [10, 11]. The aforementioned symptoms are also associated with diabetic hand syndrome which may present with limited joint mobility, palmar fibromatosis (Dupuytren's contracture), and stenosing tenosynovitis ("trigger finger") [12]. The physical exam finding known as the "prayer sign" (inability to press palmar surfaces on each hand together) may be present in patients with diabetic hand syndrome and scleroderma-like skin changes [13]. On histology, scleroderma-like skin changes reveal thickening of the dermis, minimal-to-absent mucin, and increased interlinking of collagen.

Although not fully understood, the pathogenesis is believed to involve increased fibroblast production, decrease in collagen breakdown, nonenzymatic glycosylation of collagen.

Strict glycemic control of blood sugar may result in the narrowing of thickened skin. Aldose reductase inhibitors may be efficacious. In patients with restricted ranges of motions, physical therapy can help.

11.1.2.6 Limited Joint Mobility

Limited Joint Mobility (LJM), also known as diabetic cheiroarthropathy, is a relatively common complication of long-standing diabetes mellitus. It is often associated with scleroderma-like skin changes. LJM often begins with joints of the fifth finger and then involves other joints of hand with progressive flexed contractures and hindered joint extension, most commonly involving the metacarpophalangeal and interphalangeal joints of the hand. Patients may present with an inability to press the palmar surfaces of each of their hands together ("prayer sign") or against the surface of a table when their forearms are perpendicular to the surface of the table ("tabletop sign") [14]. These changes occur as a result of periarticular enlargement of connective tissue. The pathogenesis likely involves hyperglycemia-induced formation of advanced glycation end-products, which accumulate to promote inflammation and the formation of stiffening cross-links between collagen. Patients with LJM may also be at increased risk for falls. Symptomatic patients may benefit from nonsteroidal anti-inflammatory drugs or targeted injection of corticosteroids. Improved glycemic control, as well as physical therapy, may help.

11.1.2.7 Scleredema Diabetocorum

Scleredema diabeticorum is a chronic and slowly progressive sclerotic skin disorder that is often seen in the context of diabetes. It presents with symmetric and diffuse involvement leading to indurated and thickened skin. The most commonly involved areas are the upper back, shoulders, and back of the neck. The face, chest, abdomen, buttocks, and thighs may also be involved; however, the distal extremities are classically spared. The affected areas are normally asymptomatic, but there can be reduced sensation. Patients with severe longstanding disease may develop a reduced range of motion, most often affecting the trunk. In extreme cases, this can lead to restrictive respiratory problems. The histology of scleredema displays increased collagen and a thickened reticular dermis, with a surrounding mucinous infiltrate.

The pathogenesis of scleredema may involve an interplay between non-enzymatic glycosylation of collagen, increased fibroblast production of collagen, or decreases in collagen breakdown, tissue hypoxia due to microangiopathy [15].

Improved glycemic control may be an important means of prevention. A variety of therapeutic options have been proposed which include immunosuppressants, corticosteroids, intravenous immunoglobulin, electron-beam therapy, and phototherapy. Physical therapy is an important therapeutic modality for patients with limited mobility of joints.

11.1.2.8 Necrobiosis Lipoidica

Necrobiosis lipoidica (NL) is a rare chronic granulomatous dermatologic disease that is seen most frequently in diabetics and has a female predilection. The highest comorbidity rates in patients with NL were patients with type 2 diabetes. NL begins as a single or group of firm well-demarcated erythematous papules which then form plaques characterized by red-brown borders and a firm yellow-brown waxy atrophic center containing telangiectasias. NL occurs bilaterally and exhibits Koebnerization. Lesions are almost always found on the pretibial areas of the lower extremities. Additional involvement of the forearm, scalp, distal upper extremities, thighs, popliteal regions, feet, face, or abdomen may be present on occasion. Often asymptomatic, there may be pruritus and hypoesthesia of affected areas, and pain may be associated with ulceration. Ulceration can be associated with secondary infections and squamous cell carcinoma. The histology of NL primarily involves the dermis and is marked by palisading granulomatous inflammation, necrobiotic collagen, a mixed inflammatory infiltrate, blood vessel wall thickening, and reduced mucin.

The pathogenesis of NL may involve diabetes-related microangiopathy, irregularities in collagen, autoimmune disease, and neutrophil chemotaxis [16, 17].

Corticosteroids are used in the management of active disease topically, intralesionally, or orally. Some other modalities are Calcineurin inhibitors (e.g., cyclosporine), antitumor necrosis factor inhibitors (e.g., infliximab), pentoxifylline, antimalarials (e.g., hydroxychloroquine), PUVA, granulocyte colony-stimulating factor, dipyridamole, and low-dose aspirin, hyperbaric oxygen therapy, fumaric acid esters, pulse dye laser, photodynamic therapy, thalidomide, IVIg. Patients with newly diagnosed NL should be screened for hypertension, hyperlipidemia, and thyroid dysfunction.

11.1.2.9 Bullosis Diabeticorum

Bullosis diabeticorum (BD) is an uncommon eruptive blistering condition that often occurs in long-standing diabetes along with other complications such as neuropathy, nephropathy, and retinopathy. BD is significantly more common in male patients and has an average age of onset between 50 and 70 years of age [18].

BD presents with abrupt onset of one or more nontender, firm, sterile bullae on healthy-appearing skin which increase in size and become more flaccid, ranging in size from about 0.5 to 5 cm. Bullae frequently present bilaterally involving the acral areas of the lower extremities, sometimes upper extremities and trunk. Histology typically shows an intraepidermal or subepidermal blister, spongiosis, no acantholysis, minimal inflammatory infiltrate, and normal immunofluorescence.

Various pathogenetic mechanisms have been proposed like microangiopathy, autoimmune processes, exposure to ultraviolet light, variations in blood glucose, neuropathy [19].

BD resolves without treatment within 2–6 weeks and is therefore managed by avoiding secondary infection and the corresponding sequelae (e.g., necrosis, osteomyelitis).

11.1.3 Nonspecific Dermatologic Signs and Symptoms

11.1.3.1 Ichthyosiform Changes of the Shins

Ichthyosiform changes of the shins or the fish scale-like skin present with bilateral areas of dryness and scaling. Anterior shin is most classically involved., although hands and feet may be involved (Fig. 11.5). These cutaneous changes are related to rapid skin aging, adhesion defects, reduced hydration of the stratum corneum and altered keratinocyte function [20]. The development of ichthyosiform changes of the shins is related to production of advanced glycosylation end products and microangiopathic changes. Topical emollients or keratolytic agents may be beneficial.

11.1.3.2 Xerosis

Xerosis is one of the most common skin presentations in patients with diabetes and has been reported to be present in as many as 40% of patients with diabetes. Pruritus is a common complaint (Fig. 11.6). Affected skin may present with scaling, cracks, or a rough texture, and it may precede eczema and ulceration. Diabetic microangiopathy and autonomic neuropathy are involved in the pathogenesis. To avoid complications such as fissures and secondary infections, xerosis can be managed with emollients and avoiding irritants.

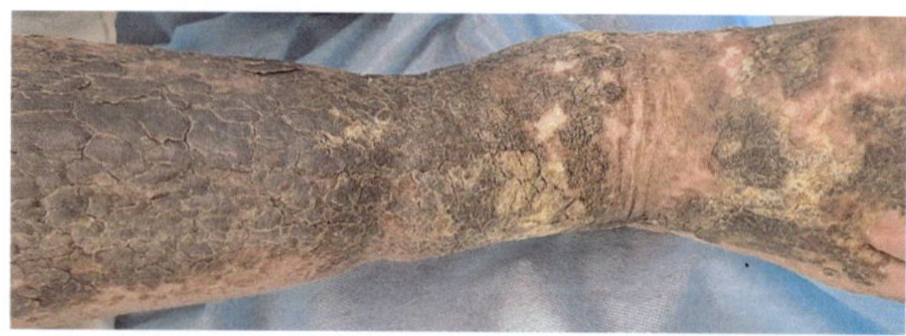

Fig. 11.5 Icthyosiform change

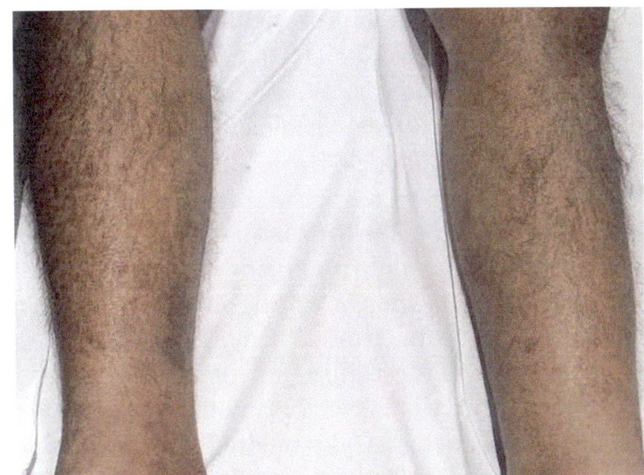

Fig. 11.6 Xerosis of the skin of legs

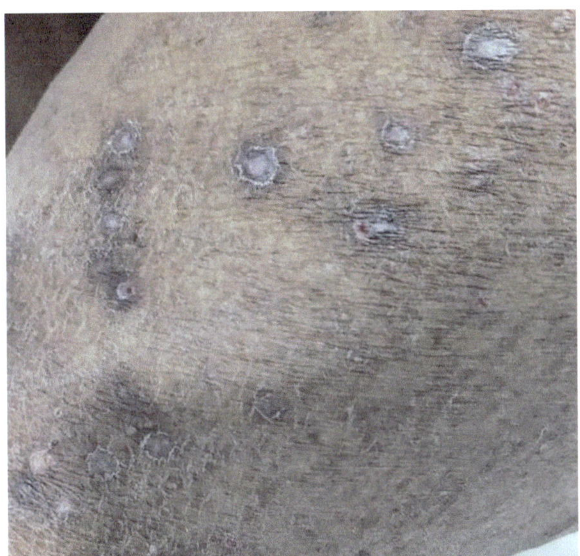

Fig. 11.7 Acquired perforating dermatosis

11.1.3.3 Acquired Perforating Dermatosis

Perforating dermatoses, a disorder of keratinisation, refers to a broad group of chronic skin disorders characterized by a loss of dermal connective tissue. Acquired perforating dermatoses (APD) is classically observed in patients with chronic renal failure or long-standing diabetes [21] (Fig. 11.7).

APD presents as groups of hyperkeratotic umbilicated-nodules and papules with centralized keratin plugs or craters over extensor surfaces of the arms, legs, and trunk. Lesions are extremely pruritic. Histologically, perforating dermatoses are characterized by a lymphocytic infiltrate, an absence or degeneration of dermal connective tissue components (e.g., collagen, elastic fibers), and transepidermal extrusion of keratotic material. The glycosylation of microvasculature or dermal component, metabolic disturbances, or the accumulation of unknown immunogenic substances that are not eliminated by dialysis has been implicated in the pathogenesis [21].

Treatment involves topical emollients, keratolytics, retinoids, and high-potency steroids. Intralesional steroids and cryotherapy help. Systemic therapy with oral antihistamines, retinoids, PUVA, allopurinol, oral antibiotics (doxycycline or clindamycin), and immunomodulating agents such as dupilumab may be effective in treating the condition.

11.1.3.4 Eruptive Xanthomas

It presents as eruptions of clusters of glossy pink-to-yellow papules, ranging in diameter from 1 to 4 mm, overlying an erythematous area. The lesions can be found on extensor surfaces of the extremities, the buttocks, and in areas susceptible to Koebnerization. It is usually asymptomatic but may be pruritic or tender. The histology reveals a mixed inflammatory infiltrate of the dermis which includes triglyceride-containing macrophages, also referred to as foam cells.

In an insulin-deficient state, such as poorly controlled diabetes, there is decreased or altered lipoprotein lipase activity resulting in the accumulation of chylomicrons and other triglyceride-rich lipoproteins which are scavenged by macrophages [22]. These lipid-laden macrophages then collect in the dermis of the skin where they can lead to eruptive xanthomas.

It can be resolved with improved glycemic control and a reduction in serum triglyceride levels.

11.1.3.5 Acrochordons

Acrochordons (also known as soft benign fibromas, fibroepithelial polyps, or skin tags) are benign, soft, pedunculated growths that vary in size and can occur singularly or in groups (Fig. 11.8). The neck, axilla, periorbital area, and intertriginous areas can be affected. It can often act as a marker for impaired glucose tolerance. Patients with acanthosis nigricans may have acrochordons overlying the affected areas of skin. Pathophysiology is attributed to the proliferative effect of increased insulin on skin epidermal cells and fibroblasts [23]. It can be excised for aesthetic reasons or if it is causing any discomfort by radiofrequency or electrocautery.

11.1.3.6 Diabetes-Associated Pruritus

Diabetes can be associated with pruritus, which can be localized or generalized. Pruritus is more likely in patients with diabetes who have xerosis, diabetic peripheral neuropathy, diabetic retinopathy, diabetic chronic kidney disease, and uncontrolled diabetes. Management includes control of dryness, topical capsaicin, antihistamines, gabapentin, or pregabalin.

11.1.3.7 Huntley's Papules (Finger Pebbles)

Huntley's papules, also known as finger pebbles, present as clusters of non-erythematous, asymptomatic, small papules on the dorsal surface of the hand, specifically affecting the metacarpophalangeal joints and periungual areas. These can be associated with hypopigmentation and induration of the skin. Huntley's papules are strongly associated with type 2 diabetes. There is no effective treatment.

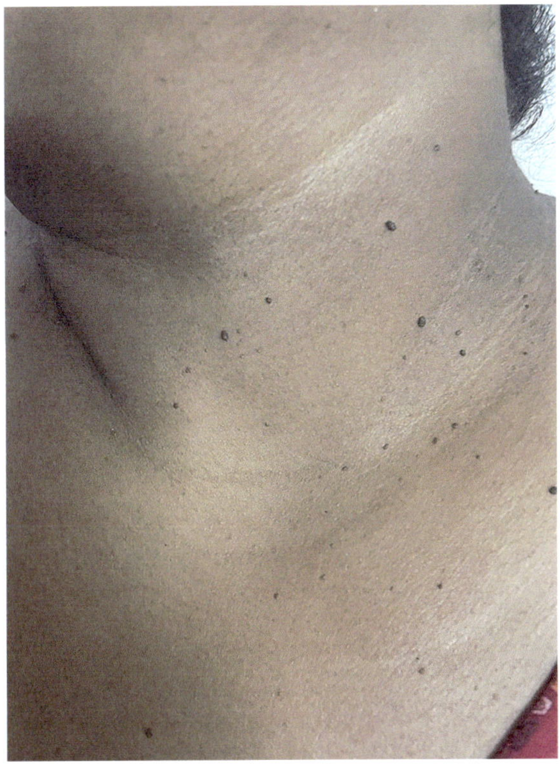

Fig. 11.8 Acrochordons

11.1.3.8 Keratosis Pilaris

Keratosis pilaris is a very common benign keratotic disorder that classically presents with areas of keratotic perifollicular papules with surrounding erythema or hyperpigmentation. The posterior surfaces of the upper arms are often affected but involvement of the thighs, face, and glutei can also be seen. Keratosis pilaris can be treated with various topical therapies, including salicylic acid, glycolic acid, retinoids, and urea-based moisturizers.

11.1.3.9 Pigmented Purpuric Dermatoses

Pigmented purpuric dermatoses (capillaritis) is associated with diabetes, more often in the elderly with cardiac issues and diabetic dermopathy. Brownish macules are seen on the pretibial areas of the legs or the dorsum of the feet. The lesions are usually asymptomatic but may be pruritic. Pigmented purpuric dermatoses occur as a result of microangiopathic damage to capillaries and sequential iron deposition due to erythrocyte breakdown. Prolonged standing aggravates this. Treatment involves strict glycemic control and emollient usage.

11.1.3.10 Palmar Erythema

Palmar erythema is a benign finding that presents with symmetric redness and warmth involving the palms. The erythema is asymptomatic and often most heavily affects the hypothenar and thenar eminences of the palms. The microvascular complications of diabetes are thought to be involved in the pathogenesis of palmar erythema [24].

11.1.3.11 Periungual Telangiectasias

Periungual telangiectasias is an early finding of diabetes. It presents asymptomatically with erythema and telangiectasias surrounding the proximal nail folds along with "ragged" cuticles and fingertip tenderness. The cutaneous findings are due to venous capillary dilatation that occurs secondary to diabetic microangiopathy, altered blood viscosity, increased erythrocyte rigidity, and dysregulation in endothelial cell function.

11.1.3.12 Rubeosis Faciei

Rubeosis faciei is persistent flushed appearance of face and neck in diabetics in which telangiectasias may also be visible. It frequently indicates poor glycemic control and might also indicate the onset of retinopathy. The flushed appearance is thought to occur secondary to small vessel dilation and microangiopathic changes. Retinopathy, neuropathy, and nephropathy are also associated with rubeosis faciei [25]. Adequate glycemic control is essential for treatment.

11.1.3.13 Yellow Skin and Nails

Asymptomatic yellow discolorations of skin or fingernails may involve the palms, soles, face, or the distal nail of the first toe. The accumulation of various substances like carotene, glycosylated proteins in patients with diabetes may be responsible for the colour.

11.1.3.14 Ingrown Toe Nails

This condition is caused by the overgrowth of the nail plate or due to trauma, leading to nail digging into the skin. This can lead to recurrent paronychia infections if left untreated.

11.1.4 Dermatologic Diseases Associated with Diabetes

11.1.4.1 Generalized Granuloma Annulare

It occurs more frequently in women than in men, and in those with type 1 diabetes. GGA initially presents with groups of skin-colored or reddish, firm papules that slowly grow and centrally involute to then form hypo- or hyper-pigmented annular rings with elevated circumferential borders. There are bilaterally symmetrical lesions over trunk and extremities. GGA is normally asymptomatic but can present with pruritus. The histology shows dermal granulomatous inflammation surrounding foci of necrotic collagen and mucin. The pathogenesis of GGA is believed to involve an unknown stimulus that leads to the activation of lymphocytes through a delayed-type hypersensitivity reaction, ultimately initiating a proinflammatory cascade and granuloma formation [26]. Corticosteroids, antimalarials, retinoids,

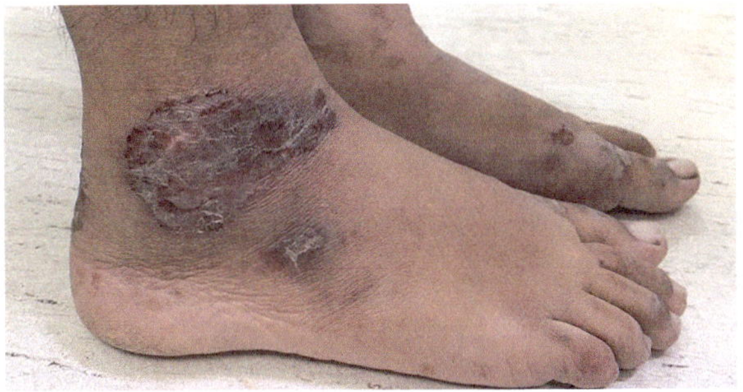
Fig. 11.9 Chronic plaque psoriasis

dapsone, cyclosporine, PUVA, and calcineurin inhibitors have been suggested as various modalities of treatment.

11.1.4.2 Psoriasis

Psoriasis is a chronic immune-mediated inflammatory disorder that may present with a variety of symptoms, including erythematous, indurated, and scaly areas of skin. Psoriasis has a strong association with metabolic syndrome, which increases the likelihood of cardiovascular disease (Fig. 11.9). TNFa is implicated in the pathogenesis of insulin resistance [27]. "Psoriatic march" whereby there is worsening of systemic chronic inflammatory loop may impact DM, obesity, atherosclerosis, thrombosis.

11.1.4.3 Lichen Planus

Lichen planus is a mucocutaneous inflammatory disorder characterized by firm, erythematous, polygonal, pruritic, papules. These papules classically involve the wrists or ankles, although the trunk, back, and thighs can also be affected. Oral LP is more implicated. Defective insulin signaling, impaired carbohydrate and lipid metabolism, autoimmune response, and impaired immune function are implicated in the pathogenesis.

11.1.4.4 Vitiligo

Vitiligo is an acquired autoimmune disorder involving melanocyte destruction. Patients with vitiligo present with scattered well-demarcated areas of depigmentation that can occur anywhere on the body. Its more common in Type 1 DM. Coinciding vitiligo and type 1 diabetes mellitus may be associated with endocrine autoimmune abnormalities of the gastric parietal cells, adrenal, or thyroid and is a result of autoreactive cytotoxic T-cell-mediated destruction.

11.1.4.5 Hidradenitis Suppurativa

Hidradenitis suppurativa (HS) also known as acne inversus is a chronic inflammatory condition (Fig. 11.10). It is characterized by inflamed nodules and abscesses, draining tracts, and fibrotic scars located in intertriginous areas such as the axilla, groin, perianal, perineal, and inframammary areas rich in apocrine glands. These lesions are often painful and malodorous. Increased prevalence of metabolic

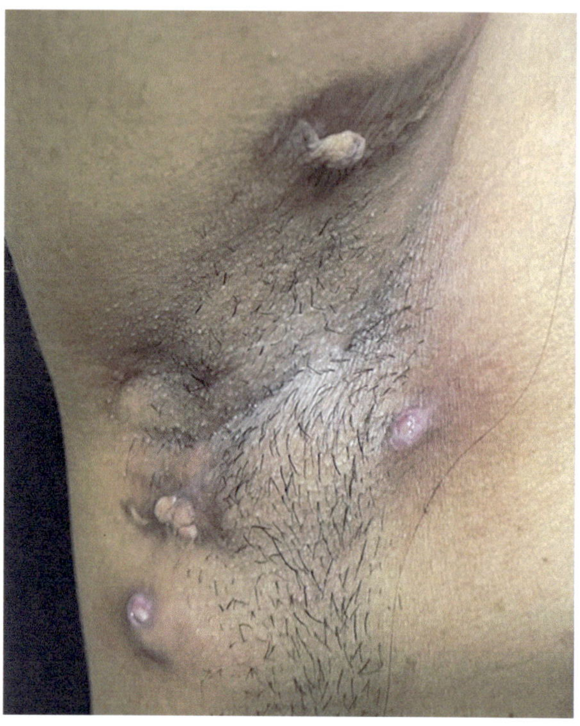

Fig. 11.10 Hidradenitis suppurativa

syndrome (MetS) has been noted in association with HS. It is recommended that patients with HS be screened for insulin resistance (IR). Treatment of HS includes the use of antibiotics, retinoids, antiandrogens, biologicals. Surgical debridement may be necessary at times.

11.1.4.6 Glucagonoma

Glucagonoma is a rare neuroendocrine tumor that most frequently affects patients in their sixth decade of life. Necrolytic migratory erythema (NME) is classically associated with glucagonoma and presents in 70–83% of patients [28, 29]. NME is characterized by erythematous erosive crusted or vesicular eruptions of papules or plaques with irregular borders. The lesions may become bullous or blistered and may be painful or pruritic. The abdomen, groin, genitals, or buttocks are frequently involved, although cheilitis or glossitis may also be present. Biopsy at the edge of the lesion may demonstrate epidermal pallor, necrolytic edema, and a perivascular inflammatory infiltrate.

11.1.4.7 Skin Infections

The prevalence of cutaneous infections in patients with diabetes is about one in every five patients. Compared with the general population, patients with diabetes mellitus are more susceptible to infections and more prone to repeated infections. A variety of factors are believed to be involved in this like angiopathy, neuropathy, hindrance of the anti-oxidant system, abnormalities in leukocyte adherence, chemotaxis, phagocytosis, disruption of the immune system, compromised skin and mucosal barrier as well as, a glucose-rich environment.

11.1.5 Cutaneous Changes Associated with Diabetes Medications

11.1.5.1 Insulin

The most common local adverse effect of subcutaneous injection of insulin is lipohypertrophy, which affects less than 30% of patients with diabetes that use insulin [30, 31]. Lipohypertrophy is characterized by localized regional accumulation of adipocytes separated by fibrous bands which present as soft dermal nodules with lipoma-like consistency. Continued injection of insulin at sites of lipohypertrophy can result in delayed systemic insulin absorption and capricious glycemic control. With avoidance of subcutaneous insulin at affected sites, lipohypertrophy normally improves over the course of a few months.

Furthermore, lipoatrophy is an uncommon cutaneous finding that occurred more frequently prior to the introduction of modern purified forms of insulin. Lipoatrophy presents at insulin injection sites over a period of months with round concave areas of adipose tissue atrophy. It may be caused by the liolytic ingredients of the mixture or an immune complex-mediated inflammatory reaction.

Allergic reactions to the injection of insulin may be idiosyncratic. It may present as life-threatening reactions like DRESS syndrome, TEN, or SJS.

11.1.5.2 Oral Medications

Oral hypoglycemic agents may cause a number of different cutaneous adverse effects. DPP-IV inhibitors, such as vildagliptin, can be associated with inflamed blistering skin lesions, including bullous pemphigoid and Stevens–Johnson syndrome, as well as, angioedema [32, 33]. Allergic skin and photosensitivity reactions may occur with sulfonylureas [34]. The sulfonylureas, chlorpropamide, and tolbutamide are associated with the development of a maculopapular rash during the initial 2 months of treatment; the rash quickly improves with the stoppage of the medication [35]. In certain patients with genetic predispositions, chlorpropamide may also cause acute facial flushing following alcohol consumption [35]. SGLT-2 inhibitors have been associated with an increased risk of genital fungal infections and Fournier's gangrene. Metformin may cause psoriasiform lesions, lichenoid eruptions, leukocytoclastic vasculitis, and erythema multiforme.

11.2 Bacterial

Erysipelas and cellulitis are cutaneous infections that occur frequently in patients with diabetes. Folliculitis is common and is characterized by inflamed, perifollicular, papules, and pustules. Uncomplicated cellulitis and erysipelas are typically treated empirically with oral antibiotics, whereas uncomplicated folliculitis may be managed with topical antibiotics. Colonization with methicillin-resistant Staphylococcus aureus (MRSA) is not uncommon among patients with diabetes.

Infection of the foot is the most common type of soft tissue infection in patients with diabetes. If left unattended can lead to sepsis, amputation, or even death. The areas between the toes and the toenails are also frequently infected in patients with diabetes. Infections can stem from monomicrobial or polymicrobial etiologies. Staphylococcal infections are the most common [36], although complications with infection by *Pseudomonas aeruginosa* are also common [37].

Necrotizing fasciitis is an acute life-threatening infection of the skin and the underlying tissue. Those with poorly controlled diabetes are at an increased risk for necrotizing fasciitis. Necrotizing fasciitis presents early with erythema, induration, and tenderness which may then progress within days to hemorrhagic bullous. Patients will classically present with severe pain out of proportion to their presentation on physical exam. Palpation of the affected area often illicit crepitus. Involvement can occur on any part of the body but most commonly affects the lower extremities. Fournier's gangrene refers to necrotizing fasciitis of the perineum or genitals, often involving the scrotum and spreading rapidly to adjacent tissues. The infection in patients with diabetes is most often polymicrobial. Complications of necrotizing fasciitis include thrombosis, gangrenous necrosis, sepsis, and organ failure. Necrotizing fasciitis has a mortality rate of around 20%. In addition, those patients with diabetes and necrotizing fasciitis are more likely to require amputation during their treatment. It is an emergency and involves extensive surgical debridement and broad-spectrum antibiotics.

Erythrasma is a chronic asymptomatic cutaneous infection, most often attributed to *Corynebacterium minutissiumum.* It presents as clearly demarcated red-brown finely scaled patches or plaques. These lesions are commonly located in intertriginous areas such as the axilla or groin. The presence of coral-red fluorescence under Wood's light can confirm the diagnosis of erythrasma. Treatment options include topical clindamycin and oral erythromycin.

Malignant otitis externa is an infection of external ear caused by Pseudomonas aeruginosa. Patients present with ear pain, ear discharge, difficulty in hearing, swelling, and redness of ear canal. The infection can spread to nearby structures and cause complications such as chondritis, osteomyelitis, meningitis, or cerebritis. Treatment involves long-term systemic antibiotics with appropriate pseudomonal coverage, hyperbaric oxygen, and possibly surgical debridement.

11.3 Fungal

Candidiasis is frequently present in patients with diabetes (type1>type 2) (Fig. 11.11). Its various mucocutaneous presentations include oral candidiasis or thrush by Candida albicans (which presents as red plaques with white adherent exudate and satellite pustules) Vulvovaginitis (Fig. 11.12), Perianal candidiasis, Angular cheilitis, intertrigo including interdigital webspace infection (which may

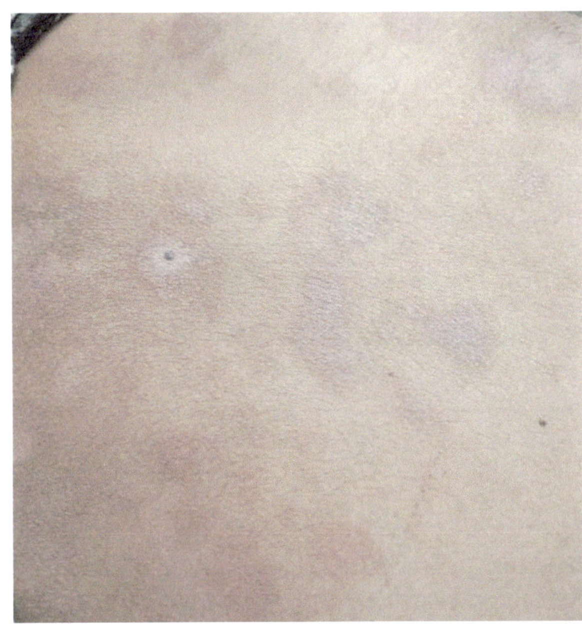

Fig. 11.11 Tinea corporis

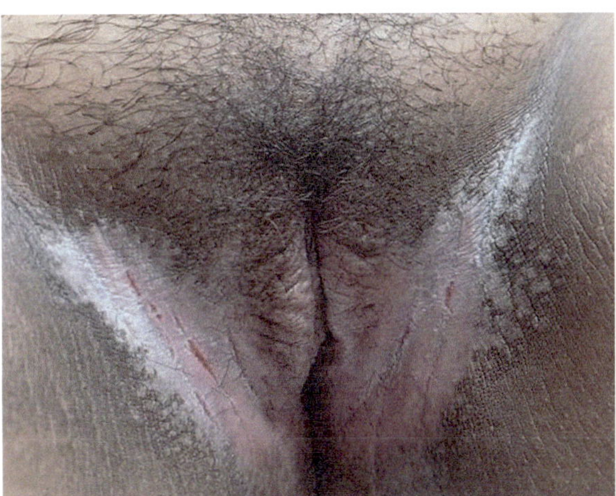

Fig. 11.12 Intertrigo

be pruritic or painful and presents with red macerated, fissured plaques with satellite vesciulopustules).

Paronychia and Onychomycosis—Involvement of the nails may present with periungual inflammation or superficial white spots.

Candidiasis is treated with topical or oral antifungal agents. Patients also benefit from improved glycemic control and by keeping the affected areas dry.

Dermatophytosis or tinea is the superficial infection of skin, hair, and nails caused by most commonly *Trichophyton rubrum*, *T. mentagrophytes*, and *T. tonsurans*. The most common infections seen are tinea corporis, tinea pedis, and tinea unguium. Treatment may include topical or systemic antifungal medications depending on the severity.

Mucormycosis is a serious infection caused by Mucor, Absidia, and Rhizopus species. It is associated with type 1 diabetes mellitus, particularly common in those who develop diabetic ketoacidosis. Mucormycosis should be treated urgently with surgical debridement and intravenous amphotericin B and voriconazole.

11.4 Conclusion

Dermatological manifestations may be the only presenting feature of underlying diabetes. It may be used as a marker for diagnosing DM and monitoring glycemic control. It may serve as a forewarning to the varied complications diabetes may present with. Early detection and prompt management will help to reduce the burden of the disease thereby improving the quality of life. It will also help to reduce microvascular complications and neurological damage.

References

1. Meurer M, Stumvoll M, Szeimies R-M. Hautveränderungen bei Diabetes mellitus. Hautarzt. 2004;55(5):428–35.
2. Labib A, Rosen J, Yosipovitch G. Skin Manifestations of Diabetes Mellitus. [Updated 2022 Apr 21]. In: Feingold KR, Anawalt B, Blackman MR, et al., editors. Endotext [Internet]. South Dartmouth (MA).
3. Stuart CA, Gilkison CR, Smith MM, Bosma AM, Keenan BS, Nagamani M. Acanthosis nigricans as a risk factor for non-insulin dependent diabetes mellitus. Clin Pediatr. 1998;37(2):73–9.
4. Panda S, Das A, Lahiri K, Chatterjee M, Padhi T, Rathi S, et al. Facial acanthosis nigricans: a morphological marker of metabolic syndrome. Indian J Dermatol. 2017;62:591–7.
5. Bustan RS, Wasim D, Yderstræde KB, Bygum A. Specific skin signs as a cutaneous marker of diabetes mellitus and the prediabetic state—a systematic review. Dan Med J. 2017;64(1):A5316.
6. Binkley GW. Dermopathy in the diabetic syndrome. Arch Dermatol. 1965;92(6):625–34.
7. Jeffcoate WJ, Harding KG. Diabetic foot ulcers. Lancet. 2003;361(9368):1545–51.
8. Lobmann R, Schultz G, Lehnert H. Proteases and the diabetic foot syndrome: mechanisms and therapeutic implications. Diabetes Care. 2005;28(2):461–71.
9. Vinik AI, Erbas T. Recognizing and treating diabetic autonomic neuropathy. Cleve Clin J Med. 2001;68(11):928. 30, 32, 34–44
10. Yosipovitch G, Hodak E, Vardi P, et al. The prevalence of cutaneous manifestations in IDDM patients and their association with diabetes risk factors and microvascular complications. Diabetes Care. 1998;21(4):506–9.
11. Brik R, Berant M, Vardi P. The scleroderma-like syndrome of insulin-dependent diabetes mellitus. Diabetes Metab Res Rev. 1991;7(2):121–8.
12. Yosipovitch G, Yosipovitch Z, Karp M, Mukamel M. Trigger finger in young patients with insulin dependent diabetes. J Rheumatol. 1990;17(7):951–2.
13. Kim RP, Edelman SV, Kim DD. Musculoskeletal complications of diabetes mellitus. Clin Diabetes. 2001;19(3):132–5.

14. Fitzgibbons PG, Weiss A-PC. Hand manifestations of diabetes mellitus. J Hand Surg Am. 2008;33(5):771–5.
15. Martin C, Requena L, Manrique K, Manzarbeitia F, Rovira A. Scleredema diabeticorum in a patient with type 2 diabetes mellitus. Case Rep Endocrinol. 2011;2011:560273.
16. Reid SD, Ladizinski B, Lee K, Baibergenova A, Alavi A. Update on necrobiosis lipoidica: a review of etiology, diagnosis, and treatment options. J Am Acad Dermatol. 2013;69(5):783–91.
17. Kota SK, Jammula S, Kota SK, Meher LK, Modi KD. Necrobiosis lipoidica diabeticorum: a case-based review of literature. Indian J Endocrinol Metab. 2012;16(4):614.
18. Larsen K, Jensen T, Karlsmark T, Holstein PE. Incidence of bullosis diabeticorum—a controversial cause of chronic foot ulceration. Int Wound J. 2008;5(4):591–6.
19. Lipsky BA, Baker PD, Ahroni JH. Diabetic bullae: 12 cases of a purportedly rare cutaneous disorder. Int J Dermatol. 2000;39(3):196–200.
20. Patel N, Spencer LA, English JC, Zirwas MJ. Acquired ichthyosis. J Am Acad Dermatol. 2006;55(4):647–56.
21. Saray Y, Seçkin D, Bilezikçi B. Acquired perforating dermatosis: clinicopathological features in twenty-two cases. J Eur Acad Dermatol Venereol. 2006;20(6):679–88.
22. Zaremba J, Zaczkiewicz A, Placek W. Eruptive xanthomas. Adv Dermatol Allergol. 2013;30(6):399.
23. Ahmed I, Goldstein B. Diabetes mellitus. Clin Dermatol. 2006;24:237–46.
24. Serrao R, Zirwas M, English JC. Palmar erythema. Am J Clin Dermatol. 2007;8(6):347–56.
25. Demirseren DD, Emre S, Akoglu G, et al. Relationship between skin diseases and extracutaneous complications of diabetes mellitus: clinical analysis of 750 patients. Am J Clin Dermatol. 2014;15(1):65–70.
26. Cyr PR. Diagnosis and management of granuloma annulare. Am Fam Physician. 2006;74(10):1729.
27. Boehncke WH, Boehncke S, Tobin AM, Kirby B. The 'psoriatic march': a concept of how severe psoriasis may drive cardiovascular comorbidity. Exp Dermatol. 2011;20:303–7.
28. Eldor R, Glaser B, Fraenkel M, Doviner V, Salmon A, Gross DJ. Glucagonoma and the glucagonoma syndrome—cumulative experience with an elusive endocrine tumour. Clin Endocrinol. 2011;74(5):593–8.
29. Wermers RA, Fatourechi V, Wynne AG, Kvols LK, Lloyd RV. The glucagonoma syndrome clinical and pathologic features in 21 patients. Medicine. 1996;75(2):53–63.
30. Richardson T, Kerr D. Skin-related complications of insulin therapy. Am J Clin Dermatol. 2003;4(10):661–7.
31. Lima AL, Illing T, Schliemann S, Elsner P. Cutaneous manifestations of diabetes mellitus: a review. Am J Clin Dermatol. 2017;18:1–13.
32. Attaway A, Mersfelder TL, Vaishnav S, Baker JK. Bullous pemphigoid associated with dipeptidyl peptidase IV inhibitors. A case report and review of literature. J Dermatol Case Rep. 2014;8(1):24.
33. Byrd JS, Minor DS, Elsayed R, Marshall GD. DPP-4 inhibitors and angioedema: a cause for concern? Ann Allergy Asthma Immunol. 2011;106(5):436–8.
34. Hitselberger JF, Fosnaugh RP. Photosensitivity due to chlorpropamide. JAMA. 1962;180(1):62–3.
35. Walker G, Slater J, Westlake E, Nabarro J. Clinical experience with tolbutamide. Br Med J. 1957;2(5040):323.
36. Casqueiro J, Casqueiro J, Alves C. Infections in patients with diabetes mellitus: a review of pathogenesis. Indian J Endocrinol Metab. 2012;16(Suppl 1):S27.
37. Driscoll JA, Brody SL, Kollef MH. The epidemiology, pathogenesis and treatment of Pseudomonas aeruginosa infections. Drugs. 2007;67(3):351–68.

12 Neurological Complications and Management in Diabetes Mellitus

Sreenivas Meenakshisundaram
and Cherin Josi Champannoor

12.1 Introduction

Diabetes mellitus is a disorder of chronic hyperglycemia that can affect all components of the nervous system—both central and peripheral. The involvement of the nervous system can be in myriad ways and can in fact be the initial presenting symptom of diabetes mellitus. Here we look at some of the different presentations of diabetic involvement in the nervous system.

Diabetes can cause involvement of the neurological system both in the short and long term.

Acute neurological manifestations in diabetes mellitus include:

12.1.1 Hyperosmolar Coma

Hyperosmolar non-ketotic coma (HONK), is a condition seen in older individuals with type 2 diabetes. Extreme hyperglycemia (40–80 mmol/L) is seen, along with hypernatremia, and this combines to produce a state of very high osmolarity. Patients can have varying levels of consciousness, with higher blood sugars being associated with poorer consciousness levels. Seizures can occur, which can be either focal or generalised. A specific type of focal epilepsy to look for is occipital lobe seizures with visual hallucinations. Epileptic nystagmus has also been reported in hyperglycemia. Abnormal dystonic movements can rarely be seen as well. The neurological findings are reversible usually and improve with correction of blood glucose and the osmolarity [1].

S. Meenakshisundaram (✉) · C. J. Champannoor
MGM Healthcare, Chennai, Tamil Nadu, India

G. Abraham et al. (eds.), *Management of Diabetic Complications*,
https://doi.org/10.1007/978-981-97-6406-8_12

12.1.2 Diabetic Ketoacidosis

This is a complication seen in people with type 1 diabetes mellitus, who are poorly controlled. This can even be the presenting symptom of diabetes mellitus. The predominant neurological symptom is altered sensorium and disorientation. This is reversible with the correction of the metabolic derangements [2].

12.1.3 Hypoglycaemia

Hypoglycaemia is a common problem encountered in patients with diabetes mellitus, on treatment, especially with insulin. Hypoglycaemia usually becomes symptomatic when the blood sugar levels drop below 3 mmol/L. The early warning signs of hypoglycaemia such as excessive sweating and palpitation can be absent if there is autonomic neuropathy as well. Neuroglycopenia can present across a spectrum, depending on the duration and severity of the hypoglycaemia. This can range from mild cognitive impairment and dysarthria to seizures and hemiplegia and even death [3].

12.1.4 Hyperglycaemic Chorea

Hyperkinetic movement disorders are not uncommon presentations of uncontrolled hyperglycaemia. Patients can present with unilateral symptoms more commonly than bilateral, which is unusual given that metabolic disorders present with bilateral symptoms. The movement disorders are usually choreiform, but they can range from athetosis to severe ballismus. The symptoms are usually reversible with correction of the hyperglycaemia, but resolution can be delayed in some cases. Occasionally the movement disorder may become permanent. This depends on the duration of hyperglycaemia before treatment is initiated. MRI imaging during the episode can reveal hyper intensities in the putamen, called ‘diabetic striatopathy’. These changes are usually reversible [4].

With long-standing diabetes, there are multiple neurological presentations that can be seen.

The different systems which can be affected include:

1. Peripheral neuromuscular system
2. Cortical function
3. Extrapyramidal system
4. Cerebrovascular system

12.2 Neuropathy in Diabetes

Neuromuscular disease is one of the most common types of neurological involvement in diabetes [5–7]. There are various types of neuropathy that can occur in diabetes. The common patterns of neuropathy seen in diabetes are:

1. Distal symmetric peripheral neuropathy
2. Asymmetric radiculoplexopathy
3. Mononeuropathy
4. Autonomic neuropathy

12.3 Distal Symmetric Peripheral Neuropathy

This is the most common type of neuropathy in diabetes. The condition presents initially as sensory symptoms. The pattern of involvement is called 'stocking and glove'. The feet are first to be involved, followed by proximal spread. The hands get involved, when the symptoms have spread up to mid-thigh in the lower limbs, causing the characteristic stocking and glove pattern. Initial sensory symptoms can be painful paresthesias or loss of sensation. This can progress over time to cause mild distal motor weakness as well. Examination can reveal absent distal deep tendon reflexes and minimal objective sensory loss distally, which is usually symmetrical. Posterior column sensations are usually involved later on, although it could be an early manifestation, leading to sensory ataxia. Pain is a common symptom, with a much higher likelihood to present if the patient has poor glycemic control, impaired renal function, or high BMI. The pain may be described as sharp, stabbing, burning, or aching in character. Painful symptoms can improve over time, with dying away of the distal neurone. Investigation with nerve conduction studies can be normal early in the presentation, even if symptomatic. Later, axonal sensorimotor neuropathy, which is diffuse and symmetrical, can be seen. Management is usually by diabetic control and nutritional support. Symptomatic management of pain and paresthesias has multiple options such as pregabalin, gabapentin, duloxetine, tricyclic antidepressants, SSRIs, etc. Severe pain might necessitate use of opioids and local pain medications such as lignocaine jelly [5–7].

12.4 Asymmetric Radiculoplexopathy

Diabetes can produce a characteristic pattern of involvement, in the form of monophasic, asymmetric, proximal weakness, associated with pain. This syndrome is known by various names such as diabetic amyotrophy, diabetic lumbosacral radiculoplexus neuropathy (DLRPN), Bruns Garland syndrome, etc. The clinical presentation can be acute or subacute in onset, with the possibility to progress to severe paraplegia. There is early proximal muscle atrophy in the lower limb, which is grossly asymmetric and associated with significant weight loss. Diabetic amyotrophy can present early in the course of the disease. Risk factors include rapid correction of hyperglycaemia. A close differential remains lumbar radiculopathy. This can be ruled out by MRI imaging of the lumbar spine. Imaging also reveals T2 hyperintensity in the lumbosacral plexus. Nerve conduction studies can show reduced amplitude of sensory and motor action potentials. CSF analysis may reveal raised protein levels and pleocytosis, which might suggest inflammation. In view of this, it has become common practice to attempt pulse steroids to look for improvement or arresting the symptom progression. Severe cases have warranted use of stronger immunosuppressive therapy such as immunoglobulins or plasma exchange. The evidence for the same is limited at the moment. Pain management with SSRIs, TCAs, anticonvulsants, NSAIDs, and opioids is also suggested based on symptoms. Another differential with inflammatory components, which can respond to immunomodulation, is a variant of chronic immune demyelinating polyradiculoneuopathy. The Nerve conduction studies might show demyelinating changes in these patients, aiding in decision-making regarding long-term immunosuppression [6–8].

12.5 Mononeuropathies

Involvement of a single nerve is less common compared to distal symmetric peripheral neuropathy or autonomic neuropathy. There can be involvement of either cranial or peripheral nerves.

Cranial neuropathy is the most common form of mononeuropathy in diabetes. The cranial nerves commonly affected include:

1. *Oculomotor nerve*—This is the most commonly affected cranial nerve in diabetes. The presentation is with double vision, preceded by unilateral pain around and above the eye. The characteristic finding of oculomotor palsy in diabetes is the sparing of the pupils. This is thought to be due to the peripheral location of the autonomic fibres in the oculomotor nerve bundle, protecting it from ischemia, which usually starts in the centre. Most patients recover spontaneously within 3 months, although some centres use anti-platelets due to the presumed thrombosis of the vasa nervosum.
2. *Abducens and Trochlear Nerve*—These are the next most commonly affected cranial nerves. The clinical presentation is with diplopia, classically horizontal when the abducens nerve is involved and vertical when the trochlear nerve is involved. There is much less chances of pain compared to oculomotor nerve involvement. Recovery usually occurs by 12 weeks. However due to the myriad other causes of involvement of these nerves, it is imperative to investigate thoroughly. Diabetic cranial nerve involvement becomes a diagnosis of exclusion.
3. *Facial Nerve*—There is a higher incidence of Bell's palsy in diabetics. There is a typical lower motor neurone type of involvement of the facial nerve, with preserved taste sensation, indicating involvement of the nerve distal to the origin of the chorda tympani.

Diabetic radiculopathy is a specific type of mononeuropathy that involved the nerve roots in the thoracic and abdominal region. The patients present with unilateral severe pain in the thorax or abdomen, which is worse at night, distributed along single or multiple dermatomes and does not cross the midline. Management is symptomatic and anti-platelets may be used. The pain usually resolves in 6–12 weeks.

Pressure sensitive or entrapment neuropathies are mono neuropathies that can occur at any of the peripheral nerves in the extremities. They are brought about due to pressure on the nerve causing impaired conduction and producing sensory and motor symptoms in the distribution. Nerve conduction studies usually show a conduction block, especially when tested across the proposed site of pressure. Diabetes makes nerves more susceptible to pressure palsy. This occurs due to damage to the myelin. In addition, glycosylation of collagen makes it stiffer and less elastic, increasing pressure on underlying nerve. Some of the common entrapment neuropathies are:

1. *Carpal tunnel syndrome*—This is the most common type of compression neuropathy. It is due to compression of the median nerve within the carpal tunnel, between the carpal bones and transverse ligaments. The symptoms are usually tingling and pain over the lateral part of the hand and the lateral 2–3 fingers. The symptoms seem to worsen at night and are relieved by dangling the hand. If untreated for a long time, there can be weakness and wasting of the muscles of the thenar eminence. Tapping over the median nerve can produce tingling, known as the 'Tinel sign'. The diagnosis is confirmed by electrophysiological studies which show a possible conduction block, especially with comparison studies with the ulnar nerve, across the wrist. Ultrasound of the wrist can also show proximal thickening of the nerve, suggesting a compression. Management is symptomatic and with proper positioning of the wrist. If symptoms are progressive or intolerable, surgical decompression might be needed.
2. *Ulnar entrapment neuropathy*—The ulnar nerve is highly susceptible to compression at the elbow in the pisohamate tunnel. Ulnar neuropathy presents with paresthesia, tingling, and numbness over medial 1/3rd of the hand, along with weakness of the medial 2 fingers. Clawing of the fingers is a characteristic finding in ulnar nerve damage. The diagnosis can be confirmed by nerve conduction testing across the elbow, which can show conduction blocks. If the weakness or muscle wasting is severe, surgical decompression may be beneficial.
3. *Peroneal entrapment neuropathy*—This is a common cause of foot drop in diabetics. The common peroneal nerve is compressed at the level of the neck of the fibula. Pain, paresthesia, and numbness occur over the dorsum of the foot. Diagnosis can be confirmed by nerve conduction testing showing a conduction block across the neck of fibula. There is spontaneous resolution in 6–12 weeks.
4. *Femoral cutaneous nerve compression*—The femoral cutaneous nerve is compressed below the inguinal ligament. The clinical symptoms include pain, paresthesia, and numbness in the anterolateral part of the thigh, leading to the syndrome called 'Meralgia paresthetica'. Management is symptomatic for

paresthesias. There is spontaneous resolution within 12 weeks. Surgical decompression is rarely needed [5–7].

12.6 Autonomic Neuropathy

Autonomic nervous system involvement is a common complication in diabetes mellitus and is usually under recognised and under reported. The thinly myelinated and unmyelinated nerve fibres are the components of the autonomic nervous system and can affected by chronic hyperglycaemia. This can be selective or a co-involvement with other types of neuropathy, especially DSPN. Autonomic neuropathy can be silent initially and may become manifest only when end-organ damage occurs as a result of this. The symptoms can be non-specific but highly disagreeable and disabling. A high degree of suspicion is necessary to detect autonomic neuropathy early.

The different organs involved with autonomic neuropathy are:

12.6.1 Cardiovascular

The cardiovascular involvement is common and manifests as orthostatic hypotension and neurogenic peripheral edema. Loss of peripheral vasoconstriction and splanchnic pooling are some of the proposed mechanisms underlying these manifestations. The symptoms are usually non-specific fatigue and dizziness, with some pain, especially around the neck and shoulders (coat hanger pain), although in severe cases it can present as blacking out and syncope on standing. Unexplained tachycardia can also be seen at times. Symptoms are usually worse when getting out of bed in the morning and fluctuate through the day, although they can get better with continuing mobility. Symptom severity does not correlate with degree of fall in systolic blood pressure on standing. Diagnosis of orthostatic hypotension can be done bedside by looking for lying and standing blood pressure. Definite diagnosis is made if there is a drop in systolic BP of >30 mmHg. Symptomatic management is made by optimising medications and avoiding drugs causing fluid loss or drop in BP. Raising the head end in bed and use of elastic stockings and abdominal binders are other options. In resistant patients, medications to help with OH, such as fludrocortisone and midodrine, can be used. However, caution should be exercised with these medications, since they have the potential to cause supine hypertension, which can lead to even hypertensive emergencies. Ephedrine has been found to be useful to relieve neurogenic peripheral edema. In the long term, orthostatic hypotension has been linked to higher rates of morbidity and mortality in diabetics. They are correlated with a higher degree of cardiovascular mortality.

12.6.2 Sudomotor

Sudomotor involvement refers to involvement of the fibres innervating the sweat glands and subcutaneous vessels. This can lead to loss of sweating, dryness of skin, and occasionally dry mouth as well. In advanced cases, there can be abnormal reinnervation leading to development of symptoms such as gustatory sweating, which is felt to be highly characteristic of diabetic autonomic neuropathy. Confirmation of sudomotor involvement can be made by electrophysiological testing such as QSART and thermoregulatory sweat testing. Treatment may be required in cases of gustatory sweating. Anticholinergics, either orally or locally, have been found to be highly effective. In certain refractory cases, botulinum toxin over the area of sweating might be an option.

12.6.3 Genitourinary

Impotence and neurogenic bladder are the features of genitourinary involvement due to autonomic neuropathy.

1. Neurogenic bladder is usually symptomatic only when involvement is severe. The findings are due to damage to innervation of the detrusor muscle. Afferent denervation leads to loss of sensation of bladder filling. Efferent denervation leads to impaired detrusor activity and leads to impaired sphincter opening and bladder emptying. The clinical symptoms include hesitancy, straining to void, feeble stream, and dribbling. Occasionally the patient can present with distended bladder and overflow incontinence. With patients with troublesome symptoms, they should be encouraged to voluntarily void every 3 h. In advanced disease, patients may require intermittent self-catheterisation.
2. Impotence is due to both sympathetic and parasympathetic denervation of the vasa vasorum supplying the dorsal penile artery. It is usually gradual in onset and progressive, leading to complete impotence 2 years after onset. This contrasts with psychogenic impotence which is sudden and total at onset, with nocturnal tumescence. Potential treatment options include intracavernous prostaglandin E, condom vacuum pump, etc. Sildenafil can be useful occasionally.

12.6.4 Gastrointestinal

1. Gastroparesis is the most common manifestation of autonomic denervation of the GI system. There is reduced motility and delayed gastric motility, leading to fullness, bloating, and early satiety. In severe cases, there can be vomiting, which is usually intermittent and rarely requires surgical intervention. Clinical evaluation can reveal a gastric splash and radiological evaluation reveals large food particles and residual gastric filling. Dopamine antagonists can alleviate some of the symptoms, especially vomiting. In patients with persistent and intolerable

vomiting, gastrectomy with Roux-en-Y loop anastomosis has been found to be beneficial.

2. At the other end of the spectrum is diabetic diarrhoea, where patients suffer from borborygmi and discomfort, followed by watery diarrhoea. Nocturnal fecal incontinence is a common problem in severe cases. Symptoms can be intermittent, lasting hours to days. Intestinal bacterial overgrowth has been postulated as one of the mechanisms of this phenomenon. Tetracycline 500 mg at the onset of an attack has been found to be a good abortive. Other medications used include codeine, loperamide, and clonidine. Somatostatin analogues have antisecretory effect and have been proposed to be effective, though definite data is still not available [5–7].

12.6.5 Management of Diabetic Neuropathy

The management of diabetic neuropathy depends on the type and presenting symptoms. The major point to note is that most diabetic neuropathy is not reversible and the deficit which occurs can be permanent. Treatment is aimed at symptom management and improving the quality of life of the patient Table 12.1.

Some general principles of management include:

- Multidisciplinary care is necessary to address different facets of neuropathy
- Supplementation with nutraceuticals might delay progression
- Most medications are targeted at managing pain

The medications approved for use in painful diabetic neuropathy include antidepressants, anticonvulsants, opioids, and similar substances. The choice of drug is highly individual and depends on physician preference. There is a lot of variability among guidelines for the same as well:

Table 12.1 Patterns of nerve involvement in diabetes mellitus

Pattern	Structures involved	Symptoms
Distal symmetric peripheral neuropathy	Small myelinated, unmyelinated, and large myelinated nerves fibres, in a length-dependent pattern	Pain, paresthesia, sensory loss, ataxia, distal weakness
Radiculoplexopathy	Lumbosacral plexus	Proximal weakness with pain and muscle wasting
Mononeuropathies	Single/multiple peripheral nerves	Sensory loss and weakness in a nerve distribution, footdrop/wrist drop
Autonomic neuropathy	Small unmyelinated fibres	Orthostatic hypotension, neurogenic bladder, gastroparesis

- AAN recommends pregabalin as Level A, followed by venlafaxine, duloxetine, gabapentin, opioids, amitryptiline, valproate, and topical capsaicin as Level B.
- Mayo Clinic recommends duloxetine, oxycodone, pregabalin, and TCAs as the first tier, and gabapentin, lamotrigine, tramadol, and venlafaxine as the second tier, along with topical capsaicin and lignocaine.
- NICE guidelines recommend duloxetine as the first line, followed by amitryptiline and pregabalin as second line.
- FDA has approved only duloxetine, pregabalin, and tapentadol for management of painful diabetic neuropathy.

Recent evidence has emerged regarding the role of nutraceuticals in relieving neuropathic pain in patients with small fibre neuropathy. The agents that have shown benefit include agamatine and palmitoylethanolamide, which have both shown improvement in pain scores and quality of life indices. These are being offered as an adjunct or alternative to the commonly used medications for neuropathic pain.

In distal peripheral neuropathy, one of the most important complications to note is the development of non-healing ulcers and Charcot's joints. This can be addressed by combined efforts of the diabetologist, neurologist, vascular surgeons, podiatrist, and orthotist by providing proper orthotics. Avoiding injury to the foot is paramount in these conditions.

Diabetic lumbar radiculoplexoneuropathy can be partially reversible and treatment with early immunosuppression has shown some benefit, although long-term outcomes might not change.

In entrapment neuropathies, relieving the compression can lead to the reversal of symptoms, unless the damage has been long standing and permanent.

Patients with autonomic neuropathy need to be careful about the high-risk complication of orthostatic syncope. This can be prevented by supportive measures such as increased fluid and salt intake, optimising medications to avoid hypotension, and getting up in a delayed manner. Crossing legs before standing is another compensatory manoeuver to relieve the symptoms. In severe cases, compression stockings or abdominal binders might be required. When such measures are not helpful, patient might require pharmacological intervention in the form of steroids or midodrine, to increase the blood pressure. However, the treating doctor needs to be aware of the risk of supine hypertension with these medications [9–12].

12.7 Diabetes and Cerebrovascular Disease

Diabetes mellitus is one of the recognised risk factors for cerebrovascular disease. Some studies have revealed a 13-fold increase of stroke in women with diabetes and a six-fold increase in men with diabetes. The most common type of stroke is lacunar, with the posterior circulation affected more commonly than the anterior. Specifically, the paramedian perforating branches of the basilar are involved, leading to the development of multiple named brainstem stroke syndromes. Thromboembolic strokes also occur, due to an increased rate of atherosclerosis of the internal carotid artery. The risk of stroke in diabetics increases due to concomitant hypertension. There has been no clear correlation between glycemic control and incidence of stroke. There is not enough evidence to propose prophylactic antiplatelet therapy in diabetics [13].

12.8 Infections of the Nervous System in Diabetes

Diabetes increases the risk of infections generally, due to compromised phagocytic function. There are two infections that are characteristic of diabetes:

1. *Rhinocereberal mucormycosis:* This is an airborne fungus found in decaying plant matter. It can invade the nasal mucosa in patients with uncontrolled diabetes and diabetic ketoacidosis. This leads to development of fungal sinusitis and invasion of the nearby neural structures in the orbit and the cavernous sinus. If untreated, this can spread to cause headaches, double vision due to involvement of cranial nerves 3,4,6, blurring of vision, and complete blindness due to optic nerve involvement in severe cases. Occasionally, it has been reported to cause the base of skull osteomyelitis, where it can affect other cranial nerves as well and can spread intracranially, causing dural venous sinus thrombosis and can be potentially fatal. Diagnosis is by endoscopy and biopsy of the paranasal sinuses. This needs aggressive treatment with debridement and antifungals such as amphotericin B. This condition is endemic in south India and there has been a sharp uptick in cases post the COVID pandemic. Early recognition and treatment can be vision and life saving in many patients [14, 15].
2. *Malignant otitis externa:* This is caused by *Pseudomonas aeruginosa* and follows procedures of the external ear such as syringing. It occurs mainly in patients with uncontrolled hyperglycaemia. This can spread and cause mastoiditis and intracranial extension in the form of meningitis, dural venous sinus thrombosis, and multiple cranial nerve palsy. This can be potentially fatal if untreated. Treatment is with antibiotics and occasionally surgical intervention for debridement [16].

Apart from these presentations, diabetes mellitus can be a part of specific genetic and acquired syndromes which can affect the neurological system as well. Here diabetes is an association, rather than a causation for the neurology. Some of the prominent such syndromes are:

12.8.1 Friedrich's Ataxia

Friedrich's ataxia is an autosomal recessive spinocerebellar ataxia, caused by a GAA repeat expansion on chromosome 9q, resulting in defective frataxin. The neurological presentation is cerebellar ataxia, with depressed distal deep tendon reflexes and evidence of some peripheral neuropathy, especially in the lower limbs. Diabetes mellitus is seen in 10–20% of patients with Friedrich's ataxia. The onset of the diabetes is always after the onset of the neurology and is usually insulin dependent [17].

12.8.2 Wolfram Syndrome

Wolfram syndrome is an autosomal recessive inherited syndrome, with predominant endocrinological abnormalities and associated neurology. The exact gene is not known, although it is known to be linked to chromosome 4. This is also known as the DIDMOAD syndrome, which stands for diabetes insipidus, diabetes mellitus, optic atrophy and deafness. Neurological involvement can also be in the form of cerebellar ataxia, psychiatric disturbances, anosmia, apnea, and excessive startle reflex [18].

12.8.3 Mitochondrial Disorders

Disorders affecting the energy production process in the mitochondria can lead to development of neurological involvement in the form of sensorineural deafness and multiaxial involvement including the cortex, cerebellum, muscle, and nerve. These disorders are maternally inherited. Diabetes mellitus has been found to be associated with a number of these conditions, including MIDD, MELAS, and Kearns Sayre syndrome. Diabetes onset is usually in the fourth to fifth decade and can present as insulin-dependent disease. Diabetic ketoacidosis has been reported in a few patients as well [19].

12.8.4 Stiff Person Spectrum Disorders

Stiff person spectrum disorders are a group of conditions where the patient presents with dynamic increased tone in skeletal muscles, especially in the paraspinal groups. The patient typically presents with back pain, stiffness, and difficulty walking and bending forward. An autoimmune aetiology has been hypothesised, and there is a high association with Anti-GAD antibodies. This antibody is also associated with autoimmune diabetes mellitus and the presence of Anti-GAD antibodies in a patient with Stiff Person Syndrome increases the risk of diabetes [20].

12.9 Conclusion

Diabetes mellitus can affect many of the components of the nervous system and can present in myriad fashion. The knowledge of the different types of presentation allows the clinician to recognise early nervous system involvement and initiate appropriate management measures, which in turn will lead to an improved quality of life for the patient.

References

1. Pasquel FJ, Umpierrez GE. Hyperosmolar hyperglycemic state: a historic review of the clinical presentation, diagnosis, and treatment. Diabetes Care. 2014;37(11):3124–31.
2. Lizzo JM, Goyal A, Gupta V. Adult diabetic ketoacidosis. In: StatPearls. Treasure Island, FL: StatPearls Publishing; 2023 [cited 2023 Nov 3]. http://www.ncbi.nlm.nih.gov/books/NBK560723/.
3. Scheen AJ. [Diagnosis and assessment of hypoglycemia in patients with diabetes mellitus]. Rev Med Liege. 2014;69(2):110–5.
4. Chua CB, Sun CK, Hsu CW, Tai YC, Liang CY, Tsai IT. "Diabetic striatopathy": clinical presentations, controversy, pathogenesis, treatments, and outcomes. Sci Rep. 2020;10:1594.
5. Watkins PJ, Thomas PK. Diabetes mellitus and the nervous system. J Neurol Neurosurg Psychiatry. 1998;65(5):620–32. Association of stiff-person syndrome with autoimmune endocrine diseases—PubMed. [cited 2023 Oct 11]. https://pubmed.ncbi.nlm.nih.gov/31624742/.
6. Charnogursky GA, Emanuele NV, Emanuele MA. Neurologic complications of diabetes. Curr Neurol Neurosci Rep. 2014;14(7):457.
7. Feldman EL, Callaghan BC, Pop-Busui R, Zochodne DW, Wright DE, Bennett DL, et al. Diabetic neuropathy. Nat Rev Dis Primers. 2019;5(1):1–18.
8. Diaz LA, Gupta V. Diabetic amyotrophy. In: StatPearls. StatPearls Publishing; 2023 [cited 2023 Oct 12]. https://www.ncbi.nlm.nih.gov/books/NBK560491/.
9. Brocco E, Ninkovic S, Marin M, Whisstock C, Bruseghin M, Boschetti G, et al. Diabetic foot management: multidisciplinary approach for advanced lesion rescue. J Cardiovasc Surg. 2018;59(5):670–84.
10. Cohen K, Shinkazh N, Frank J, Israel I, Fellner C. Pharmacological treatment of diabetic peripheral neuropathy. P T. 2015;40(6):372–88.
11. Rosenberg ML, Tohidi V, Sherwood K, Gayen S, Medel R, Gilad GM. Evidence for dietary agmatine sulfate effectiveness in neuropathies associated with painful small fiber neuropathy. A pilot open-label consecutive case series study. Nutrients. 2020;12(2):576.
12. Schifilliti C, Cucinotta L, Fedele V, Ingegnosi C, Luca S, Leotta C. Micronized palmitoylethanolamide reduces the symptoms of neuropathic pain in diabetic patients. Pain Res Treat. 2014;2014:849623.
13. Chen R, Ovbiagele B, Feng W. Diabetes and stroke: epidemiology, pathophysiology, pharmaceuticals and outcomes. Am J Med Sci. 2016;351(4):380–6.
14. Singh V, Singh M, Joshi C, Sangwan J. Rhinocerebral mucormycosis in a patient with type 1 diabetes presenting as toothache: a case report from Himalayan region of India. BMJ Case Rep. 2013;2013:bcr2013200811.
15. Rhinocerebral mucormycosis in a patient with type 1 diabetes presenting as toothache: a case report from Himalayan region of India. BMJ Case Rep. [cited 2023 Oct 16]. https://casereports.bmj.com/content/2013/bcr-2013-200811#.
16. Yang TH, Xirasagar S, Cheng YF, Wu CS, Kao YW, Shia BC, et al. Malignant otitis externa is associated with diabetes: a population-based case-control study. Ann Otol Rhinol Laryngol. 2020;129(6):585–90.
17. Reetz K, Dogan I, Hohenfeld C, Didszun C, Giunti P, Mariotti C, et al. Nonataxia symptoms in Friedreich Ataxia: report from the Registry of the European Friedreich's Ataxia Consortium for Translational Studies (EFACTS). Neurology. 2018;91(10):e917–30.
18. Urano F. Wolfram syndrome: diagnosis, management, and treatment. Curr Diab Rep. 2016;16(1):6.
19. Karaa A, Goldstein A. The spectrum of clinical presentation, diagnosis, and management of mitochondrial forms of diabetes. Pediatr Diabetes. 2015;16(1):1–9.
20. Association of stiff-person syndrome with autoimmune endocrine diseases—PubMed. [cited 2023 Oct 11]. https://pubmed.ncbi.nlm.nih.gov/31624742/.

13 Comprehensive Care for Women with Diabetes Mellitus and Gynecological Complications

Pallavi Khanna and Maithrayie Kumaresan

13.1 Introduction

13.1.1 Significance of Managing Obstetrical and Gynecological Issues in Diabetes Patients

Diabetes mellitus, a chronic metabolic disorder characterized by high blood glucose levels, affects millions of women worldwide. Among its various complications, the management of obstetrical and gynecological issues in diabetes patients holds paramount importance. Diabetes confers a substantial risk to women's reproductive health, encompassing not only preconception, pregnancy, and childbirth but also a broader spectrum of gynecological conditions [1]. With the global diabetes epidemic showing no signs of abating, the significance of addressing these issues has become increasingly pressing.

To underscore this significance, epidemiological evidence consistently reveals a heightened prevalence of obstetrical complications, such as preeclampsia, gestational diabetes, preterm birth, and congenital anomalies, in women with diabetes [2]. Moreover, gynecological concerns like polycystic ovary syndrome (PCOS) and recurrent urinary tract infections are disproportionately prevalent in this population [3]. Unmanaged diabetes during pregnancy can also lead to long-term consequences for both the mother and her offspring, including an increased risk of type 2 diabetes in the child [1].

P. Khanna (✉)
Obstetrics and Gynecology, College of Medicine, University of Tennessee Health Science Center, Memphis, TN, USA
e-mail: pkhanna1@uthsc.edu

M. Kumaresan
Royal Free Hospital, London, UK

G. Abraham et al. (eds.), *Management of Diabetic Complications*,
https://doi.org/10.1007/978-981-97-6406-8_13

13.1.2 Scope and Objectives of the Chapter

This chapter aims to provide a comprehensive overview of the scope and objectives related to managing obstetrical and gynecological issues in diabetes patients. Specifically, we will delve into the latest research, guidelines, and clinical practices relevant to diabetes and women's health. The chapter's primary objectives include:

1. Highlighting the epidemiological landscape of diabetes in women and the associated obstetrical and gynecological complications.
2. Presenting the latest insights on preconception care, prenatal management, and postpartum care for diabetic women.
3. Discussing the impact of diabetes on common gynecological conditions and exploring tailored management strategies.
4. Offering U.S.-specific evidence-based recommendations for healthcare providers, emphasizing the importance of a multidisciplinary approach to provide holistic care.

13.1.3 Overview of Diabetes and Its Impact on Women's Health

To understand the intricacies of managing obstetrical and gynecological issues in diabetes patients, it is crucial to grasp the broader context of diabetes and its specific impact on women's health. In the following sections, we will delve into the physiological underpinnings of diabetes, its epidemiology among women, and the multifaceted ways in which it affects their reproductive and gynecological health.

13.2 Diabetes Types and Their Relevance

13.2.1 Types of Diabetes (Type 1, Type 2, Gestational)

Diabetes mellitus encompasses various types, including type 1 diabetes, type 2 diabetes, and gestational diabetes. Type 1 diabetes is an autoimmune condition where the body's immune system attacks and destroys insulin-producing beta cells in the pancreas [4]. In contrast, type 2 diabetes primarily results from insulin resistance and relative insulin deficiency [4]. Gestational diabetes, specific to pregnancy, involves elevated blood sugar levels that develop during gestation, often resolving after childbirth [4]. These diabetes types differ in etiology, pathophysiology, and management.

13.2.2 How the Type of Diabetes Influences Obstetrical and Gynecological Issues

The type of diabetes significantly influences obstetrical and gynecological concerns. Women with type 1 diabetes may face challenges related to pregnancy planning, as they require meticulous blood glucose control to minimize risks.

Complications can include preeclampsia, preterm birth, and congenital anomalies [4]. Women with type 2 diabetes mellitus are at a higher risk of developing polycystic ovary syndrome (PCOS), impacting fertility and gynecological health [5].

Gestational diabetes directly affects pregnancy, increasing the risk of macrosomia and other complications [4]. Additionally, women with a history of gestational diabetes are at a higher risk of developing type 2 diabetes in the future [4]. The interplay between diabetes type and obstetrical/gynecological issues necessitates personalized care approaches and risk assessment.

13.2.3 Prevalence and Demographic Trends

Diabetes is a growing public health concern in the United States, with an estimated 34.2 million people living with diabetes [4]. Type 2 diabetes is higher among older adults and certain ethnic groups, including Hispanic, African American, and Native American populations [4]. Gestational diabetes affects approximately 6–9% of pregnancies in the United States., and its incidence is rising due to increasing obesity rates and maternal age [4]. Demographic trends are crucial for healthcare planning, early intervention, and addressing healthcare disparities.

13.3 Preconception Care and Family Planning

13.3.1 Importance of Preconception Counseling

Preconception counseling is a critical component of healthcare for women with diabetes. It serves as an essential step in optimizing maternal and fetal health outcomes. This counseling involves discussions and interventions aimed at assessing and improving the health of women before they become pregnant.

Preconception counseling is vital for several reasons. It provides an opportunity to assess and manage pre-existing medical conditions and lifestyle factors that can impact pregnancy. For women with diabetes, it offers a platform to evaluate glycemic control, adjust medication regimens, and address any diabetes-related complications. This proactive approach can help prevent complications during pregnancy, such as gestational diabetes and preeclampsia, and reduce the risk of congenital anomalies in the baby. Moreover, it allows women to make informed decisions regarding family planning, ensuring they are physically and emotionally prepared for pregnancy.

13.3.2 Managing Diabetes Before Pregnancy

Effective management of diabetes before conception is a cornerstone of preconception care. Glycemic control is paramount, as uncontrolled diabetes during pregnancy can lead to adverse outcomes, including preterm birth, macrosomia, and birth defects. It's essential for women with diabetes to optimize their blood glucose levels, adhere to a healthy diet, maintain regular physical activity, and, if necessary, adjust medication regimens. Additionally, addressing any diabetes-related complications, such as diabetic retinopathy or nephropathy, is critical to reduce the risk of complications during pregnancy.

13.3.3 Contraceptive Options and Considerations

Family planning and the choice of contraception are integral components of preconception care. Women and their partners should consider contraceptive options during preconception counseling to make informed choices about when to start or expand their family. This period allows for a comprehensive evaluation of readiness for parenthood, considering factors like age, financial stability, and personal goals. Discussing birth control methods in preconception care ensures that pregnancy occurs at the right time for each individual or couple, and it can help prevent unintended pregnancies.

Women with diabetes should carefully consider contraceptives to ensure their reproductive health while managing their medical condition. According to the Centers for Disease Control and Prevention (CDC) Medical Eligibility Criteria for Contraceptive Use, most contraceptive methods are generally safe and appropriate for women with diabetes. Both hormonal and nonhormonal, intrauterine devices (IUDs) are highly effective and suitable. Additionally, contraceptive implants, birth control pills, patches, and barrier methods like condoms are often appropriate. However, women with diabetes need to consult with healthcare providers to determine the most suitable contraceptive option based on their specific health status and any potential drug interactions with their diabetes medications. A healthcare provider's guidance can help women with diabetes make informed decisions about contraception, considering both their reproductive goals and overall health [6].

In conclusion, preconception counseling and family planning are essential for women with diabetes. By optimizing diabetes management before pregnancy and considering contraceptive options, healthcare providers can support healthy pregnancies and improve maternal and child health outcomes.

13.4 Management of Diabetes during Pregnancy

Diabetes Management During Pregnancy Is a Critical Aspect of Prenatal Care, and It Is Guided by Recommendations from the American College of Obstetricians and Gynecologists (ACOG) and the Society for Maternal-Fetal Medicine (SMFM) in the United States.

13.4.1 Blood Glucose Monitoring and Targets

According to ACOG and SMFM guidelines, rigorous blood glucose monitoring is fundamental during pregnancy for women with preexisting diabetes or gestational diabetes. The recommended blood glucose targets typically include fasting glucose levels below 95 mg/dL and postprandial levels below 140 mg/dL. These targets aim to maintain adequate glycemic control while minimizing the risk of hypoglycemia and adverse pregnancy outcomes.

13.4.2 Medications, Insulin Therapy, and Gestational Diabetes

For women with gestational diabetes, the initial approach often involves dietary and lifestyle modifications. If blood glucose targets cannot be achieved through these measures alone, insulin therapy may be initiated. ACOG and SMFM guidelines underscore the importance of individualized treatment plans, tailored to each patient's needs, which may include the use of insulin or oral antidiabetic agents if necessary, while ensuring fetal safety [3, 7].

13.4.3 Nutrition and Meal Planning

Both ACOG and SMFM emphasize the significance of nutritional therapy in managing diabetes during pregnancy. Women are advised to work with registered dietitians or nutrition specialists to create meal plans that meet their specific dietary needs. A focus on a balanced diet, consisting of complex carbohydrates, lean proteins, and healthy fats, is encouraged to help stabilize blood glucose levels.

13.4.4 Exercise and Lifestyle Modifications

Lifestyle modifications, including regular physical activity, are key components of diabetes management during pregnancy. ACOG and SMFM guidelines recommend at least 150 min of moderate-intensity exercise per week for most pregnant women with diabetes. Tailored exercise regimens, under the guidance of healthcare providers, can aid in maintaining appropriate weight gain and improving insulin sensitivity.

In summary, adherence to ACOG and SMFM guidelines is crucial for effectively managing diabetes during pregnancy. These guidelines provide a comprehensive framework for blood glucose monitoring, medication usage, nutrition, and lifestyle modifications to ensure optimal maternal and fetal outcomes.

13.5 Obstetrical Complications

Obstetrical complications in women with diabetes are a critical concern, and healthcare providers rely on various assessments and interventions to manage these issues effectively.

13.5.1 Pregestational Diabetes and Its Implications

Pregestational diabetes, particularly type 1 and type 2 diabetes, can increase the risk of complications during pregnancy. Uncontrolled hyperglycemia in the preconception period and early pregnancy is associated with an elevated risk of congenital anomalies. Tight glycemic control before and throughout pregnancy is essential to minimize these risks.

13.5.2 Preeclampsia and Diabetes

Women with pregestational diabetes face an increased risk of developing preeclampsia during pregnancy. Preeclampsia can further complicate diabetes management and pregnancy outcomes. It is crucial to closely monitor blood pressure and renal function in these cases, as well as to ensure well-controlled blood glucose levels.

13.5.3 Preterm Labor and Diabetes

Diabetes, especially when poorly managed, is linked to a higher likelihood of preterm labor. Chronic hyperglycemia can trigger inflammation and uterine contractions, leading to preterm birth. Managing diabetes through glycemic control and addressing any associated risk factors is crucial for preventing preterm labor.

13.5.4 Role of Ultrasound in Monitoring Fetal Development

Ultrasound plays a vital role in monitoring fetal development in pregnancies complicated by diabetes. It helps assess fetal growth, detect congenital anomalies, and monitor amniotic fluid levels. Regular ultrasound examinations allow healthcare providers to make informed decisions about timing and mode of delivery, ensuring the best possible outcomes for both mother and baby [8].

13.6 Pregnancy and Diabetes-Related Complications

Pregnancy in women with diabetes presents a complex interplay of factors that can lead to various complications, and healthcare providers aim to mitigate these challenges to ensure the best possible maternal and fetal outcomes.

13.6.1 Hypoglycemia and Hyperglycemia During Pregnancy

Maintaining optimal blood glucose levels is crucial. Hypoglycemia, if not appropriately managed, can result in maternal discomfort and potential harm to the fetus.

Conversely, hyperglycemia can lead to excessive fetal growth and a higher risk of birth complications.

13.6.2 Diabetic Ketoacidosis and Pregnancy

Diabetic ketoacidosis is a severe complication of uncontrolled diabetes. During pregnancy, it poses a significant threat to both the mother and the fetus. Timely recognition and prompt intervention are essential to prevent adverse outcomes.

13.6.3 Impact on Maternal and Fetal Health

The impact of diabetes-related complications during pregnancy extends to maternal health, as it increases the risk of conditions such as preeclampsia and gestational hypertension. Additionally, uncontrolled diabetes can lead to macrosomia and respiratory distress in the newborn.

13.6.4 Strategies to Reduce Complications

Healthcare providers employ a combination of strategies to reduce complications. These include meticulous blood glucose monitoring, individualized insulin regimens, and close monitoring of maternal and fetal well-being through regular prenatal care.

13.7 Medications and Medical Interventions

Effective diabetes management during pregnancy involves medication adjustments, advanced monitoring technologies, and a multidisciplinary healthcare team to ensure optimal maternal and fetal health.

13.7.1 Medication Adjustments During Pregnancy

Medication regimens for women with diabetes often require adjustment during pregnancy. These changes may include transitioning from oral antidiabetic agents to insulin therapy to maintain tight glycemic control, given the potential risks associated with certain medications during pregnancy.

13.7.2 Continuous Glucose Monitoring and Insulin Pumps

Continuous glucose monitoring (CGM) and insulin pumps have revolutionized diabetes management during pregnancy. CGM provides real-time data on blood glucose levels, enabling more precise insulin dosing. Insulin pumps offer precise control of insulin delivery, minimizing the risk of hypoglycemia. Both technologies are integral to achieving stable blood glucose levels during pregnancy.

13.7.3 Role of a Multidisciplinary Healthcare Team

Managing diabetes during pregnancy requires a multidisciplinary approach. A healthcare team, including maternal-fetal medicine, obstetricians, dietitians, and diabetes educators, collaborates to tailor treatment plans, provide education, and ensure comprehensive care. This approach is vital to address the unique challenges and complexities of diabetes in pregnancy.

13.8 Delivery and Postpartum Care

Delivery and postpartum care for women with diabetes necessitate a comprehensive approach to ensure the well-being of both mother and child.

13.8.1 Birth Options and Considerations

Women with diabetes should explore birth options, including vaginal delivery or cesarean section, and timing of delivery, in consultation with their healthcare providers. These decisions are often influenced by maternal glycemic control, obstetrical factors, and fetal well-being. Individualized birth plans are crucial to address the unique needs of women with diabetes.

13.8.2 Labor Management for Diabetes Patients

During labor, close monitoring of blood glucose levels and the administration of intravenous fluids with appropriate glucose concentrations are essential to maintain stable glycemic control. For women on insulin pumps, modifications may be needed. Healthcare providers closely supervise labor to prevent hypoglycemia and hyperglycemia, adjusting insulin doses as necessary.

13.8.3 Postpartum Diabetes Control

Postpartum diabetes management is critical for women with diabetes. Blood glucose levels may fluctuate following childbirth, necessitating ongoing monitoring and adjustment of medication or insulin regimens. Healthcare providers play a crucial role in guiding women through this transition period to ensure stable glycemic control.

13.8.4 Neonatal Care and Breastfeeding

Newborns of mothers with diabetes require specialized neonatal care to monitor for hypoglycemia and other potential complications. Additionally, breastfeeding is encouraged, as it can support neonatal glycemic control and provide numerous health benefits. Healthcare providers offer guidance on breastfeeding and neonatal care, fostering a healthy start for both mother and baby.

13.9 Gynecological Issues

Gynecological issues in women with diabetes encompass a range of conditions that necessitate careful monitoring and management.

13.9.1 Menstrual Irregularities and Diabetes

Diabetes, especially uncontrolled diabetes, can lead to menstrual irregularities in women. Fluctuating blood glucose levels can affect hormonal balance, leading to variations in the menstrual cycle. These irregularities can affect fertility and underscore the importance of maintaining stable glycemic control for women seeking to conceive [1].

13.9.2 Polycystic Ovary Syndrome (PCOS)

Women with diabetes are at a higher risk of developing polycystic ovary syndrome (PCOS), a condition characterized by irregular periods, hyperandrogenism, and multiple cysts on the ovaries. PCOS often complicates diabetes management due to insulin resistance and hormonal imbalances. Addressing both conditions is crucial for optimal health and fertility outcomes [9].

13.9.3 Menopause and Diabetes Management

The onset of menopause in women with diabetes can pose unique challenges. Hormonal changes during menopause can impact insulin sensitivity and glycemic control, necessitating adjustments to diabetes management plans. Healthcare providers should carefully monitor and adapt treatment strategies to address these changes effectively [10].

13.9.4 Diabetes and Gynecological Cancer Risk

Studies have shown that women with diabetes may face an elevated risk of certain gynecological cancers, such as endometrial cancer. Hyperinsulinemia and estrogen imbalances associated with diabetes can contribute to these increased risks. Regular gynecological screenings and early detection are essential to mitigate these risks [11].

13.10 Gynecological Screenings and Diabetes

Gynecological screenings play a crucial role in the comprehensive care of women with diabetes.

13.10.1 Regular Gynecological Care for Diabetes Patients

Women with diabetes should prioritize regular gynecological care to address their unique healthcare needs. Routine check-ups provide an opportunity to assess overall health, manage diabetes-related gynecological issues, and monitor for potential complications. These visits offer a platform for discussing family planning, contraceptive options, and addressing menstrual irregularities related to diabetes.

13.10.2 Cervical Cancer Screenings

Regular cervical cancer screenings, such as Pap smears, are essential for women with diabetes, as they are at a slightly higher risk for cervical cancer. Close monitoring and early detection through these screenings can significantly reduce the risk of cervical cancer and ensure timely intervention if abnormalities are detected.

13.10.3 Mammograms and Breast Health

Breast health is paramount for women with diabetes. Mammograms are recommended for breast cancer screening, as women with diabetes may face a higher risk of developing this cancer. Regular mammograms, along with breast self-exams, are integral to early detection and improving breast health outcomes.

Engaging in regular gynecological screenings not only enhances overall well-being but also plays a critical role in the holistic healthcare management of women with diabetes.

13.11 Emotional and Psychological Well-being

Emotional and psychological well-being is a critical aspect of healthcare for women with diabetes and gynecological issues, given the substantial impact of these conditions on a woman's life.

13.11.1 Coping with Diabetes and Gynecological Issues

The challenges of managing diabetes and dealing with gynecological concerns can take a toll on a woman's emotional well-being. Coping strategies are essential to navigate the physical and emotional complexities that may arise. This includes finding ways to manage the stress and uncertainty associated with diabetes, as well as addressing the emotional aspects of gynecological conditions such as PCOS or menstrual irregularities.

13.11.2 Support Systems and Counseling

Having a robust support system and access to counseling services is crucial. Family, friends, and support groups can provide emotional assistance and practical help. Professional counseling can address psychological challenges and provide valuable coping strategies, particularly in the context of chronic illnesses like diabetes and gynecological issues.

13.11.3 Mental Health Considerations

Mental health is an integral component of a woman's overall well-being. Managing diabetes and gynecological conditions necessitates an awareness of the potential impact on mental health. Anxiety, depression, and stress are common concerns, and healthcare providers should be attentive to these issues and offer referrals for mental health support when needed.

Balancing emotional and psychological well-being with the demands of managing diabetes and addressing gynecological issues is crucial for women's overall health and quality of life. A comprehensive approach to care should encompass the psychological and emotional aspects, alongside the medical management of these conditions.

13.12 Conclusion

In conclusion, the care of women with diabetes and related obstetrical and gynecological complications is a multifaceted endeavor that necessitates a comprehensive approach, as highlighted in the preceding sections.

Key takeaways include the importance of preconception counseling and family planning, meticulous diabetes management during pregnancy, and the critical role of gynecological screenings and emotional well-being. To ensure the best possible outcomes for patients with these conditions, healthcare professionals must remain vigilant in adapting clinical guidance to the specific needs of each patient. Individualized care plans that encompass blood glucose monitoring, medication adjustments, and lifestyle interventions are crucial. Additionally, healthcare providers should recognize the value of support systems, counseling, and mental health considerations in the holistic care of women with diabetes and gynecological issues.

Furthermore, community-directed interventions, such as education and awareness campaigns, can greatly improve outcomes for women with diabetes. Collaborative efforts among healthcare providers, communities, and patients can lead to enhanced prevention, management, and support systems, ultimately promoting the well-being and health of women with diabetes and related gynecological complications.

References

1. American Diabetes Association. Standards of medical care in diabetes—2021. Diabetes Care. 2021;44(Suppl 1):S1–S230.
2. Dabelea D, Crume T. Maternal environment and the transgenerational cycle of obesity and diabetes. Diabetes. 2011;60(7):1849–55.
3. American College of Obstetricians and Gynecologists. ACOG Practice Bulletin No. 190: gestational diabetes mellitus. Obstet Gynecol. 2018;131(2):e49–64.
4. American Diabetes Association. Classification and diagnosis of diabetes: standards of medical care in diabetes-2021. Diabetes Care. 2021;44(Suppl 1):S15–33.
5. Legro RS, Arslanian SA, Ehrmann DA, et al. Diagnosis and treatment of polycystic ovary syndrome: an endocrine society clinical practice guideline. J Clin Endocrinol Metab. 2013;98(12):4565–92.
6. Centers for Disease Control and Prevention. U.S. medical eligibility criteria for contraceptive use, 2016. MMWR Recomm Rep. 2016;65(3):1–104.
7. SMFM Publications Committee. SMFM statement: pharmacological treatment of gestational diabetes. Am J Obstet Gynecol. 2018;218(5):B2–4.
8. Salvesen KÅ, Lees C. Ultrasound in the management of women with diabetes and intrauterine growth restriction. Ultrasound Obstet Gynecol. 2011;38(2):125–35.
9. Legro RS, Arslanian SA, Ehrmann DA, et al. Diagnosis and treatment of polycystic ovary syndrome: an endocrine society clinical practice guideline. J Clin Endocrinol Metabol. 2013;98(12):4565–92.
10. American Diabetes Association. Diabetes and reproductive health: a position statement of the American Diabetes Association. Diabetes Care. 2019;42(12):2286–99.
11. Boyle P, Boniol M, Koechlin A, et al. Diabetes and breast cancer risk: a meta-analysis. Br J Cancer. 2012;107(1):160–6.

Sexual Dysfunction in Diabetes Mellitus 14

A. V. Raveendran and Peedikakkal Rajini

14.1 Introduction

Diabetes mellitus, its associated risk factors, complications, and associated co-morbidities and psychological stress have a significant negative impact on the normal sexual function of both men and women resulting in an increased risk of development of sexual dysfunction (SD). In men, the most established diabetes-related SD is erectile dysfunction (ED). In men, DM is also associated with ejaculatory and desire disorders. Females with diabetes can have dysfunction in all the phases of the sexual response cycle including desire, arousal, lubrication, orgasm, and satisfaction. In this chapter, we are briefly reviewing the sexual problems in people with diabetes.

The stages of normal sexual response include desire and excitement, plateau, orgasm, and resolution. Depending upon the stages of the sexual response cycle involved, it is classified.

14.1.1 Male Sexual Dysfunction in Diabetes

Various sexual dysfunction (SD) seen in men with diabetes include erectile dysfunction, ejaculatory, and desire disorders.

14.1.1.1 Erectile Dysfunction

ED is the most commonly described sexual dysfunction in males. ED is characterized by the persistent and recurring inability to achieve or maintain penile erection with sufficient rigidity and duration for satisfactory sexual activity [1]. Prevalence of ED increases with age and at 40 years around 40% report ED, whereas it increases

A. V. Raveendran (✉) · P. Rajini
Badr Al Samaa, Barka, Sultanate of Oman

G. Abraham et al. (eds.), *Management of Diabetic Complications*,
https://doi.org/10.1007/978-981-97-6406-8_14

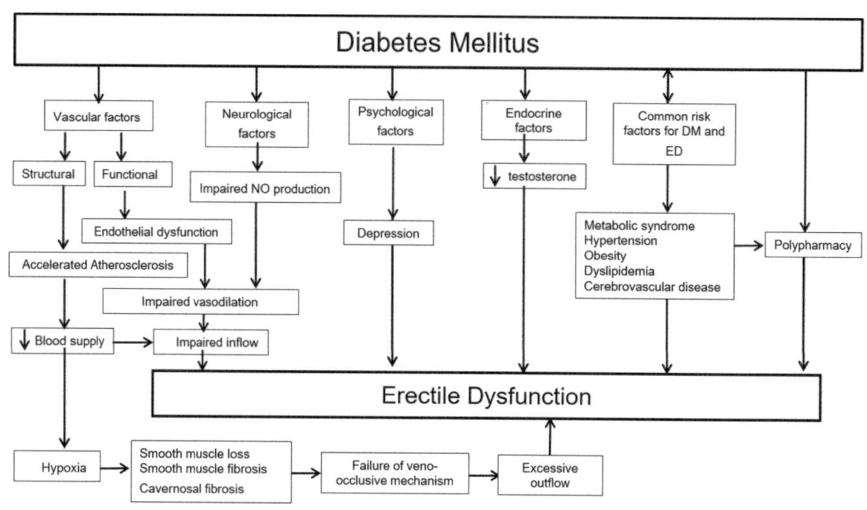

Fig. 14.1 Pathophysiological mechanisms in the development of ED in people with diabetes

to 70% for the age group of 70 years [2]. People with diabetes have ED 3.5 times higher than those without ED, and it can be a presenting symptom of DM [3]. ED frequently precedes adverse cardiovascular events by 3–5 years indicating the need for cardiovascular evaluation in all those presenting with ED [4]. The "artery size" hypothesis of atherosclerosis connecting ED and CVD proposes that arteries smaller in diameter manifest occlusive symptoms earlier than larger vessels, and penile atherosclerotic symptoms precede coronary arteries occlusive symptoms as coronary arteries (3–4 mm) are slightly larger in diameter than penile arteries (1–2 mm) [5]. ED is considered as "tip of the iceberg" of systemic atherosclerotic disease (Fig. 14.1) [6].

A detailed history including sexual history and physical examination will give valuable clues to the etiology and severity of ED. Drug history requires special emphasis as drug-induced ED is a common problem in clinical practice.

There are validated questionnaires (like the International Index of erectile function questionnaire—IIEF) to assess the severity of ED. A simple way to assess the severity of ED is to ask the patient to grade his erectile rigidity with 100% being the best and hardest erection, 0% completely flaccid, and 50% just hard enough for penetration (M1). The onset of ED (sudden or gradual), the status of morning erection, associated sexual problems like ejaculatory problems, sexual desire disorder, and the presence of other diseases like hypertension, and atherosclerotic vascular diseases add valuable clinical information. Genital examination to assess the testicular size (Hypogonadism), hair distribution, penile fibrosis or plaque (Peyronie's disease) signs of infection (balanoposthitis), and phimosis. A detailed physical examination and genital examination are helpful in identifying the etiology of ED.

In people with diabetes, presenting with ED, assess the level of control of diabetes, associated co-morbidities, and complications. In people with ED, there is indirect evidence of underlying endothelial dysfunction and vascular disease especially atherosclerotic vascular disease warranting a thorough evaluation for underlying coronary artery diseases [5, 6].

Investigations There is no specific test required for the evaluation of ED. In addition to routine blood testing, liver and kidney function tests and electrolytes, HbA_1C and lipid profile, TSH, morning (8–11 AM, as testosterone levels are highest in the morning hours) testosterone, sex hormone binding globulin and albumin measurement are usually done. In those with low testosterone, measure other pituitary hormones like FSH, LH, and prolactin to rule out central hypogonadism. Hypogonadism is usually diagnosed if total testosterone <320 ng/dL and free testosterone <64 pg/ml [7].

In penile biothesiometry, with the help of a vibrating probe, the vibrational threshold sensitivity can be assessed which is a simple office screening test for penile neuropathy [8]. People with abnormal biothesiometry can have an increased response to intra-cavernosal injection therapy due to denervation hypersensitivity.

Nocturnal penile tumescence testing (NPT) involves assessing the frequency, tumescence duration, and maximal rigidity of nocturnal erection during REM sleep. In a normal individual, usually, 3–6 erection with a mean duration greater than 30 minutes with maximal rigidity of more than 70% occurs during nocturnal erection. The penile circumference increases by more than 3 cm at the base and more than 2 cm at the tip. NPT helps to differentiate psychogenic ED from organic ED. In people with hypogonadism, the rigidity decreases [9].

Penile duplex Doppler ultrasound helps to access vascular flow and is usually performed after intra-cavernosal injection of vasoactive drug (20 micrograms of prostaglandin E1). Peak systolic velocity (PSV) > 35 cm/s is normal, and a value of <25 cm/sec indicates vascular insufficiency [10]. Failure of penile corporal rigidity with normal arterial inflow indicates veno-occlusive disease or insufficiency. In other words, rapid detumescence despite consistently normal peak systolic and end-diastolic velocities (EDV > 5 cm/s) or a vascular resistive index <0.75 [RI = (PSV − EDV) ÷ PSV] indicate veno-occlusive disease.

Dynamic infusion cavernosometry and cavernosography were done to identify the site of the venous leak before corrective surgery. Pudendal arteriography is done to study the vasculature of the penis which will be useful before corrective/revascularization surgery. Endothelial dysfunction can be demonstrated by various tests including penile nitric oxide release test, peripheral arterial tonometry and flow-mediated dilatation, and various serum markers like endothelin-1, vascular cell adhesion molecule-1, and endothelial progenitor cells and microparticles. However, the demonstration of endothelial dysfunction is mainly of academic interest and with limited clinical utility.

Treatment Control of diabetes and other risk factors is important in the treatment of erectile dysfunction. It improves both ED and cardiovascular risk profiles. Control of blood pressure, dyslipidemia, increase in physical activity, diet control, and quitting smoking all help to improve ED. Improvement in ED is seen with dietary manipulation and lifestyle modification. Any medication-inducing ED has to be modified after considering the general condition of the patient if possible.

L-arginine is an amino acid supplement that is a substrate of nitric oxide synthase enzyme and is useful in mild to moderate ED (1500 mg to 5000 mg) [11].

Oral phosphodiesterase-5 inhibitors (PDE-5 inhibitors) act by inhibiting the phosphodiesterase enzyme, thereby reducing the degradation of C-GMP resulting in the relaxation of cavernosal smooth muscles and increased cavernosal blood flows. PDE-5 inhibitors do not initiate erectile response as sexual stimulation is essential for the release of nitric oxide from vascular endothelium and penile nerve ending to initiate an erectile response. Commonly used PDE 5 inhibitors are Sildenafil, vardenafil, tadalafil, and avanafil and are used on demand or on a daily basis. New evidence suggests that daily use of PDE 5 inhibitors can reduce or even reverse penile tissue damage, improve vascular function reduce inflammation and oxidative stress.

Side effects are usually mild like headache, nasal stuffiness, and bluish coloration of vision. Rarely it can cause permanent blindness due to non-arteritic anterior ischemic optic neuropathy and unilateral deafness. PDE-5 inhibitors should not be used in people on nitrates and be cautious with antihypertensives and alpha blockers because of the risk of profound hypotension.

Release of nitric oxide from the neuronal and endothelial cells is impaired in people with neuropathy and endothelial dysfunction results in blunted response to PDE-5 inhibitor in people with DM.

In PDE-5 nonresponders, try another PDE-5 inhibitor, which may work sometimes. Also, check for testosterone deficiency, and if found supplement testosterone along with PDE-5 inhibitors [12]. The overall success rate of PDE5 is 76%.

Testosterone supplementation is useful in people with ED and hypogonadism who failed on initial PDE-5 inhibitors therapy. It improves libido in those with hypogonadism and low libido. In addition to sexual function improvement, testosterone therapy also improves insulin sensitivity and lean body mass [12]. The overall success rate of testosterone supplementation is 35% [11].

External vacuum devices create negative pressure around the penis helping the engorgement of corpora with blood resulting in an artificial erection. The efficiency rate is about 70–80%.

Medicated urethral system for erection (MUSE) involves intraurethral insertion of prostaglandin $E_{1,}$ which gets absorbed through the urethra and results in smooth muscle relaxation of corpora cavernosa resulting in erection. Its efficiency is 50–65%.

Intra-cavernosal injections of medicines causing smooth muscle relaxation and vasodilatation like papaverine, prostaglandin E1 (A1prostadil), phentolamine, and atropine are useful in those who fail with PDE-5 inhibitors. It is effective in up to 94% of patients (P19-108). Intra-cavernosal injections using combinations like trimix (Papaverine 30 mg + phentolamine 1 mg + Prostaglandin E, 20 mcg/cc) or Quadrimix (trimix +0.2 mg atropine) are commonly used. The initial dose is 0.2 to

0.25 cc. Failure of intra-cavernosal injection indicates vasculogenic ED. One of the serious complications of this is priapism, which can cause permanent damage to the corpora if not treated in time (Priapism antidote phenylephrine). If the erection lasts for more than 4 h, people are advised to report to the nearest emergency department.

Combination therapy: Combination of intra-cavernosal injections or MUST plus PDE-5 inhibitor act synergistically as all these use different chemical mediators (CAMP for intra-cavernosal injection & CGMP for PDE-5).

Priapism with PDE 5 inhibitor is about 3%, and penile injection therapy is 88% [13]. Drug indeed priapism treatment includes intermittent intra-cavernosal injection of diluted phenylephrine solution 200 mcg at a time, about 5–10 min apart until detumescence or a maximum dose of 1 mg of phenylephrine. If this fails, surgical shunting procedure has to be done. Intra-cavernosal stem cell installation and platelet-rich plasma therapy are under clinical trial.

Penile prosthesis is used when other treatment fails. The prosthesis is surgically inserted into the corpora cavernosa to improve erection artificially. Two types of prosthesis are used—malleable and inflatable. Erosion, infection, leakage, and mechanical failures are the complications associated with penile prostheses. The penile prosthesis is associated with high patient satisfaction scores about 90%.

Penile revascularization surgery involves anastomosing the inferior epigastric artery to the dorsal artery of the penis or directly to the corpora cavernosa, which is usually done for young people with ED and isolated vascular injury. Arterial balloon angioplasty is useful in those with focal stenosis of pudendal or penile arteries. Venous ligation surgery or embolization can be done for veno-occlusive or insufficiency (of penial vein like deep dorsal vein).

Low-intensity shock wave therapy improves cavernosal hemodynamics, induction of endothelial cell proliferation, and activation of endogenous stem cells and penile revascularization. 3000 pulses per session give better results. In people with diabetes, having ED not responding to PDE-5 inhibitors was found to respond to PDE-5 inhibitors after low-intensity shock ware therapy. But long-term results are not satisfactory. The overall success rate at 30 months is about 40%.

ED has to be differentiated from hypogonadism, lack of desire, depression, or other psychological issues. It has to be differentiated from other sexual dysfunctions. The outcome of ED treatment depends upon the underlying cause and its severity.

14.1.1.2 Ejaculatory Disorders

In people with diabetes involvement of nerves involved in normal ejaculation leads to ejaculatory disorders.

Premature ejaculation (PE) or early ejaculation is common in people with diabetes mellitus. Those with PE usually ejaculate early. The inability to control ejaculation, leading to early ejaculation results in psychological distress affecting the quality of life. In people with early ejaculation, see the onset of symptoms. Is it from the onset of sexual life (lifelong) or after a period of normal sexual life (acquired) and is it always present (global) or not (situational)? Is it associated with erectile dysfunction (complicated PE)? [14, 15] There are validated questionnaires like the index of PE, PE profile, PE diagnostic tool, Arabic index of PE, and Chinese index of sexual function for PE. Clinical examination is usually normal in people with PE. Rectal examination is usually done if PE is associated with painful ejaculation. The time interval between vaginal penetration and intravaginal ejaculation, i.e., Intravaginal Ejaculatory Latency Time (IELT) used to get objective evidence of early ejaculation. PE is a clinical diagnosis. Raveendran's proposed diagnostic criteria is useful for diagnosing PE [16].

Investigations in PE depend upon contributing factors identified during clinical evaluation. Low serotonin levels shorten the ejaculatory time. Various non-pharmacological treatment options include psycho-sexual counseling, the "stop-start" technique, the squeeze technique, pre-coital masturbation, pelvic floor exercise, extended foreplay, and interval sex. Topical anesthetic creams, tramadol, TCA like clomipramine, and SSRIs like Paroxetine Fluoxetine, sertraline, and dapoxetine are useful in the treatment of PE. Various procedures like Dorsal Penile nerve cryoablation, neuromodulation, hyaluronic acid gel glans augmentation, and botulinum toxin injection are useful in the treatment of PE.

Retrograde ejaculation (RE) occurs when semen moves backward into the bladder, instead of out through the penis. Cloudy urine after sexual activity or demonstration of sperms in the post-orgasmic urine sample confirms the diagnosis [17]. It can cause subfertility. Stimulating the sympathetic activity or blocking the parasympathetic stimulation helps in the treatment of RE by increasing the tone of the bladder neck. Sympathomimetics like synephrine, pseudoephedrine, ephedrine, phenyl propanol amine, midrodrin, and anticholinergic like brompheniramine, and imipramine are useful in people with RE. For improving fertility urinary or surgical sperm retrieval can be done.

Delayed ejaculation (DE)/ anejaculation (AE) is a relatively less common sexual dysfunction. People with diabetic autonomic neuropathy are at increased risk of ejaculatory dysfunction [18]. Various drugs like SSRIs, TCA, MAO inhibitors, Alpha-1 blockers, and antihypertensives can delay ejaculation. Cognitive behavioral therapy psychotherapy, masturbatory retraining, couple sex therapy, testosterone, cabergoline, bupropion, amantadine, cyproheptadine, midodrine, imipramine, ephedrine, pseudoephedrine, Yohimbine, buspirone, oxytocin, and bethanechol are used to treat delayed ejaculation.

14.1.1.3 Desire Disorder

Male hypoactive sexual desire disorder is characterized by persistent or recurrent deficient sexual or erotic thoughts, fantasies, and desire for sexual activity. Low sexual desire is also common in people with diabetes. HSDD in men is often misdiagnosed as erectile dysfunction [19]. Hypogonadism and hyperprolactinemia can cause diminished sexual desire. Various psychological issues also cause sexual desire disorders. Treatment depends upon the underlying cause. Cognitive-affective-behavioral therapy is useful in this condition.

14.1.2 Female Sexual Dysfunction in Diabetes

Sexual dysfunction is common in females with diabetes but is least addressed in clinical practice. The global prevalence of SD in women with diabetes varies from 20 to 80%. Various sexual problems seen in females with diabetes include desire disorders, arousal disorders, orgasmic disorders, problems with lubrication, pain during sexual intercourse, and disorders of satisfaction [20].

Decreased sexual arousal with slow or inadequate lubrication is common in people with diabetes. Reduced vaginal lubrication in people with diabetes varies from 10 to 34% which is higher than those without diabetes. Decreased desire varies between 11 and 45%, orgasmic problems between 11% and 14%, and dyspareunia between 10 and 12% in people with diabetes [21]. Decreased lubrication, estrogen deficiency, arterial insufficiency, and tactile insensitivity cause arousal disorder in females. Reduced sexual fantasies and desire for sexual activity is termed as female hypoactive sexual desire disorder. Increased risk of vaginal infection and decreased vaginal lubrication increase the risk of sexual pain disorders in people with diabetes. Neuropathy, vascular complications, and associated increased the risk of sexual dysfunction, decreased desire, and arousal increase the risk of sexual pain disorders in people with diabetes (Fig. 14.2).

Clinical Approach Most of the time, females suffering from sexual dysfunction do not seek medical help due to various reasons. So, the clinician should build rapport with the patient and ask about sexual problems during routine diabetes follow-up. To find out the exact nature of the problem ask about the desire, orgasm, lubrication, pain and inability to relax the pelvic muscles during sex which will give a clue to the underlying problem. A detailed sexual history and any associated psychological issues also have to be obtained. Detailed menstrual history, sexual fantasies, and

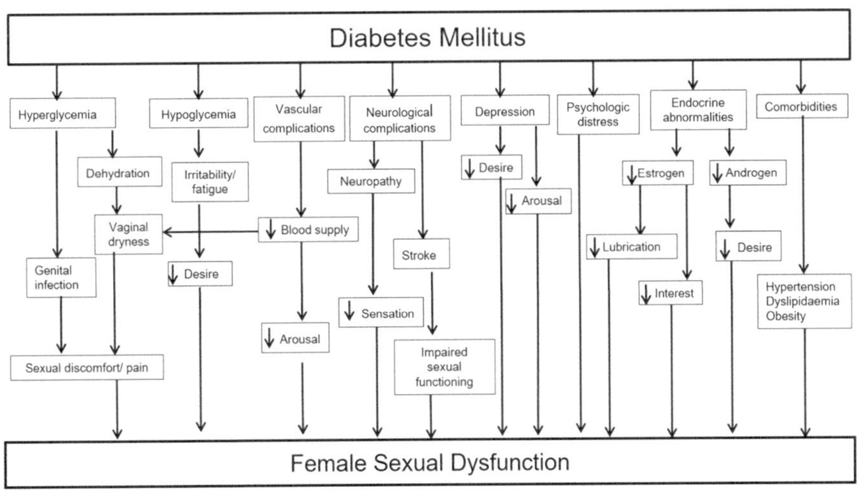

Fig. 14.2 Pathophysiological mechanisms in the development of female sexual dysfunction

sexual behavior, religious beliefs related to sexuality need to be included in the history. History from the partners also will give important clues to the diagnosis. There are validated questionnaires to assess female dysfunctions like Female Sexual Function Index (FSFI), Brief Index of Sexual Functioning for Women (BISF-W), Derogatis Interview for Sexual Function (DISF/DISFSR), and Female Sexual Distress Scale (FSDS). Relevant medical and surgical history including pelvic surgery and gynecological procedures is also important.

A complete physical examination and pelvic examination are important in women with SD. Evidence of atherosclerotic vascular disease gives a clue regarding vascular etiology. The presence of galactorrhea may be a manifestation of underlying prolactinoma, which can cause decreased sexual desire. Enlargement of thyroid may be a manifestation of underlying hypothyroidism which results in abnormalities of sexual desire and arousal. Look for evidence of neuropathy, anemia, etc. which can cause sexual dysfunction in females. Underlying musculoskeletal issues and associated pain also interfere with sexual activity leading to SD.

Gynecological abnormalities like uterine prolapse, retroverted uterus, vaginal discharge, tenderness of vulvar vestibules, and dermatological abnormalities of valvar skin can result in sexual dysfunction in females. Hypertonicity of pelvic muscles may be indicative of vaginismus. Low pubic hair may be indicative of low androgen levels which can impair sexual desire. Vaginal or labial atrophy may be due to estrogen deficiency leading to decreased arousal and dyspareunia [22].

There are various models for addressing sexual health with the patient which include the PLISSIT model (Permission, Limited Information, Specific Suggestions, Intensive Therapy) and the ALLOW model (Ask, Legitimize, Limitations, Openup, Work together).

Investigations depend upon the clinical examination findings. In addition to the routine blood test, cholesterol level, HbA_1C, Liver function test, and ultrasound of pelvis or transvaginal ultrasound, various hormone assays like thyroid function test, sex steroids, prolactin, and adrenal precursors are done. In special situations, vulvoscopy, vaginal photoplethysmography, functional MRI, biothesiometry, and perineometry are done.

Treatment of FSD There are various challenges in the management of FSD. Lack of single causative factors, physicians' unfamiliarity and limited expertise in the treatment of FSD, limited treatment options, and barriers from the patient side are important challenges in the management.

Control of diabetes, healthy diet, regular physical exercise, and control of other risk factors like hypertension, and dyslipidemia are important in the treatment of FSD.

Nonpharmacological therapies like psychoeducation, sex therapy, mindfulness training, cognitive behavioral therapy, sensate focusing exercise, communication training, sexual fantasy training, directed masturbation, and self and or partner exploration are the various non-pharmacological modalities tried in FSD.

Hypoactive Sexual Desire Disorder The non-pharmacological treatment includes education, stress management, and psycho-sexual support, in addition to diet control and exercise. Identification of contributing factors and their management is also important for successful treatment. Pharmacological agents used to treat include testosterone, topical and systemic estrogen, phosphodiesterase 5 inhibitors, bupropion, DHEA, and flibanserin [23]. Omega 3 fatty acids improve desire. Testosterone improves desire, increases blood flow to genitalia, and improves sexual gratification. In females with hypoactive sexual desire disorder on testosterone transdermal patch, if no improvement after 6 months, therapy may be stopped. During treatment monitor for adverse effects like acne, hirsutism, and virilization. DHEA increases androgen levels and decreases the sex hormone binding globulin. It improves sexual thoughts, interest, and sexual satisfaction. PDE-5 inhibitors increase the blood flow to the vagina, clitoris, and female genitalia and improve sexual arousal and lubrication. Flibanserine is a serotonin 1A receptor agonist and 2A receptor antagonist, useful in the treatment of generalized acquired hypoactive sexual desire in premenopausal women. The dose is 100 mg daily at bedtime. If there is no response after 8 weeks, it is discontinued. It can cause sedation, dry mouth, hypotension, and syncope. It is contraindicated in people with hepatic impairment and should not be used along with alcohol and moderate or strong CYP3A4 inhibitors. Tibolone improves vaginal lubrication and sexual desire. Yohimbine is an indole alkaloid. It is a selective competitive alpha 2 adrenergic blocker. Bremelanotide is a melanocortin receptor agonist that is found useful in female hypoactive sexual desire disorders. The exact mechanism of action is not known. It stimulates the release of dopamine. Bupropion is a dopamine and norepinephrine reuptake inhibitor and nicotinic acetylcholine receptor antagonist which increases sexual desire and is useful in the treatment of SSRI-induced sexual dysfunction in premenopausal women.

Sexual arousal disorder treatment includes education, phosphodiesterase inhibitors, and Eros clitoral therapy devices. Alprostadil is a potent vasodilator and on local application, it increases the blood flow to the female genital tract and improves sexual arousal. Eros is a battery-operated suction device, which fits around the clitoris and facilitates engagement.

Female Orgasmic Disorder Treatment includes various non-pharmacological measures like directed masturbation, penetrative and non-penetrative vibrating six aids, psychosexual support, clitoral therapy devices, cognitive behavior therapy, and sensate focus exercise [24]. Pharmacological agents used include PDE 5 inhibitors, bupropion, and yohimbine.

Sexual Pain Disorders Identification and treatment of underlying pathophysiological mechanisms producing dyspareunia is an important step in the treatment. For example, Oestrogen for vaginal atrophy, lubricants for vaginal dryness, antifungal for vulvovaginal candidiasis, tricyclic antidepressants, and anticonvulsants for vulvar vestibulitis. Sex education, education regarding genital hygiene, cognitive behavior therapy, pelvic floor electrical stimulation, educational pelvic examination, systemic desensitization, and use of vaginal dilators are other treatment options [25].

Postmenopausal Vulvovaginal Atrophy Treatment includes the use of vaginal lubricants and moisturizers, vaginal estrogen therapy, systemic hormone therapy, and ospemifene. Ospemifene is a selective estrogen receptor modulator useful in the treatment of vulvovaginal atrophy and dyspareunia in postmenopausal women. It is contraindicated in people with estrogen-dependent neoplasia, DVT, PE, or thromboembolic disorder.

14.2 Conclusion

Sexual dysfunction is common in both men and women with diabetes mellitus. Control of diabetes and other risk factors are important components of the management of SD in people with diabetes. Lifestyle modification improves both cardiovascular outcomes and sexual dysfunction. Contrary to popular belief, effective treatment options are available for various sexual dysfunctions currently.

References

1. Kocjancic E, Chung E, Garzon JA, Haylen B, Iacovelli V, Jaunarena J, Locke J, Millman A, Nahon I, Ohlander S, Pang R, Plata M, Acar O. International Continence Society (ICS) report on the terminology for sexual health in men with lower urinary tract (LUT) and pelvic floor (PF) dysfunction. Neurourol Urodyn. 2022;41:140–65. https://doi.org/10.1002/nau.24846.
2. Feldman HA, Goldstein I, Hatzichristou DG, Krane RJ, McKinlay JB. Impotence and its medical and psychosocial correlates: results of the Massachusetts Male Aging Study. J Urol. 1994;151(1):54–61.
3. Kouidrat, et al. High prevalence of erectile dysfunction in diabetes: a systematic review and meta-analysis of 145 studies. Diabet Med. 2017;34:1185–92.
4. Hodges LD, Kirby M, Solanki J, O'Donnell J, Brodie DA. The temporal relationship between erectile dysfunction and cardiovascular disease. Int J Clin Pract. 2007;61:2019–25. https://doi.org/10.1111/j.1742-1241.2007.01629.x.
5. Montorsi P, Ravagnani PM, Galli S, Rotatori F, Briganti A, Salonia A, Rigatti P, Montorsi F. The artery size hypothesis: a macrovascular link between erectile dysfunction and coronary artery disease. Am J Cardiol. 2005;96(12B):19M–23M. https://doi.org/10.1016/j.amjcard.2005.07.006. Epub 2005 Nov 4
6. Sangiorgi G, Cereda A, Benedetto D, Bonanni M, Chiricolo G, Cota L, Martuscelli E, Greco F. Anatomy, pathophysiology, molecular mechanisms, and clinical management of erectile dysfunction in patients affected by coronary artery disease: a review. Biomedicines. 2021;9(4):432. https://doi.org/10.3390/biomedicines9040432.
7. Wu F, et al. Identification of late-onset hypogonadism, in middle-aged and elderly men. N Engl J Med. 2010;363(2):123–35.
8. Breda G, Xausa D, Giunta A, Tamai A, Silvestre P, Gherardi L. Nomogram for penile biothesiometry. Eur Urol. 1991;20(1):67–9.

9. Fenwick PB, Mercer S, Grant R, Wheeler M, Nanjee N, Toone B, Brown D. Nocturnal penile tumescence and serum testosterone levels. Arch Sex Behav. 1986;15(1):13–21.
10. Jung DC, Park SY, Lee JY. Penile Doppler ultrasonography revisited. Ultrasonography. 2018;37(1):16–24.
11. Shindel AW, Lue TF. Sexual dysfunction in diabetes. [updated 2021 Jun 8]. In: Feingold KR, Anawalt B, Blackman MR, et al., editors. Endotext [internet]. South Dartmouth (MA): MDText.com, Inc.; 2000. Available from: https://www.ncbi.nlm.nih.gov/books/NBK279101/.
12. Foresta C, Caretta N, Rossato M, Garolla A, Ferlin A. Role of androgens in erectile function. J Urol. 2004;171(6 Pt 1):2358–62. quiz 2435
13. Rezaee ME, Gross MS. Are we overstating the risk of priapism with oral phosphodiesterase type 5 inhibitors? J Sex Med. 2020;17(8):1579–82.
14. Raveendran AV, Agarwal A. Premature ejaculation—current concepts in the management: a narrative review. Int J Reprod Biomed. 2021;19(1):5–22. https://doi.org/10.18502/ijrm.v19i1.8176. PMID: 33553999; PMCID: PMC7851481
15. Raveendran VA. Premature ejaculation-emerging concepts and a novel classification. Balkan Med J. 2023;40:454–5.
16. Raveendran AV. Premature ejaculation: proposed diagnostic criteria, a letter to editor. Men's Health Journal. 2022;6(1):e9. https://doi.org/10.22037/mhj.v6i1.37851.
17. Parnham A, Serefoglu EC. Retrograde ejaculation, painful ejaculation and hematospermia. Transl Androl Urol. 2016;5(4):592–601. https://doi.org/10.21037/tau.2016.06.05. PMID: 27652230; PMCID: PMC5002007
18. Abdel-Hamid IA, Ali OI. Delayed ejaculation: pathophysiology, diagnosis, and treatment. World J Mens Health. 2018;36(1):22–40. https://doi.org/10.5534/wjmh.17051. PMID: 29299903; PMCID: PMC5756804
19. Montgomery KA. Sexual desire disorders. Psychiatry (Edgmont). 2008;5(6):50–5. PMID: 19727285; PMCID: PMC2695750
20. Doruk H, Akbay E, Cayan S, Akbay E, Bozlu M, Acar D. Effect of diabetes mellitus on female sexual function and risk factors. Arch Androl. 2005;51(1):1–6. https://doi.org/10.1080/014850190512798.
21. Enzlin P, Mathieu C, Van den Bruel A, Bosteels J, Vanderschueren D, Demyttenaere K. Sexual dysfunction in women with type 1 diabetes: a controlled study. Diabetes Care. 2002;25(4):672–7. https://doi.org/10.2337/diacare.25.4.672.
22. Barbagallo F, Mongioì LM, Cannarella R, La Vignera S, Condorelli RA, Calogero AE. Sexual dysfunction in diabetic women: an update on current knowledge. Diabetology. 2020;1(1):11–21. https://doi.org/10.3390/diabetology1010002.
23. Pachano Pesantez GS, Clayton AH. Treatment of hypoactive sexual desire disorder among women: general considerations and pharmacological options. Focus (Am Psychiatr Publ). 2021;19(1):39–45. https://doi.org/10.1176/appi.focus.20200039. Epub 2021 Jan 25. PMID: 34483765; PMCID: PMC8412154
24. Meston CM, Hull E, Levin RJ, Sipski M. Disorders of orgasm in women. J Sex Med. 2004;1(1):66–8. https://doi.org/10.1111/j.1743-6109.2004.10110.x.
25. Phillips NA. Female sexual dysfunction: evaluation and treatment. Am Fam Physician. 2000;62(1):127–36. 141-2

Conservative Management of Diabetic Kidney Disease

15

Georgi Abraham, Arpita Roy Choudhary, Padmini Sirkanungo, and Vivek Kute

15.1 Introduction

A 67-year-old male diabetic for 15 years on oral hypoglycemic agent (OHA) presents with diabetic kidney disease (DKD) stage 3B, his blood pressure is 173/94 mmHg on sitting, and 144/88 mmHg on standing. He has frothy urine, he is not a smoker, but takes 3 pegs of whisky for 30 years and consumes a nonvegetarian diet 3 times a week. BMI is 21 kg/m^2. His electrolytes are Na—139 mmol/L, K—4.18 mmol/L, Cl—102 mmol/L and HCo_3—24.8 mmol/L. His UACR is 3792 mg/g of cr, HbA1c—6%, Total protein—6.4 g/dL, albumin—3.9 g/dL, USG RK—9.4 × 4.1 cm, LK—9.8 × 4.6 cm, no post-void residual, prostate is 41 cc, 2D ECHO of heart showed mild concentric LV hypertrophy, normal LV systolic function with EF 63%, No RWMA. His retina examination is not done for over 3 years. Last eye examination was done 5 years ago. As his HbA1c is appropriate, his blood sugar by continuous glucose monitoring should be 100–180 mg/dL. OHA which is long acting should be avoided to prevent hypoglycemic episodes which happen once with blood sugar declines to 32 mg/dL. However, his SBP is >144 mmHg on standing position with nifidipine 20 mg twice a day. He has swelling in the legs which is attributed to nifidipine and proteinuria. He has received COVID-19 vaccine (Covaxin 3 doses), influenza, and pneumococcal vaccine. What should be the future treatment for him?

G. Abraham (✉)
Department of Nephrology, MGM Healthcare, Chennai, Tamil Nadu, India

A. R. Choudhary
IPGMER & SSKM Hospitals, Kolkata, West Bengal, India

P. Sirkanungo
MGM Medical college Superspeciality Hospital, Indore, Madhya Pradesh, India

V. Kute
Institute of Kidney Disease and Research Center, Ahmedabad, India

G. Abraham et al. (eds.), *Management of Diabetic Complications*, https://doi.org/10.1007/978-981-97-6406-8_15

Diabetic kidney disease (DKD) is the leading cause of chronic kidney disease world over and the Indian scenario is not different as reported by several investigators, it amounts to 30–40% of the chronic kidney disease (CKD) population. (ICKD Study) [1–3]. Indian Council of Medical Research ICMR-INDIAB study report identifies a sharp rise in the prevalence of diabetes mellitus in both urban and rural populations alike. In diabetic patients, 30–40% may develop end-stage kidney disease (ESKD), and disease progression may be effectively delayed by early intervention. Altered metabolic milieu, specific changes in glomerular hemodynamics, inflammation, and fibrosis are the primary mediators of kidney tissue damage, although the relative contribution of these mechanisms may vary among individuals and over the course of the natural history of DKD. The presence of DKD is also strongly associated with cardiovascular (CV) morbidity and mortality and has a major influence on survival. This review will cover the following issues to increase awareness and early intervention in course of the disease.

1. Natural history of Type 1 and Type 2 diabetes mellitus (DM).
2. Pathogenesis of Diabetic Kidney Disease (DKD): addressing the three pathways, namely, hemodynamic, metabolic, and inflammatory.
3. Possible microvascular and macrovascular complications.

Renal involvement in diabetes mellitus can be diabetic kidney disease, nondiabetic kidney disease (NDKD), or NDKD superimposed on DKD. "Diabetic nephropathy" is a diagnosis that refers to specific pathologic structural and functional changes seen in the kidneys of patients with DM (both T1/T2DM). Histological changes (Fig. 15.1) are described as predominant glomerular changes in kidney while the clinical counterpart is characterized by persistent albuminuria and a progressively declining renal function. Though traditionally the above glomerular findings are considered the hallmark of DKD changes, hyalinosis in both afferent and efferent arterioles, tubular atrophy and interstitial fibrosis with inflammatory changes in the glomerulus from the full spectrum of diabetic nephropathy. On the other hand, DKD is a clinical syndrome characterized by overt proteinuria. Albumin excretion level measured as UACR mg of albumin/gram of creatinine, with values >30 mg/gm of creatinine suggest excessive albumin excretion in urine, a hallmark of DKD and declining kidney function.

Pathological changes on biopsy include GBM thickening, to mesangial expansion, nodular glomerulo-sclerosis, global glomerulosclerosis, glomerulomegaly, vascular lesions, Interstitial Fibrosis tubular atrophy (IFTA), and tubular resorption droplets are all commonly seen (Fig. 15.1a, b, c, d).

In the early stages of DKD (stages 1 to 3), the kidneys on ultrasound examination are normal in size and shape unlike other kidney diseases.

DKD is a clinical diagnosis based on the decreased estimated glomerular filtration rate (eGFR) in diabetic patients and proteinuria, either or both, it does not indicate a specific pathological type. It can be from diverse causes, including hypertensive nephrosclerosis and unresolved acute kidney injury. The likelihood that DN is the cause of DKD varies widely depending upon the clinical circumstances.

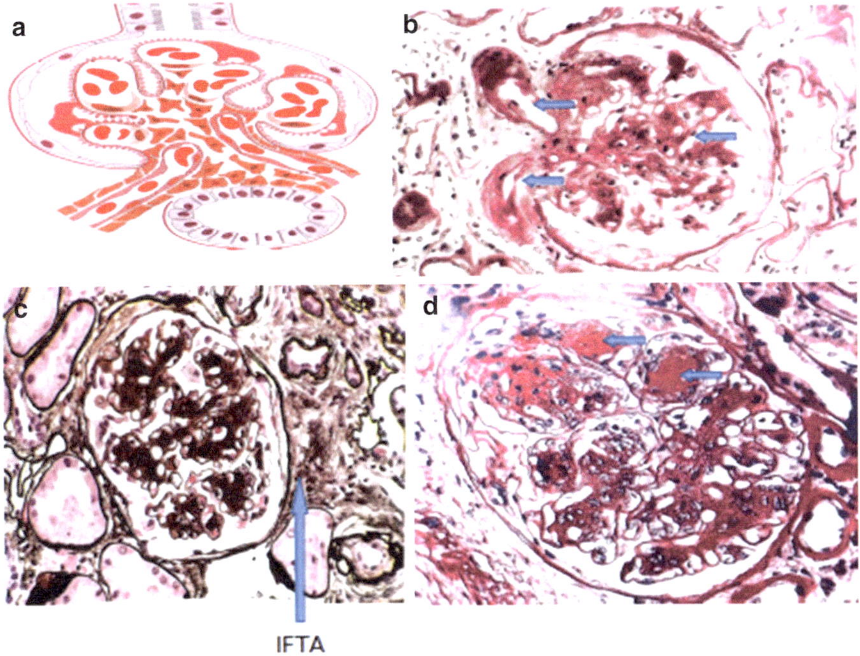

Fig. 15.1 (**a**) Normal glomerulus (**b**) Hyalinosis and glomerulosclerosis (**c**) Interstitial fibrosis tubular atrophy (**d**) Nodular glomerulosclerosis

Increased duration of diabetes particularly in Type 1 DM and to a lesser extent in T2DM, which is associated with micro or macroangiopathic complications, increases the likelihood that DN is the cause of DKD in that patient. Another subset of diabetic patients from 14% to 25% may have nonproteinuric DKD due to drugs such as RAAS-Blockers or unresolved acute kidney injury interstitial nephritis or coexistent obstructive component.

15.2 Natural History

Observations revealed that proteinuria appeared 11–23 years after the T1DM diagnosis, serum creatinine begins to increase 13–25 years later, and ESRD develops after 18–30 years. Over time, more sensitive assays to detect urinary albumin excretion were developed, which helped in detecting microalbuminuria; 30–300 mg/g creatinine. The development of overt proteinuria (macroalbuminuria > 300 mg/g creatinine) in most patients, occurs 5–10 years after the diagnosis of DM (Fig. 15.2). Presently, micro-albuminuria and macroalbuminuria are referred to A2 and A3, respectively, by the KDIGO (Kidney Disease: Improving Global Outcomes) chronic kidney disease (CKD) guideline (Fig. 15.2a, b).

a

Prognosis of CKD by GFR and albuminuria categories: KDIGO 2012				Persistent albuminuria categories, description and range		
				A1	A2	A3
				Normal to mildly increased	Moderately increased	Severely increased
				<30 mg/g <3 mg/mmol	30–300 mg/g 3–30 mg/mmol	>300 mg/g >30 mg/mmol
GFR categories (ml/min/1.73 m^2), description and range	G1	Normal or high	≥90	green	yellow	orange
	G2	Mildly decreased	60–89	green	yellow	orange
	G3a	Mildly to moderately decreased	45–59	yellow	orange	red
	G3b	Moderately to severely decreased	30–44	orange	red	red
	G4	Severely decreased	15–29	red	red	red
	G5	Kidney failure	<15	red	red	red

green, low risk (if no other markers of kidney disease, no CKD); yellow, moderately increased risk; orange, high risk; red, very high risk.

b

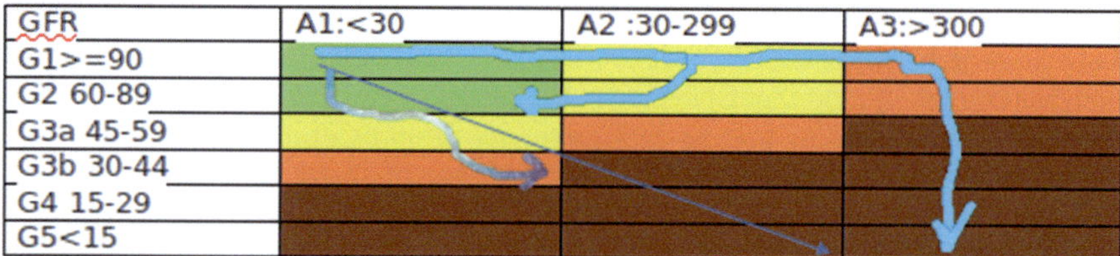

NOTE: GFR in ml/min/1.73m2 of BSA (body surface area)

DKD

NDKD

KIDNEY FAILURE

Fig. 15.2 (**a**) Heat map showing CKD stages and albuminuria. (**b**) Progression of Albuminuria and CKD in DKD

The natural history of diabetic nephropathy (Fig. 15.2) in longitudinally studied population of T2 DM was documented to have essentially similar pathology as in Type 1 DM, but as disease onset cannot be ascertained outside a study cohort situation, the patients of T2 DM can have established pathological changes of diabetic nephropathy even at diagnosis. Another important difference is in the cardiovascular (CV) mortality and morbidity spectrum, this macrovascular complication hardly appears before established renal failure in Type 1 DM patients, while it is common to have CV complication in T2DM patients even before renal disease has appeared. Kusmanns study also helped to capture a timeline of progression of diabetic nephropathy overt proteinuria to kidney function decline, and ultimately to ESRD. These stages of disease progression and the critical role of proteinuria assessment both for the purpose of diagnosis and prediction of likelihood of disease worsening have been subsequently confirmed by several international studies. The single best predictor of kidney function deterioration and diabetic nephropathy progression is proteinuria, which when combined with kidney function decline (eGFR) can be comfortably used for risk prediction and intensive target-based management is warranted. High proteinuria and apparently preserved Egfr may predict hyperfiltration injury, one form of hemodynamic insult to precipitate the earliest stage of diabetic nephropathy (Fig. 15.2a, b).

Based on studies of untreated patients with T1DM and Pima Indians with T2DM, the rate of GFR loss can be of the order of 7–12 mL/min/1.73 m^2/year. Treatment with renin-angiotensin system (RAS) inhibitors has reduced this rate of decline to 3–6 mL/min/1.73 m^2/year. Two large international trials in 1980 and 1990 have shown that T2DM cohorts with no nephropathy, early nephropathy and late nephropathy are likely to have, more CV deaths compared to renal disease progression.

In patients with CKD stage 3 (eGFR $\leq$ 60 mL/min/1.73 m^2), the risk of death is more than 10 times higher than the risk of progression to ESRD. Once on dialysis, the 5-year survival is less than 40% in these patients, predominantly owing to CVD-associated morbidity and mortality. Also, it has been observed that CKD patients have 13-fold more chance of dying from other causes rather than progression of ESRD accounting for death, the risk of death from CV is six-fold more.

15.3 Pathogenesis

A complex interaction of multiple mechanisms contributes to the development and progression of DN, which include interaction between hyperglycemia-induced metabolic and hemodynamic changes, the oxidative stress, and release of several inflammatory cytokines like TNF Alpha and TGF Beta together with genetic predisposition, ultimately setting the stage for kidney injury. In patients with type 1 or type 2 diabetes, the likelihood of developing diabetic nephropathy is markedly increased in those who have a sibling or parent with diabetic nephropathy. The likelihood of the offspring developing overt proteinuria was 14% if neither parent had proteinuria, 23% if one parent had proteinuria, and 46% if both parents had proteinuria [4–7].

15.3.1 Metabolic Factor

Hyperglycemia is crucial, but not a single causative factor. Hyperglycemia can increase VEGF, which can alter the podocyte permeability and may cause proteinuria. Three mechanisms have been postulated:

1. Nonenzymatic glycosylation-based advanced glycation end products (AGEs) formation: Their tissue deposition is initially reversible, later irreversible, they get deposited in mesangium and are responsible for increased mesangial matrix expansion and interact with the AGE receptor to reduce nitric oxide production. AGEs act to alter the soluble signal transduction like cytokines, hormones, and free radicals.
2. Activation of protein kinase C (PKC): Hyperglycemia activates PKC through DAG and oxidative stress. PKC when activated also activates Mitogen-Activated Protein Kinase (MAPK), and together act to increase the vasodilatory prostanoids leading to hyperfiltration injury, activating TGF Beta 1 it increases the mesangial cells and matrix, hallmark of DN on renal biopsy.
3. Acceleration of Aldose reductase pathway activation.

15.3.2 Hemodynamic Factor

The renal hemodynamic changes of hyperperfusion and hyperfiltration result from decreased vascular resistance in both afferent and efferent arterioles, more in afferent. The defective autoregulation is mediated by several vasoactive hormones mainly angiotensin, endothelin, and the action is enhanced by other cytokines like vascular endothelial growth factor A (VEGF-A), Transforming growth factor-β (TGF Beta), prostanoids, and nitric oxide. Albumin leakage from the glomerular capillaries is facilitated by these hemodynamic changes and released cytokines with overproduction of mesangial cell matrix and podocyte injury, and the associated increased mechanical strain from these hemodynamic changes result in pathological changes and clinical consequences.

15.4 Inflammation and Diabetic Nephropathy

Upregulation of kidney MCP-1 is documented in early human DN associated with macrophage recruitment, albuminuria, tubulointerstitial injury, and disease progression. Type 2 DM documented that aldosterone induces MCP-1 overproduction in intrinsic renal cells. Fidelio and Figaro-DKD trial showed the beneficial effect of finerenone as an adjuvant in diabetic nephropathy management [8]. Pathological changes in the tubule-interstitium are also described with typical diabetic nephropathy description.

Finerenone is a Novel Non-Steroidal Mineralocorticoid Receptor Antagonist (nSMRA) and is indicated for CKD and Type 2 diabetes (diabetic kidney disease/

DKD) to delay the progression of DKD [8]. Unlike other MRAs finerenone has exhibited better safety, potency, selectivity to the MR receptor. The passive antagonism forms a unstable receptor-ligand complex that blocks the cofactor recruitment which in turn prevents the transcription of proinflammatory and profibrotic genes hence attenuating the inflammation and fibrosis pathway. *FIDELITY which is a pre-specified pooled analysis of complementary Studies FIDELIO-DKD and FIGARO-DKD was done to perform individual patient-level analysis across the spectrum of CKD to provide more robust estimates of safety and efficacy of finerenone* versus *placebo. This analysis covered all the spectrum of CKD from Stage 1 to Stage 4.*

Finerenone reduced CV Composite outcome by 14% *(HR = 0.86 p = 0.0018)* which was driven by 22% risk reduction of hospitalization for heart failure and kidney composite endpoint was reduced by 23% *(HR = 0.77 p = 0.0002)*, this was predominantly driven by 20% reduction in ESKD events *and 30% reduction in ≥ 57% decrease in eGFR*. Finerenone has reduced Urinary Albumin to Creatinine Ratio (UACR) by 32% in fourth month from baseline. *Finerenone had reduced risk of New Onset of Heart Failure by 32% (HR = 0.68 p = 0.016) and new onset of atrial fibrillation by 29% (HR = 0.71 p = 0.0164) The CV and kidney benefits of finerenone were consistent irrespective of SGLT-2i use at baseline* Finerenone demonstrated good safety profile. In the trial, there was no reported mortality from study-related hyperkalemia. Finerenone is now recommended by ADA 2023, KDIGO guidelines 2022, ESH 2023 [8], ERA–ERBP and ESC 2023 for patients with T2DM and eGFR ≥25 mL/min/1.73 m^2, normal serum [K+], and albuminuria (ACR ≥ 30 mg/g) ESC 2023 has given Level 1A recommendation to prevent or reduce the risk of HF hospitalization.

15.4.1 Hyporeninemic Hypoaldosteronism

This is present in mild kidney injury due to dysfunction of the juxtaglomerular apparatus (JGA) due to hyalinosis of the blood vessels by diabetes mellitus [9]. It can present as hyperkalemia ($K \geq 5.5$ mmol/L) and symptoms due to depolarization, repolarization, and muscle defects such as cardiac arrhythmias and skeletal muscle weakness. Potassium homeostasis is maintained by urinary excretion of potassium which is equal to the quantity ingested minus fecal excretion. Potassium secretion by the distal convoluted tubule and cortical collecting duct and the later segment is predominantly responsible for potassium excretion. HH is a syndrome due to reduced aldosterone production from the adrenal gland and the release of renin from JGA. Autonomic insufficiency and increase in renal salt retention due to volume expansion contributes to the pathogenesis of HH while using K^+ retaining drugs such as RAAS blockade, aldosterone antagonist, beta-blockers, and insulin deficiency may lead to significant hyperkalemia. Caution should be exercised by treating doctors to be aware of HH. Management involves dietary advice, avoidance of drugs, monitoring of serum potassium, and use of loop diuretics along with potassium binding resins to maintain potassium ≥ 5 mmol/L.

15.4.2 Management of Diabetes Mellitus

KDIGO guidelines for management of diabetes mellitus including lifestyle modification, in addition to RAAS blockade, **SGLT2**i the introduction of mineralocorticoid receptor antagonist, and finerenone 10–20 mg dosage as an anti-inflammatory molecule have enabled many patients to improve or preserve GFR in addition to alleviation of albuminuria in author's experience (Fig. 15.3).

In addition to lifestyle changes, medical nutrition therapy and hypoglycemic agents are the mainstay in the treatment of diabetes mellitus (Fig. 15.4a, b). Antihypertensive therapy in patients with DKD typically consists of RAAS blockade with either an angiotensin-converting enzyme (ACE) inhibitor or angiotensin receptor blocker (ARB) titrated to maximally tolerated doses but not both simultaneously. Hyperkalemia is a potential adverse effect as DKD progresses. Calcium channel blockers, diuretics, centrally acting drugs, beta blockers, and vasodilators can be added to the therapy. Implement blood pressure lowering in patients with DKD to levels below 130/80 mmHg. On every hospital visit blood pressure should be checked as per the guidelines preferably using a digital BP monitoring apparatus both in supine and standing position. Many DKD patients may have significant postural hypotension, this should be recorded and appropriately advised. Home blood pressure (HBP) monitoring in the morning and evening is recommended.

As DKD progresses, hypoglycemia may ensue; therefore, the target of tight blood sugar control is inadvisable. Continuous glucose monitoring to maintain blood sugar between 100 mg/dl and 180 mg/dl is a good sustainable goal. It is better to avoid long-acting insulin as the pharmacokinetics and pharmacodynamics vary in progressive CKD. Glucagon indicated for severe hypoglycemic reactions in patients with diabetes treated with insulin 1 mg (1 unit) IM/SC/IV if no IV for dextrose. Repeat q15min once or twice; give high concentration dextrose as soon as it is available and if no response. Administer supplemental carbohydrates to replete glycogen stores. Frequent blood sugar measurements are mandatory while continuing

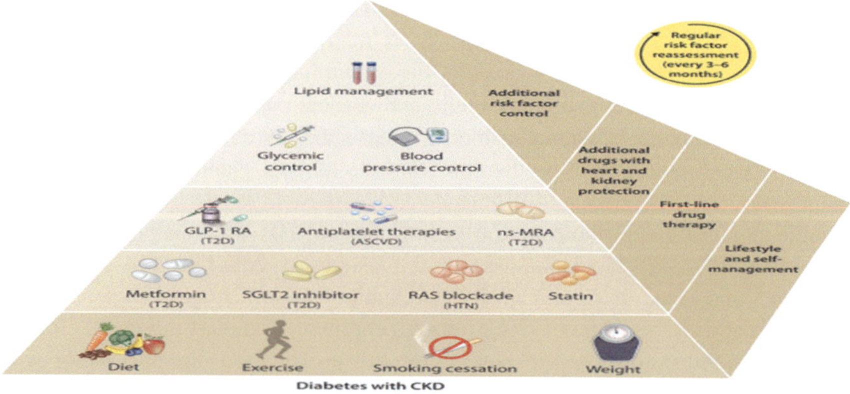

Fig. 15.3 Management algorithm for type 2 DM

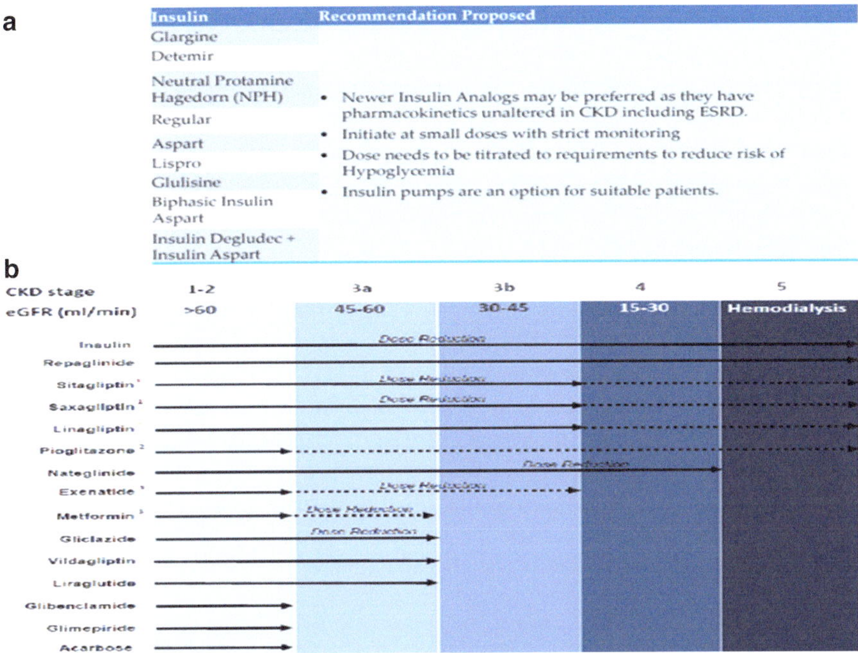

Fig. 15.4 (**a**) Injectable insulin analogs. (**b**) Dosage adjustment of hypoglycaemic agents with CKD

glucagon and high-concentration glucose infusion in DKD patients to avoid neuroglycopenia.

SGLT2i are new molecules in the treatment of DKD. However, caution should be exercised with regard to the following.

Diabetic ketoacidosis, head injury, volume depletion, hypotension, critical illness, emergency surgery, recurrent genital mycotic infections, lower limb amputation, and electrolyte imbalance.

Empagliflozin, Canagliflozin, and Dapagliflozin are commonly used SGLT2i, and their use is contraindicated for renoprotection below an eGFR 30 ml/min GLP1 analogs can be used upto an eGFR 15–29 mL/min (Dulaglutide).

The KDIGO 2022 guideline recommended initiation of an SGLT2i for patients with T2D and CKD who have eGFR ≥20 mL/min/1.73 m^2 (a change from ≥30 mL/min/1.73 m^2 in the 2020 guideline), and the ADA has also updated this threshold to ≥20 mL/min/1.73 m^2 in its living Standards of Care (from ≥25 mL/min/1.73 m^2 in the initial issue of the 2022 Standards of Care).

An SGLT2i with proven kidney or cardiovascular benefit is recommended for patients with T2D, CKD, and eGFR ≥ 20 mL/min/1.73 m^2. Once initiated, the SGLT2i can be continued at lower levels of eGFR.

15.5 Non-Proteinuric Diabetic Kidney Disease (NPDKD)

Non-proteinuric diabetic kidney disease/nonalbuminuric diabetic kidney disease (NADKD) is a phenotypic variant of DKD that is diagnosed in patients with a urine albumin creatinine ratio (UACR) of <30 mg/g. The prevalence of this phenotype is rising, ranging from 20% to 40% in patients with T2DM. It remains unclear whether nonproteinuric patients finally develop proteinuria and progress to ESKD (Fig. 15.5).

15.5.1 Pathogenesis

Remains to be fully elucidated and proposed to be multifactorial. It may involve age-associated renal senescence, hypertension, dyslipidemia, obesity, renal hypertensive and interstitial fibrosis, vascular disease, arteriosclerosis, cholesterol microemboli, lipid toxicity, inflammation, and masking of albuminuria by RAAS inhibitors. It has been hypothesized that tubulointerstitial injury contributes to the development of NADKD through the actions of liver fatty acid binding protein (L-FABP), a protein expressed in the proximal tubule.

15.5.2 Clinical Characteristics

It is more commonly diagnosed in females than males and associated with an older population group, non-smokers, and those who have had a shorter duration of diabetes mellitus [10]. They have lower levels of systolic blood pressure, diastolic blood pressure and normal levels of HbA1C, total cholesterol, low-density lipoprotein (LDL) and raised levels high-density lipoprotein (HDL). Lower prevalence of microangiopathy (represented as diabetic retinopathy).

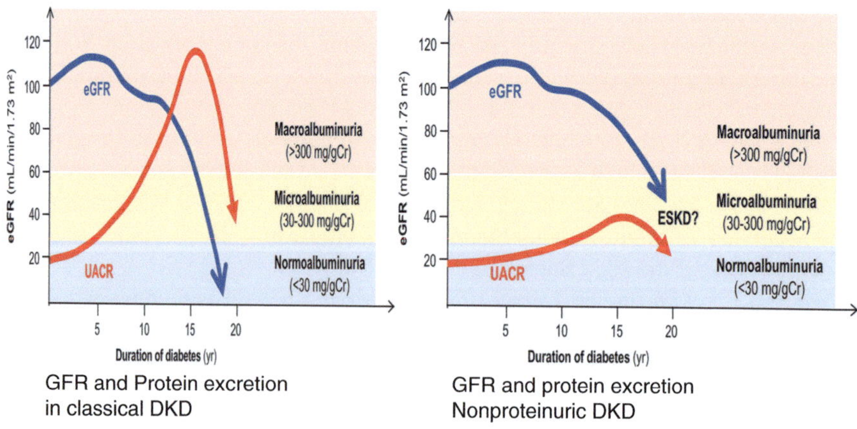

Fig. 15.5 Progression of proteinuric and nonproteinuric DKD

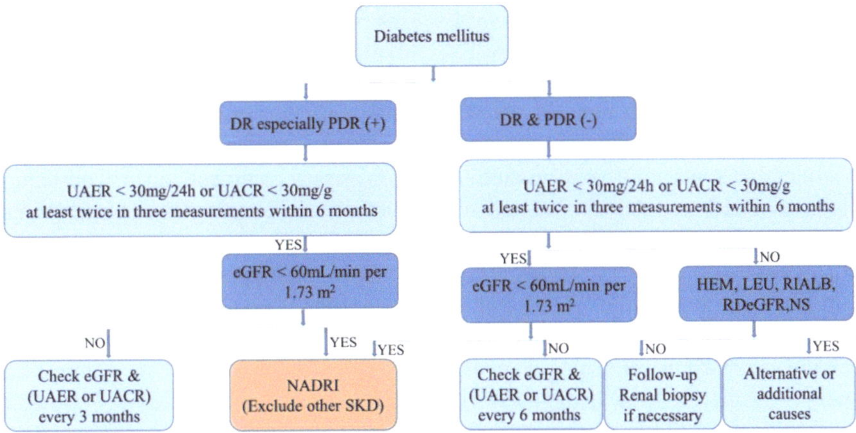

Fig. 15.6 Algoritham for diagnosis of urine albumin excretion in diabetic kidney disease

15.5.3 Proposed Diagnostic Criteria of Normoalbuminuric Diabetic with Renal Insufficiency (NADRI)

Diabetes diagnostic standards of the World Health Organization or American Diabetes Association (ADA) are applied to test and prove within 6 months, UACR < 30 mg/g, at least twice in three measurements and to avoid confounding by transient increases in conditions, such as exercise, fever, hematuria, urinary tract infection, and congestive heart failure. Detect within 6 months, eGFR < 60 mL/min/1.73 m^2 at least twice in three measurements, and exclude eGFR reduction caused by AKI and other reasons. Exclude other secondary nondiabetic kidney diseases.

15.5.4 Management and Prognosis

Currently, no clear guidelines on the management of NADKD different from albuminuric diabetic kidney disease. NADKD exhibits lower mortality and reduced risk of developing cardiovascular disease or ESKD compared with those diagnosed with albuminuric diabetic kidney disease, but higher mortality compared to diabetic patients with no kidney disease. It is possible that patients with nonproteinuric will become proteinuric or vice versa.

NADKD is a distinctive phenotypic variant of DKD, that typically presents with macrovascular complications, rather than microvascular complications. Underlying pathology of NADKD is different from the classical phenotype of DKD. It carries a better prognosis compared with patients with albuminuric diabetic kidney disease. Prevalence of NADKD is rising and more studies investigating the pathophysiological mechanisms are needed to allow for treatment options.

Avoidance of nephrotoxic agents such as NSAIDs, alternate medicines, and presence of obstructive uropathy requires careful attention in DKD patients.

Local or systemic infections are a concern in DKD patients. An appropriate investigation including system-specific care and antimicrobial dosing as per eGFR is necessary.

Tolerable physical activity including exercises is recommended for well-being [11]. As DKD progresses, anemia occurrence is not uncommon. This requires assessment of inflammatory state by measuring CRP, estimation of iron and vitamin B12 (vegans) and judicious use of erythropoiesis-stimulating agents (ESA) to maintain a hemoglobin level of 10–12 g/dl.

As DKD reaches stage IV CKD appropriate counseling with multi-tasking professionals regarding renal replacement therapy should be discussed. Access creation such as arterio-venous fistula (AVF) or permanent peritoneal dialysis catheter implantation should be undertaken. Preserve an upper limb with good-sized veins for AVF creation avoiding Intravenous injections and phlebotomy.

Vaccinations for prevention of hepatitis B, influenza, and pneumococcal infections are important components of patient care. Ophthalmology examination and necessary interventions to prevent vision loss are must. Protection of lower limbs and feet from infections and ulcers is mandatory. All patients with cardiovascular disease should have an assessment of heart functions with 12 lead ECG and 2D ECHO.

Divalent and trivalent cation and anion homeostasis become direnged as the CKD progresses. Hyperphosphatemia with serum inorganic phosphorus level > 4 mg/dL needs to be addressed with diet and phosphorus binders to reduce secondary hyperparathyroidism. Mineral bone disease (MND) is progressively increasing in prevalence due to dietary indiscretion. Assessment of parathyroid abnormality by estimation of fasting iPTH along with Ca^{+}, $PO4^{-}$, alkaline phosphatase is necessary as CKD progress beyond stage III. Progressive diabetic neuropathy along with neuropathy due to CKD may produce burning, pain, and numbness in the distal part of the limbs. Use of pregabalin, gabapentin, and amytriptyline may help to a certain extent. However, serum B12 deficiency should be managed as a reversible cause. While addressing metabolic acidosis (HCo_3^{-}) treatment with oral soda bicarbonate therapy (1 tea spoon full baking soda mixed in 1 glass of water) will alleviate effects of metabolic acidosis on body homeostasis by maintaining serum bicarbonate level ≥ 22 mmol/L. Dietary protein restriction to 1 g/kg body weight to 0.7 g/kg may be necessary along with K^{+} restriction to ≤1 mmol/kg/body weight, cholesterol intake 200 mg/day, salt <5 g/day, fiber 20 g/day, kilo calories 30/kg body weight (depends on the blood sugar), phosphorus minimum of 800 mg/day (reduce food with high phosphorus protein ratio), fluid intake as per daily weight, urine output and other fluid losses (50% of the solid food intake is converted to water). A wearable body composition monitoring device (BCM) by Inbioz is a useful tool that can be done in 1 minute to give estimation of water and nutritional status. Malnutrition is frequently seen in DKD patients as the CKD progresses and hence nutritional counseling is mandatory.

References

1. Umanath K, Lewis JB. Update on diabetic nephropathy: core curriculum 2018. Am J Kidney Dis. 2018;71(6):884–95. https://doi.org/10.1053/j.ajkd.2017.10.026.
2. Remuzzi G, et al. Nephropathy in patients with type 2 diabetes. NEJM. 2002;346:1145–51.
3. Kussman MJ, Goldstein HH, Gleason RE. The clinical course of diabetic nephropathy. JAMA. 1976;236(16):1861–3. https://doi.org/10.1001/jama.1976.03270170027020.
4. Mogensen CE, Christensen CK, Vittinghus E. The stages in diabetic renal disease. With emphasis on the stage of incipient diabetic nephropathy. Diabetes. 1983;32(Suppl 2):64–78. https://doi.org/10.2337/diab.32.2.s64.
5. Packham DK, Alves TP, Dwyer JP, Atkins R, de Zeeuw D, Cooper M, Shahinfar S, Lewis JB, Lambers Heerspink HJ. Relative incidence of ESRD versus cardiovascular mortality in proteinuric type 2 diabetes and nephropathy: results from the DIAMETRIC (diabetes mellitus treatment for renal insufficiency consortium) database. Am J Kidney Dis. 2012;59(1):75–83. https://doi.org/10.1053/j.ajkd.2011.09.017. Epub 2011 Nov 3
6. Maqbool M, Cooper ME, Jandeleit-Dahm KAM. Cardiovascular disease and diabetic kidney disease. Semin Nephrol. 2018;38(3):217–32. https://doi.org/10.1016/j.semnephrol.2018.02.003.
7. Trevisan R, Viberti G. Genetic factors in the development of diabetic nephropathy. J Lab Clin Med. 1995;126:342–9.
8. Agarwal R, Filippatos G, Pitt B, Anker SD, Rossing P, Joseph A, Kolkhof P, Nowack C, Gebel M, Ruilope LM, Bakris GL, FIDELIO-DKD and FIGARO-DKD investigators. Cardiovascular and kidney outcomes with finerenone in patients with type 2 diabetes and chronic kidney disease: the FIDELITY pooled analysis. Eur Heart J. 2022;43(6):474–84. https://doi.org/10.1093/eurheartj/ehab777.
9. Sondheimer JH. Hyporeninemic hypoaldosteronism, Medscape Jan 20, 2022.
10. Yamanouchi M, Furuichi K, Hoshino J, Ubara Y, Wada T. Nonproteinuric diabetic kidney disease. Clin Exp Nephrol. 2020;24(7):573–81. Published online 2020 Mar 31. https://doi.org/10.1007/s10157-020-01881-0.
11. Hussain S, Jamali MC, Habib A, Hussain MS, Akhtar M, Najmi AK. Diabetic kidney disease: an overview of prevalence, risk factors, and biomarkers. Clin Epidemiol Glob Health. 2021;9:2–6.

Acute Kidney Injury in Diabetes Mellitus

16

Priyanka Govindan, Milly Mathew, and Ashlin Shafi Rajesh

16.1 Introduction

Diabetes is the principal etiology for chronic kidney diseases (CKD) and end stage renal disease (ESRD) in the world. A multicenter study from India reported a composite prevalence of diabetic-CKD of around 62.3% [1] The incidence and prevalence of diabetes mellitus (DM) are exponentially increasing with the globalization of fast-food chains, adaptation of a sedentary lifestyle and increase in the prevalence of low-fiber high-calorie diets. Acute kidney injury (AKI) is unfortunately common and has serious clinical implications on mortality and morbidity. Worldwide, AKI is estimated to affect 13.3 million individuals in a year, a number which includes 5–10% of hospitalized patients, and 60% of intensive care patients, and >85% of this burden is contributed by developing countries [2–4].

This chapter aims to highlight the pathophysiology and factors involved in AKI in diabetics. By understanding these factors, the clinician will ultimately improve outcomes in patient care.

16.2 Classification of AKI

Several systems of classification have been used for AKI with KDIGO being the most widely accepted and used. The KDIGO classification is a clinical practice guideline modifying the RIFLE and AKIN criteria to provide a single unifying definition and staging system for AKI.

P. Govindan (✉)
Department of Nephrology, The Nephrology Clinic, Fort Collins, CO, USA

M. Mathew · A. S. Rajesh
MGM Healthcare, Chennai, India

G. Abraham et al. (eds.), *Management of Diabetic Complications*,
https://doi.org/10.1007/978-981-97-6406-8_16

Table 16.1 Natural course of AKI

	AKI	AKD
Duration	Within 7 days	≤3 months
Functional criteria	Increase in SCr by 50% within 7 days (or) Increase in SCr by 0.3 mg/dL (26.5 μmol/L) within 2 days (or) Oliguria for ≥6 hours	AKI (or) GFR < 60 ml/min/1.73 m² (or) Decrease in GFR by ≥35% (or) Increase in SCr by >50%
And /or		And /or
Structural criteria	Not defined	Marker of kidney damage (albuminuria, haematuria or pyuria are most common)

Lameire NH, Levin A, Kellum JA, Cheung M, Jadoul M, Winkelmayer WC, Stevens PE; Conference Participants. Harmonizing acute and chronic kidney disease definition and classification: report of a Kidney Disease: Improving Global Outcomes (KDIGO) Consensus Conference. Kidney Int. 2021 Sep;100(3):516–526. doi: 10.1016/j.kint.2021.06.028. Epub 2021 Jul 9. PMID: 34252450

The KDIGO guidelines define AKI as follows:

- Increase in serum creatinine by ≥0.3 mg/dL (≥26.5 micromole/L) within 48 h.
- Increase in serum creatinine to ≥1.5 times baseline, which is known or presumed to have occurred within the prior 7 days.
- Urine volume < 0.5 mL/kg/h for 6 h.

This classification should be used after adequate fluid resuscitation and the exclusion of urinary obstruction.

In 2020, KDIGO defined acute kidney disease as a term to define AKI lasting 7–90 days. AKI is included specifically within AKD, thus capturing all patients who have functional and/or structural abnormalities with implications for long- and short-term health (Table 16.1).

KDIGO Staging of AKI:

Stage 1—Increase in serum creatinine to 1.5 to 1.9 times baseline or increase in serum creatinine by ≥0.3 mg/dL (≥26.5 micromol/L), or reduction in urine output to <0.5 mL/kg/h for 6–12 h
Stage 2—Increase in serum creatinine to 2.0–2.9 times baseline, or reduction in urine output to <0.5 mL/kg/hour for ≥12 h
Stage 3—Increase in serum creatinine to 3.0 times baseline, or increase in serum creatinine to ≥4.0 mg/dL (≥353.6 micromol/L), or reduction in urine output to <0.3 mL/kg/h for ≥24 h, or anuria for ≥12 h, or the initiation of kidney replacement therapy, or, in patients <18 years, decrease in estimated glomerular filtration rate (eGFR) to <35 mL/min/1.73 m²

16.3 Pathophysiology

The pathophysiology of AKI is traditionally taught as prerenal, renal, and postrenal. Broadly speaking, DM causes AKI through the first two categories. In the setting of DM, AKI increases the risk of advanced CKD by more than threefold,

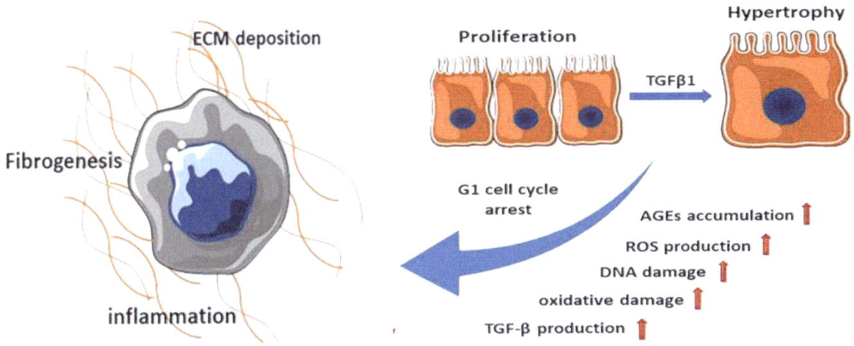

Fig. 16.1 Tubular injury showing normal inflammation and fibrosis in diabetes mellitus

independent of other risk factors of progression. Each episode of AKI has a cumulative dose-response association and doubles the risk of reaching stage 4 CKD [5].

Girman et al. reported that patients with type 2 diabetes have an increased risk for acute renal failure compared with patients without diabetes, even after adjustment for known risk factors, particularly in the elderly and those with other comorbidities such as chronic kidney disease, congestive heart failure, and hypertension [6].

There are several proposed mechanisms explaining how DM can contribute to AKI (Fig. 16.1):

1. Hyperglycemia causes an increase in oxidative stress and worsens the ischemia-reperfusion injury.
2. Cellular glucose overload induces mitochondrial dysfunction and kidney injury.
3. Hyperglycemia increases IL-6, TNF alpha, and IL 18.
4. Hyperglycemia can also induce endothelial dysfunction.

A more detailed description of molecular pathophysiology of specific scenarios is discussed below.

16.4 Diabetic Ketoacidosis and AKI

Patients suffering with DKA are prone to developing AKI. Factors that can predispose patients to AKI in the setting of DKA include older age, increased glucose, serum uric acid, white blood cell count (WBC), and hyperchloremia, heart rate (HR); decreased pH, serum albumin, bicarbonate, sodium; combined with coma on admission and preexisting chronic kidney diseases (CKD).

In pediatric patients, there is a higher frequency of AKI with DKA. Additionally, DKA-associated AKI episodes are correlated with long-term development of diabetic kidney disease [7].

16.5 Glucose Control and AKI in the ICU

There have been many studies done that compared glucose control in the intensive care unit by either conventional or intensified insulin therapy as it pertains to AKI incidence and outcomes. These studies were unable to conclude that stricter protocols improved outcomes. One of the larger studies conducted was the NICE-SUGAR [8] trial compared ICU patients receiving glucose control in a strict (81–108 mg/dL) versus a liberal (>108 and below 180 mg/dL) manner. Three thousand fifty-four patients were assigned to the first and 3050 individuals to the second group in a prospective manner. As a matter of fact, AKI incidence did not differ between the two categories, but survival was significantly lower in those receiving stricter insulin therapy (n = 829—27.5% versus 751—24.9% with $p = 0.02$). This in part was due to the higher occurrence of Hypoglycemia in the first group. The 2012 published version of the "KDIGO clinical practice guidelines for acute kidney injury" [9] therefore recommended target glucose levels of 110–149 mg/dL to be achieved in ICU patients.

16.6 CABG, AKI, and DM

Acute kidney injury is one of the most frequent postoperative complications after CABG. The AKI that develops after surgery can develop into CKD and thus have long-term implications for patients. More than 80 cohort studies have described the relationship between AKI and the risk of CKD and cardiovascular effects and mortality.

The TRIBE-AKI consortium evaluated plasma concentrations of pro-and anti-angiogenic markers in 1444 patients undergoing cardiac surgery and demonstrated that high postoperative levels of the anti-angiogenic factor vascular endothelial growth factor receptor 1 (VEGFR1) were associated with a high risk of AKI and mortality. By contrast, high levels of the pro-angiogenic factors VEGF and placental growth factor were associated with lower risk of AKI (31%) and mortality (54%) [10].

A study done by Wang et al. showed that independent of baseline renal function and cardiac function, DN was associated with an increased risk of AKI using the AKIN classification after CABG. The rate and severity of AKI were remarkably higher in patients treated with Insulin compared to those on oral hypoglycemics alone. A single measurement of A1c of more than 6% was also associated with an increased risk of AKI after CABG [11].

16.7 Drugs Associated with DM and AKI

Medications can vary in how they cause renal damage, either by directly causing nephrotoxicity or indirectly by causing renal hypoperfusion. Lapi et al. showed that the combination of ACEi/ ARB, diuretics, and NSAIDs was associated with the increased risk of AKI admissions to the hospital [12].

16.8 NSAIDS

NSAIDs block the COX 2 pathways decreasing prostacyclin synthesis thereby causing afferent arteriolar vasoconstriction and this coupled with the preferential vasodilation of the efferent arteriole impairs renal autoregulative ability. This renders the kidney to low renal perfusion and ischemic injury. The addition of a diuretic further worsens the situation causing it to be perfect storm for AKI.

16.9 SGLT2 Inhibitors

Among medications prescribed for DM, Metformin and SGLT-2 inhibitors have more renal consequences compared to others. The SGLT2 is a high-capacity, low-affinity transporter responsible for the bulk of glucose reabsorption in the proximal tubule. Under normal physiological conditions about 180 mg/dl of glucose of freely filtered by the tubule and is reabsorbed completely. This renders the urine for glucose if the blood sugar is at or below 180 mg/dL. In DM, this threshold for absorption of glucose increases to 250 mg/dL due to hypertrophy of the proximal tubule and increase in SGLT2 expression. These changes lead to a doubling in the percentage of filtered sodium reabsorbed thereby causing sodium-related volume expansion. This causes low renin hypertension and pseudo-hypoaldosteronism-related hyperkalemia associated with DM.

Naturally inhibiting the SGLT 2 receptor causes a 50% reduction in the absorbed glucose. This is less than the expected 805 due to the compensatory increase in the downstream SGLT1.

The increase in sodium delivery to the macula densa causes a tubuloglomerular feedback and afferent arteriolar vasoconstriction. This causes a decrease in intraglomerular pressure especially in patients on a RAAS blockade. This explains the 3–6 mL/min decrease in GFR noted in the first 2–3 weeks of initiation of therapy.

A decline of less than 30% GFR can be observed without interventions. A decline of greater than 30% GFR warrants evaluation for volume depletion as an osmotic diuresis causing toxic ATN can occur. In that scenario, a decrease in diuretic dose is recommended. In general, given the many benefits of SGLT 2 inhibitors, every effort should be taken to continue the drug. It is advisable to hold SGLT2i in the setting of volume depletion [13].

In a meta-analysis by Zhao et al., SGLT2 inhibitors were significantly associated with a lower risk of AKI than placebo. Moreover, SGLT2 inhibitors were significantly associated with a lower risk of AKI than both GLP-1RAs and DPP-4 inhibitors. Among these three novel glucose-lowering drugs, the results from the meta-analysis indicated that there was an 83.5 probability of SGLT2 inhibitors being the safest intervention for risk of AKI, followed by GLP-1RAs and DPP-4 inhibitors [14].

16.10 Metformin

Metformin remains the initial drug of choice for DM. Metformin is a biguanide oral antihyperglycemic agent used primarily for the treatment of diabetes. Metformin is excreted and filtered unchanged by the kidneys. Metformin inhibits mitochondrial glycerol-3 phosphate dehydrogenase (GPD2). This increases the accumulation of Cytosolic NADH. This decreases the conversion of lactate thereby causing lactic acidosis. Metformin can therefore cause lactic acidosis particularly in patients with a GFR of less than 30 mL/min.

There have been several studies demonstrating that the risk of lactic acidosis with Metformin is low [9, 15, 16]. The lactic acidosis that sometimes occurs with patients on metformin is more likely related to other etiologies rather than being due to metformin alone.

16.11 Metformin and Contrast Use

Due to the concern for AKI associated with contrast and the subsequent risk of metformin causing lactic acidosis in the setting of AKI, the ACR has issued guidelines for its use. These guidelines are as follows:

The Committee recommends that patients taking metformin be classified into one of two categories based on the patient's renal function (as measured by eGFR).

Category I consists of patients with no evidence of AKI and with eGFR ≥30 mL/min/1.73 m^2. In these patients, metformin may be continued as long as it is dosed appropriately for renal disease.

Category II consists of patients on metformin who are known to have acute kidney injury or severe chronic kidney disease (stage IV or stage V) or are undergoing arterial catheter studies that might result in emboli (atheromatous or other) to the renal arteries. In these patients, metformin should be temporarily discontinued at the time of or prior to the procedure, and withheld for 48 hours.

It is not necessary to discontinue metformin prior to contrast medium administration when the amount of gadolinium-based contrast material administered is in the usual dose range of 0.1–0.3 mmol/kg of body.

16.12 Contrast-Induced AKI and DM

Contrast-induced AKI is the third most common etiology of AKI. It is usually mild and reversible but, in some cases, can necessitate renal replacement therapy [17]. Due to often co-existing co-morbidities, diabetic patients more frequently require imaging studies.

The Contrast Media Safety Committee (CMSC) of the European Society of Urogenital Radiology (ESUR) made a most common renal function definition for CI-AKI: serum creatinine increases (sCr) ≥0.5 mg/dL (44.2 μmol/L) or ≥ 25% from baseline within 3 days after intravascular injection of iodine contrast media, while other causes of AKI are excluded.

The contrast administration causes AKI through different mechanisms. It can cause a direct toxicity causing decreased renal perfusion leading to hypoxia and ischemia. While this can happen in any patient, diabetics in particular are at risk due to endothelial dysfunction. This dysfunction creates an inability to counter the vasoconstriction caused by the contrast [18] thus accentuating the ischemia. The administered contrast also gets reabsorbed in the proximal convoluted tubule thereby causing an increase in Reactive oxygen species (ROS), mitochondrial dysfunction, and decreased ATP. This can lead to an increase in damage-associated molecular patterns [19, 20] and an increase in markers of inflammation like chemokines, interleukins, and TNF alpha. The chronic inflammation from innate immune response that is present in DM can worsen the contrast-induced nephropathy [21, 22].

16.13 Sepsis

In DM, the host's immune response is defective, predisposing those affected to infections. Sepsis causes a very robust SIRS reaction causing multi-organ damage. This causes stress induced hyperglycemia on top of preexisting impaired glucose tolerance leading to an increase in mitochondrial reactive oxygen species production. This ultimately leads to inactivation of antioxidants like eNOS and prostacyclin. The ensuing endothelial dysfunction in both micro and macrovascular beds and along with sepsis-induced increase in ROS disrupts homeostasis. The resulting hypoperfusion causes renal damage. Venot et al. reported that, although not associated with occurrence of AKI or need for renal replacement therapy (RRT), diabetic patients with severe sepsis or septic shock who experience acute kidney injury during the ICU stay more often required RRT, had higher serum creatinine values and had less often recovered to a creatinine level of less than 1.25 fold the baseline creatinine [23].

16.14 Oxalate Nephropathy in DM

Acute oxalate nephropathy is a rare entity that is characterized by massive deposition of oxalate in the renal parenchyma that presents clinically as AKI (Fig. 16.2). It can be from primary and secondary oxaluria. Primary oxaluria is from autosomal recessive disorders and causes recurrent stone disease. Secondary oxaluria is from excess oxalate absorption from the GI tract. Some oxalate precursors have been found with increased circulating levels in patients with DM, which are also identified as potential metabolite markers of DM in recent studies. A study by Bao et al. found that diabetic patients have higher oxalate excretion in the urine leading to higher rates of oxalate nephropathy in this population [24].

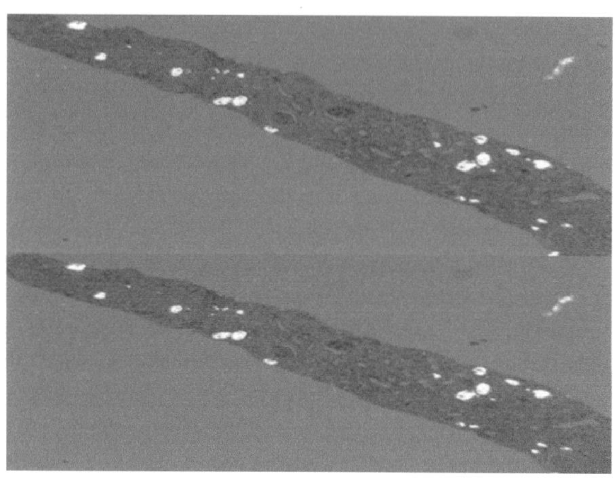

Fig. 16.2 Extensive oxalate deposition noted in a renal parenchyma in a diabetic patient

16.15 Markers of AKI

As established earlier, diabetes can predispose patients to AKI. AKI is often identified later in its clinical course and as such, the identification of early marks of AKI is an area of robust research (Fig. 16.3). These markers can be categorized by the compartment of the kidney that they affect. Glomerular biomarkers include molecules such as transferrin, immunoglobulin G, Ceruloplasmin, Type IV collegen, Laminin, glycosaminoglycans, Lipocalin-type prostaglandin D synthase, fibronectin, podocalyxin, and VEGF. These markers are freely filtered by the kidneys, but uptake is impaired due to decreased endocytosis by tubular cells during AKI. Tubular Biomarkers include nGAL, alpha 1 microglobulin, kidney injury molecule 1 (KIM-1), N-acetyl-β-D glucosaminidase, angiotensinogen, Cystatin C, liver type fatty binding protein, Nephrine, heat fatty binding protein, and advanced glycosylation end products. These products are expressed in tubular cells either constitutively or only during AKI but are released into the urine in that situation. A study by V. Williams et al. looked at the expression of urinary nGAL in pediatric patients presenting with DKA. They found that patients who responded to fluids had lower NGAL levels than those who did not respond. The NGAL levels correlated well with creatinine [25]. In 2013, a new biomarker of AKI was found. This marker is the arithmetic product of tissue inhibitors of metalloproteases 2 (TIMP2) and Insulin-like Growth Factor Binding Protein 7 (IGFBP7). This biomarker outperformed the above-listed markers [26] and is available commercially in the US and select countries in Europe as NephroCheck (Table 16.2).

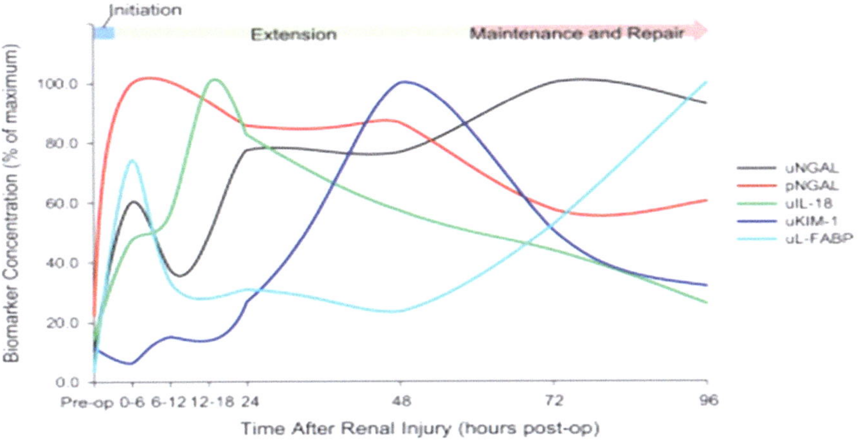

Fig. 16.3 AKI biomarker concentration after renal injury in cardiac surgery patients

Table 16.2 Different biomarkers of glomerular and tubular origin

Glomerular biomarkers	Tubular biomarkers
Transferrin	nGAL
Immunoglobulin G	Alpha 1 microglobulin
Ceruloplasmin	Kidney injury molecule 1
Type IV collagen	N-acetyl-β-D glucosaminidase
Laminin	Angiotensinogen
Glycosaminoglycans	Cystatin C
Lipocalin-type prostaglandin D synthase	Liver-type fatty binding protein
Fibronectin	Nephrine
Podocalyxin	Heat fatty binding protein
VEGF	Advanced glycosylation end products

16.16 Complications of AKI

AKI episodes cause both renal and nonrenal complications. CVS, mortality, risk of procedures. Renal complications include progression of CKD, ESRD, electrolyte and acid-base, and elevations in BP. Proteinuria is a complication of AKI and can result in incomplete renal recovery and sclerosis. Albuminuria at 90 days after a hospitalization complicated by AKI is a strong predictor of progressive decline in kidney function.

In a meta-analysis involving >1 million participants, low estimated glomerular filtration rates (eGFRs) and high urine albumin-to-creatinine ratios (ACRs) were associated with an increase in the risk of AKI, with hazard ratios (HRs) being generally higher among individuals with diabetes for any level of eGFR or ACR [27].

In one study by Harding et al., rates of dialysis-requiring AKI were approximately five times higher among persons with diabetes than among persons without diabetes [28], and whereas dialysis-requiring AKI rates appeared to plateau among individuals without diabetes, they have continued to increase in patients with diabetes.

The STARRT-AKI trial demonstrated that early initiation of kidney replacement therapy for patients with AKI in intensive care units did not improve outcomes.

16.17 Conclusion

In conclusion, AKI is a complication of DM with long-term renal complications. Several factors such as glucose control, medications, and infection both positively and adversely affect outcomes. The treating physician's understanding of the pathophysiology and knowledge of studies are crucial in improving outcomes for the patient. This knowledge will also help clinicians come up with strategies that will reduce the healthcare burden from these two common entities that often co-exist.

References

1. Dash SC, Agarwal SK, Panigrahi A, Mishra J, Dash D. Diabetes, hypertension and kidney disease combination "DHKD syndrome" is common in India. J Assoc Physicians India. n.d.; https://pubmed.ncbi.nlm.nih.gov/30341865/
2. Priyamvada PS, Jayasurya R, Shankar V, Parameswaran S. Epidemiology and outcomes of acute kidney injury in critically ill: experience from a tertiary care center. Indian J Nephrol. 2018;28:413–20.
3. Mehta R, Bagga A, Patibandla R, Chakravarthi R. Detection and management of AKI in the developing world: the 18th acute disease quality initiative (ADQI) international consensus conference. Kidney Int Rep. 2017;2:515–8.
4. Moore PK, Hsu RK, Liu KD. Management of acute kidney injury: core curriculum 2018. Am J Kidney Dis. 2018;72:136–48.
5. Thakar CV, Christianson A, Himmelfarb J, Leonard AC. Acute kidney injury episodes and chronic kidney disease risk in diabetes mellitus. Clin J Am Soc Nephrol. 2011;6(11):2567–72. https://doi.org/10.2215/CJN.01120211. Epub 2011 Sep 8. PMID: 21903988; PMCID: PMC3359576
6. Girman CJ, Kou TD, Brodovicz K, Alexander CM, O'Neill EA, Engel S, Williams-Herman DE, Katz L. Risk of acute renal failure in patients with type 2 diabetes mellitus. Diabet Med. 2012;29(5):614–21. https://doi.org/10.1111/j.1464-5491.2011.03498.x. PMID: 22017349
7. Huang JX, Casper TC, Pitts C, et al. Association of acute kidney injury during diabetic ketoacidosis with risk of microalbuminuria in children with type 1 diabetes. JAMA Pediatr. 2022;176:169.
8. NICE-SUGAR Study Investigators, Finfer S, Chittock DR, Su SY, Blair D, Foster D, Dhingra V, Bellomo R, Cook D, Dodek P, Henderson WR, Hébert PC, Heritier S, Heyland DK, McArthur C, McDonald E, Mitchell I, Myburgh JA, Norton R, Potter J, Robinson BG, Ronco JJ. Intensive versus conventional glucose control in critically ill patients. N Engl J Med. 2009;360(13):1283–97. https://doi.org/10.1056/NEJMoa0810625. Epub 2009 Mar 24
9. Richy FF, Sabido-Espin M, Guedes S, Corvino FA, Gottwald-Hostalek U. Incidence of lactic acidosis in patients with type 2 diabetes with and without renal impairment treated with metformin: a retrospective cohort study. Diabetes Care. 2014;37:2291–5.
10. Mansour SG, et al. The association of angiogenesis markers with acute kidney injury and mortality after cardiac surgery. Am J Kidney Dis. 2019;74:36–46. https://doi.org/10.1053/j.ajkd.2019.01.028.

11. Wang R, Zhang H, Zhu Y, Chen W, Chen X. The impact of diabetes mellitus on acute kidney injury after coronary artery bypass grafting. J Cardiothorac Surg. 2020;15(1):289. https://doi.org/10.1186/s13019-020-01312-x. PMID: 33004056; PMCID: PMC7528489
12. Lapi F, Azoulay L, Yin H, Nessim SJ, Suissa S. Concurrent use of diuretics, angiotensin converting enzyme inhibitors, and angiotensin receptor blockers with non-steroidal anti-inflammatory drugs and risk of acute kidney injury: nested case-control study. BMJ. 2013;346:e8525. https://doi.org/10.1136/bmj.e8525. PMID: 23299844; PMCID: PMC3541472
13. Palmer BF, Clegg, Deborah J. Kidney-protective effects of SGLT2 inhibitors. CJASN. 2023;18(2):279–89. https://doi.org/10.2215/CJN.09380822.
14. Zhao M, Sun S, Huang Z, Wang T, Tang H. Network meta-analysis of novel glucose-lowering drugs on risk of acute kidney injury. Clin J Am Soc Nephrol. 2020;16(1):70–8. https://doi.org/10.2215/CJN.11220720. Epub 2020 Dec 29. PMID: 33376101; PMCID: PMC7792639
15. Inzucchi SE, Lipska KJ, Mayo H, Bailey CJ, McGuire DK. Metformin in patients with type 2 diabetes and kidney disease: a systematic review. JAMA. 2014;312:2668–75.
16. Salpeter SR, Greyber E, Pasternak GA, Salpeter EE. Risk of fatal and nonfatal lactic acidosis with metformin use in type 2 diabetes mellitus. Cochrane Database Syst Rev. 2010;14:CD002967.
17. Nash K, Hafeez A, Hou S. Hospital-acquired renal insufficiency. Am J Kidney Dis. 2002;39(5):930–6. https://doi.org/10.1053/ajkd.2002.32766.
18. Calvin AD, Misra S, Pflueger A. Contrast-induced acute kidney injury and diabetic nephropathy. Nat Rev Nephrol. 2010;6(11):679–88.
19. Jensen H, Doughty RW, Grant D, Myhre O. A modified model of gentamicin induced renal failure in rats: toxicological effects of the iodinated X-ray contrast media ioversol and potential usefulness for toxicological evaluation of iodinated X-ray contrast media. Exp Toxicol Pathol. 2013;65(5):601–7. https://doi.org/10.1016/j.etp.2012.06.003.
20. Andreucci M, Faga T, Serra R, De Sarro G, Michael A. Update on the renal toxicity of iodinated contrast drugs used in clinical medicine. Drug Healthc Patient Saf. 2017;9:25–37. https://doi.org/10.2147/DHPS.S122207.
21. Navarro-Gonzalez JF, Mora-Fernandez C, Muros de Fuentes M, Garcia-Perez J. Inflammatory molecules and pathways in the pathogenesis of diabetic nephropathy. Nat Rev Nephrol. 2011;7(6):327–40. https://doi.org/10.1038/nrneph.2011.51.
22. Pichler R, Afkarian M, Dieter BP, Tuttle KR. Immunity and inflammation in diabetic kidney disease: translating mechanisms to biomarkers and treatment targets. Am J Physiol Renal Physiol. 2017;312(4):F716–F31. https://doi.org/10.1152/ajprenal.00314.2016.
23. Venot M, Weis L, Clec'h C, Darmon M, Allaouchiche B, Goldgran-Tolédano D, Garrouste-Orgeas M, Adrie C, Timsit JF, Azoulay E. Acute kidney injury in severe sepsis and septic shock in patients with and without diabetes mellitus: a multicenter study. PLoS One. 2015;10(5):e0127411. https://doi.org/10.1371/journal.pone.0127411. PMID: 26020231; PMCID: PMC4447271
24. Bao D, Wang Y, Yu X, Zhao M. Acute oxalate nephropathy: a potential cause of acute kidney injury in diabetes mellitus—a case series from a single center. Front Med (Lausanne). 2022;9:929880. https://doi.org/10.3389/fmed.2022.929880. PMID: 36133577; PMCID: PMC9484473
25. Williams V, Jayashree M, Nallasamy K, et al. Serial urinary neutrophil gelatinase associated lipocalin in pediatric diabetic ketoacidosis with acute kidney injury. Clin Diabetes Endocrinol. 2021;7:20. https://doi.org/10.1186/s40842-021-00133-8.
26. Kashani K, Al-Khafaji A, Ardiles T, et al. Discovery and validation of cell cycle arrest biomarkers in human acute kidney injury. Crit Care. 2013;17:R25.
27. James MT, Grams ME, Woodward M, et al. CKD prognosis consortium. A meta-analysis of the association of estimated GFR, albuminuria, diabetes mellitus, and hypertension with acute kidney injury. Am J Kidney Dis. 2015;66:602–12.
28. Harding JL, Li Y, Burrows NR, Bullard KM, Pavkov ME. US trends in hospitalizations for dialysis-requiring acute kidney injury in people with versus without diabetes. Am J Kidney Dis. 2020;75:897–907.

17 Renal Replacement Therapy in Patients with Diabetic Kidney Disease

Santosh Varughese and Georgi Abraham

17.1 Introduction

According to the American Diabetic Association, screening of all persons in the community is expected to be initiated at the age of 45 years, considered the average onset age for type II diabetes mellitus [1]. This effort to detect diabetes early and prevent complications of diabetes in patients is not uniform in many parts of the world, especially developing countries. In fact, over 50% of patients with chronic kidney disease stage 5 (CKD G5), i.e., estimated glomerular filtration rate (eGFR) less than 15 ml/min/1.73 m^2 present with this low eGFR at their initial hospital visit itself [2]. It, therefore, becomes crucial that early planning for renal replacement therapy (RRT) is done for patients with diabetic kidney disease (DKD) that are worsening relentlessly despite optimal medical care or nearing end-stage kidney disease (ESKD), i.e., requirement of RRT.

17.2 Planning and Choice of Renal Replacement Therapy

17.2.1 Arterio-Venous Fistula Construction

In general, construction of an arterio-venous fistula (AVF) is recommended when the eGFR drops below 15–20 ml/min/1.73 m^2 as part of the "Patient First: ESKD Life-Plan." [3] The primary objective of early vascular access creation is to avoid

S. Varughese (✉)
Department of Nephrology, Christian Medical College Vellore, Vellore, Tamil Nadu, India
e-mail: santosh@cmcvellore.ac.in

G. Abraham
Department of Nephrology, MGM Healthcare, Chennai, Tamil Nadu, India

G. Abraham et al. (eds.), *Management of Diabetic Complications*, https://doi.org/10.1007/978-981-97-6406-8_17

urgent/"crash-start" (i.e., without prior pre-dialysis education) dialysis via a cuffed or uncuffed intravascular dialysis catheter. There may be also an additional unforeseen benefit of early AVF construction. A propensity score matched retrospective study from Canada showed that early construction of AVF slows the progression of eGFR decline. The crude annual eGFR decline decreased from −4.1 ml/min/m^2 per year before AVF creation to −2.5 ml/min/m^2 per year after AVF creation [4]. The physiology behind this observation and its universality is a subject of debate in the nephrology community and more studies are awaited. While the debate rages on regarding the purported benefit of an AVF on eGFR deadline, the benefit of an early AVF in avoiding urgent necessity of a jugular or femoral dialysis catheter is incontrovertible and recommended to all who are eligible.

17.2.2 Peritoneal Dialysis Verses Hemodialysis

The pros and cons of peritoneal dialysis (PD) and hemodialysis (HD) need to be discussed by CKD educators, nurses, or physicians so that the patient can make an early, informed choice.

Initial data seemed to suggest that initiation of RRT with peritoneal dialysis (PD) was superior with mortality benefit lasting at least the first 2 years and hemodialysis (HD) offering a better likelihood of survival thereafter [5]. It was subsequently found that the data was fraught with residual confounding [6] and the mortality was similar when elective, outpatient, and incident dialysis patients are compared. Survival analysis of the Canadian Organ Replacement Register and the United States Renal Data System showed similar survival [7].

Most incident dialysis patients worldwide are started on HD via an internal jugular venous temporary access and are at risk of high mortality within the first 3 months [8]. "Crash start" patients are at a risk of increased mortality and risk of hospitalization and usually have a poor blood biochemistry at RRT initiation [9]. Patients initiating on "crash start" HD are at a higher risk of infections (including bacteremia and septicemia) than if they opt for PD. They have similar peritonitis rates compared to those with planned PD initiation but have more mechanical complications [10]. When patients present in the emergency department and need initiation of RRT, most patients are suitable candidates for a "crash start" with PD except in certain patients i.e. those with pulmonary edema, severely uncontrolled hypertension, uremic pericarditis/colitis, or severe hyperkalemia. Table 17.1 lists the advantages of

Table 17.1 Benefits of initiating RRT with peritoneal dialysis (modified) [11]

• Most ESKD patients are eligible for PD
• Similar survival between PD and HD
• Effective solute and water removal
• Slower decline in residual kidney function compared to HD
• Declining risk in PD-related peritonitis over the last decades
• Technically simple
• Greater autonomy and independence for patients compared to facility-HD
• Lower actual cost compared to HD in most countries

Table 17.2 Contraindications to RRT modalities (modified) [10]

Peritoneal dialysis	Hemodialysis
Absolute	*Absolute*
• Loss of peritoneal function producing inadequate clearance • Adhesions blocking dialysate flow • Surgically uncorrectable abdominal hernia • Abdominal wall stoma • Diaphragmatic fluid leak • Inability to perform exchanges in absence of suitable assistant	• No vascular access possible
Relative	*Relative*
• Recent abdominal aortic graft • Ventriculoperitoneal shunt • Intolerance of intraabdominal fluid • Large muscle mass • Morbid obesity • Severe malnutrition • Skin infection • Bowel disease	• Difficult vascular access • Needle phobia • Cardiac failure • Coagulopathy

initiating RRT with PD [11] and patients with DKD are to be counseled with respect to both HD and PD and patients are to make an informed choice.

While most patients with DKD could choose either RRT modality, patients with severe vascular access issues or severe congestive heart failure will benefit from being initiated on PD. Similarly, patient with multiple abdominal surgery scars and peritoneal adhesins will need to choose HD as RRT modality. Table 17.2 lists the contraindications of either RRT modality [10].

17.3 Transitioning to Dialysis

In the setting of multiple comorbidities and complications, transition from pre-dialysis to dialysis can be a difficult period for patients with diabetic kidney disease. Of late, nephrologists believe that initiation of dialysis slightly earlier in patients with DKD may have helped to decrease their morbidity and risk of mortality [12]. Integration of a multidisciplinary approach to deal with microvascular and macrovascular complications helps in rehabilitation of patients with DKD in coping with dialysis initiation. Whenever possible, maximal effort must be made to ensure that an AVF is constructed and available for use at least 1–2 months before HD initiation, to allow for the proper AVF maturation [13]. Patients with DKD are at a higher risk of atherosclerotic vascular disease and this may predispose to fistula function. Arterio-venous fistulas are preferred to be arterio-venous grafts (AVGs) as the former have greater longevity and AVG are at a higher risk of infections, though with better maturation rate compared to AVFs. AVGs have a lower risk of maturation failure and may be a better choice in certain patients [14].

17.4 Predictors of Mortality

The predictors of mortality in patients with DKD on dialysis are:

(a) **History of Smoking**

Smoking increases the risk of development and progression of macrovascular, and microvascular complications increase the risk of cardiovascular mortality and morbidity [15].

(b) **Known Coronary Artery Disease**

Prior coronary artery disease increases mortality risk in patients with DKD on dialysis. Within 2 years of dialysis imitation, the mortality in this population may be as high as 40% in patient with coronary artery disease verses 0% in though without coronary artery disease [16].

(c) **Autonomic Neuropathy and Orthostatic Hypotension**

Patients with DKD, especially while on hemodialysis, are at risk of signifiable orthostatic hypotension, and resulting fluid overload and increased risk of sudden cardia death and cerebrovascular accidents [17]. Autonomic neuropathy compounds vascular disease in patient with DKD [18]. Severe orthostatic hypotension can result in decreased cerebral perfusion and ischemic brain damage during or after a hemodialysis session [19].

(d) **Increased Inter-dialytic Weight Gain in Hemodialysis**

High inter-dialytic weight gain is a risk factor of mortality in patients with DKD [19].

(e) **Uncontrolled Hypertension**

Hypertension is more frequent in dialysis patients with DKD compared to nondiabetics. Over half of these patients require antihypertensive drugs for blood pressure (BP) control compared to a little over a quarter of nondiabetic dialysis patients [19, 20].

(f) **Degree of Blood Glucose Control**

Strict blood glucose control in diabetes has long been known to reduce the risk of microvascular complication of nephropathy, neuropathy, and retinopathy [21]. This is especially true in patients with type 1 diabetes mellitus. In type II diabetes, patients with DKD are being initiated on hemodialysis, uncontrolled blood sugars have been shown to be strong predictor of both cardiovascular mortality and long-term survival [22].

17.5 Survival of Patients with DKD on Dialysis

In the early days of RRT availability, patients with DKD had very poor survival [23]. This has doubtless improved through the years but their survival is significantly lower than their nondiabetic counterparts [24]. The five-year survival in these patients varies between 20% and 50% (in different countries) compared to 35% to 70% in nondiabetics [25]. Cardiovascular disease contributes to 23–54% of mortality in patients with DKD on hemodialysis [25]. Another major contributor to mortality is occurrence of infections and over three-fourths of infection-related deaths occur due to septicemia [26]. Catheter-associated blood-stream infections and infected diabetic foot ulcers, compounded by impaired cellular and humoral immunity and malnutrition are important contributors [27–29]. Traditional risk factors of mortality are not to be forgotten and these are ever present. Dyslipidemia, uncontrolled hypertension, left ventricular hypertrophy, hypoalbuminemia, and advanced age (with increasing longevity) all contribute to mortality in these patients [12].

Early initiation of dialysis and rehabilitation of patients with DKD is impeded by the presence of coronary artery disease (36% in type I diabetes mellitus and 40% in type II diabetes mellitus) [30], other cardiovascular complications of left ventricular hypertrophy cardiac failure and peripheral vascular disease (present in 31% of type I diabetics and 41% in type II diabetics) [31], amputation of lower limbs (up to 18% in DKD) and ophthalmological complications of retinopathy and blindness, which are present in up to 97% [32] and 30% [33, 34], respectively.

South Asian data suggest a 5-year survival of only 20.7% compared to 38.2% in nondiabetic dialysis DKD patients ($p < 0.001$) and this is greater in those with a poor socio-economic background [35].

Typically, hemodialysis is offered as twice or thrice weekly sessions of 4 h each. In patients with DKD who are being initiated on HD with indications of fluid overload or hyperkalemia rather than uremia, per se, one may be able to attempt incremental dialysis [36], where HD hemodialysis is offered with lower intensity in order to achieve symptom relief, electrolyte correction, and reasonable RRT for bodily functions to proceed normally. There is scheduled transition as required to thrice-weekly HD sessions when residual kidney function declines. There is also the provision of long-duration, daily nocturnal home HD or nocturnal in-centre HD which provide the additional benefits of normalization of serum phosphate, better correction of anemia, improved quality of life, and regression of left ventricular hypertrophy.

In initiating patients on PD, a chronic PD catheter made of silicone rubber is inserted surgically into the abdomen connecting the peritoneal cavity to the outside. The catheter forms the conduit for filling up the potential space of the peritoneal cavity with dextrose (or other substance) containing fluid. The osmotic gradient generated by the dextrose dissolved in the PD fluid causes ultrafiltration. There is a shift of osmoles from the peritoneal capillaries across the semipermeable barrier of the peritoneal membrane to the indwelling PD fluid. This results in a decrease in uremic solutes, abnormally high electrolytes like potassium and H^+ ions and increase in HCO_3 ions, etc. Peritoneal dialysis is usually done as continuous ambulatory peritoneal dialysis (CAPD) in which PD fluid exchanges are done typically three to four times daily. One may also opt for automated peritoneal dialysis (APD) in which exchanges are driven by a pump (part of a cycler device) and occur while the patient is asleep unlike CAPD when the exchanges are included by gravity. The long day dwell may be a higher concentration of dextrose (2.5% or 4.25%) to maintain the gradient longer. Icodextrin, a glucose polymer, that is poorly absorbed and thus enables the gradient to remain, is another alternative for use as a long day or night dwell.

Initiation of PD may be done by insertion of the chronic PD catheter via percutaneous method (either blind or with fluoroscopy visualization), mini-laparotomy or by advanced laparoscopy. The International Society of Peritoneal Dialysis (ISPD) guideline suggests that any of the techniques may be adopted depending on local expertise. The ISPD guideline suggests that a break-in period (between catheter insertion and start of regular exchanges) of 2 weeks be adopted whenever feasible. However, it has been shown that urgent-start PD with an ultra-short break-in period of 2 ± 2 days [37] could safely become the norm. Incidentally, patients with DKD being initiated on PD appear to be at a lower risk for catheter migration (1.5% vs. 9.7%, $p = 0.004$) and primary catheter non-function (5.3% vs. 15%, $p = 0.01$) compared to nondiabetics [37].

In patients with DKD and ESKD, PD offers the advantages of maintenance of residual kidney function, lower risk of hyperkalemia, less BP fluctuations (compared to HD), and preservation of vascular access. There is also the theoretical benefit of potentially adding insulin in the PD fluid instead of subcutaneous administration. However, this is only rarely, if ever, practiced clinically. These advantages of using PD for RRT come at a price of metabolic complications secondary to systemic glucose absorption from the PD fluid. Higher glucose levels in blood need to be controlled to avoid complications that result from hyperglycemia. The lipid profile of patients on PD is atherogenic and there may be increased risk of accelerated coronary artery disease. There also exists the risk of hyperglycemic increasing anorexia and secondary malnutrition. Gastroparesis is also observed to be worse in patients with DKD who are on PD. These patients have been observed to have at baseline, a less vascularized and thicker peritoneal membrane which may affect continuance of PD longer term [38].

17.6 Management of Diabetes Mellitus in Dialysis Patients

In up to a third of DKD patients on dialysis, spontaneous resolution of hyperglycemia and apparent normalization of glycosylated hemoglobin (HbA1C) is seen to occur. This is called "burnt-out diabetes." [39, 40] Multiple etiologies contribute to this phenomenon: (1) reduced clearance of exogenous insulin with renal dysfunction resulting in increased half-life of insulin in circulation, (2) reduced hepatic clearance of insulin that often improves after initiation of RRT, (3) increase in Guanidino compounds (as uremic toxins) act similar to the pharmacologic action of biguanides like metformin, (4) presence of protein energy malnutrition and (5) diabetic gastroparesis. Hence, the control of blood sugars is to be balanced against the risk of hypoglycemia and with target HbA1c <7.0% is deemed sufficient [41, 42]. HbA1c may be erroneous in patient with DKD on dialysis. Both metabolic acidosis and uremic toxins decrease the erythrocyte life-span and spuriously increase the HbA1c. Similarly, a spuriously low value of HbA1c is seen in the presence of severe anemia, requirement of multiple blood transfusions, use of erythropoiesis-stimulating agents (ESAs) and malnutrition. Fructosamine and glycated albumin are suggested alternatives to HbA1c but are not used in routine clinical practice, their main limitation being that the target range in CKD has yet to be established [22]. Insulin, and, when needed, oral hypoglycemic agents are used for blood sugar control in patients with DKD on dialysis. Commonly used classes of drugs like bigaunides, thiazolidinediones, dipeptidyl peptidase-4 (DPD4) inhibitors, glycogen-like peptide–1 (GLP1) analogs, alpha-glucosidase inhibitors, and sodium-glucose cotransporter-2 (SGLT2) inhibitors are avoided in patients with DKD and ESKD, or are used only rarely [22].

The dextrose-containing PD fluid has glucose concentration between 1.36 and 3.6 g/dl of glucose [38] and delivers up to 30% of daily calorie intake [43].

17.7 Kidney Transplantation in ESKD Patients with Diabetic Kidney Disease

In general, kidney transplantation is considered the best RRT modality with lower morbidity and modality, compared with chronic HD or PD [44]. In all patients with DKD who are eligible, transplantation is recommended as it offers improved survival with a mortality risk at 4 years almost 70% lower compared to those who are continued as dialysis [45], with a projected increase in longevity of 11 years. The mortality benefit of transplantation stems from reduced risk of cardiovascular events [46–49]. Preemptive transplantation, i.e. transplantation surgery before the requirement of dialysis initiation, has a mortality benefit compared to those who undergo transplantation after being on chronic dialysis for a while [50]. The benefit of preemptive transplantation extends to a decrease in death-censored graft survival as well.

An Indian study looking at kidney transplantation in DKD found similar in the 40–60 age group (DKD-43%) and age group 60 years and above (DKD-59%) (Fig. 17.1) [51].

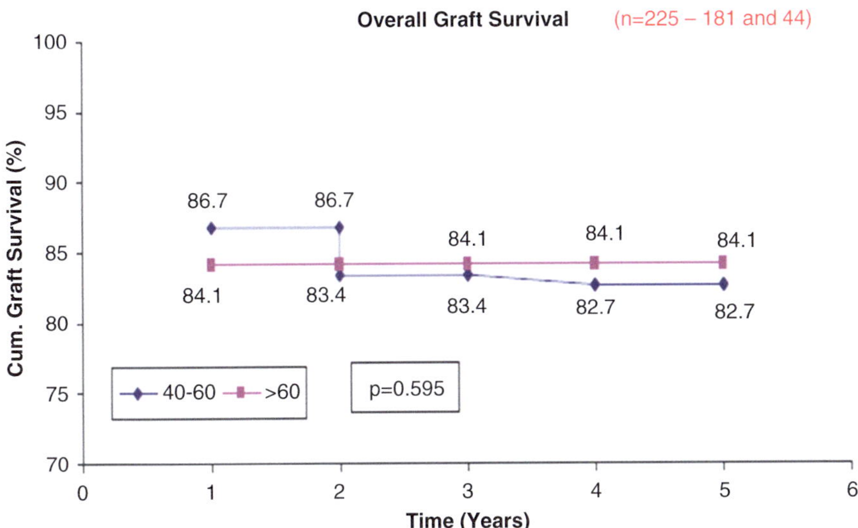

Fig. 17.1 Overall graft survival between ages 40 and 60 years and > 60 years

Living-donor transplantation results are better outcomes compared to decreased-donor transplantation. High kidney profile index (KDPI) deceased-donor transplantation has increased short-term but decreased longer-term mortality risk and is advised for consenting wait-listed DKD ESKD patients as it reduces waiting time considerably [52].

Kidney transplantation in diabetics requires detailed pre-transplant evaluation to look for occult cardiovascular disease, apart from the meticulous evaluation that all prospective renal allograft recipients are subjected to. Evaluation using a stress test or a coronary angiogram is needed to avoid resurgence of accelerated coronary artery disease in the post-transplant period with increased morbidity and mortality risk and also the antecedent risk of contrast-induced nephropathy when percutaneous coronary angiogram/angioplasty becomes necessary.

Similarly, evaluation of bladder capacity and compliance is necessary to decrease the risk of urinary tract infections (UTIs).

Post-transplant hyperglycemic needs to be strictly controlled as in the general population. This will reduce the risks of infections (especially UTIs), recurrence of DKD in the allograft, and other complications of uncontrolled diabetes. Dietary advice and nutritional counseling, as well as oral hypoglycemic agents and/or insulin is provided to all diabetic transplant recipients with frequent self-monitoring of capillary blood glucose and medication adjustment as needed for meticulous control of sugars.

A south Asian study of kidney transplantation in which nearly 60% of those above the age of 60 years and 45.3% in the age group 40–59 years were diabetic, the mortality was significantly higher in the more than 60 years age group [51].

17.8 Pancreas-Kidney Transplantation in Diabetic Kidney Disease

In select patients DKD on dialysis, simultaneous pancreas-kidney (SPK) transplantation is being offered with increasing success worldwide. A few sequential pancreas after kidney (PAK) transplants are also being done.

Usual candidates for SPK are patients with type 1 diabetes and advanced DKD/ESKD. Some type II DKD patients may be eligible candidates for SPK. In general, DKD patients with severe insulin resistance are not considered appropriate candidates for SPK. While the criteria to choose eligible patients with type II diabetes very between transplant centers, the generally accepted criteria for patient selection are:

1. Age less than 60 years.
2. Body mass index (BMI) <30 kg/m^{2}.
3. Insulin requiring status for a minimum of 3 years with a total daily insulin requirement <1 unit/kg/day.
4. Fasting C-peptide level < 10 mg/ml.
5. Presence of complicated or hyperlabile diabetes.

Where both renal and pancreas allografts survive beyond the first year following transplantation, SPK may confer superior long-term survival compared to kidney transplantation alone [53, 54]. The other potential advantage of SPK is a shorter waiting time for deceased-donor transplantation by virtue of a shorter list and prioritization for multi-organ transplantation, compared to those waiting for kidney transplantation alone.

Apart from patient selection, surgical skill and close follow up is paramount in these patients.

17.9 Conclusion

Diabetic kidney disease is major contributor to end-stage kidney disease worldwide. Either peritoneal dialysis or hemodialysis may be offered to all patients requiring renal replacement therapy. Kidney transplantation is an excellent option for these patients after pre-transplant cardiovascular and bladder evaluation in addition to routine evaluation. Preemptive kidney transplantation may confer some benefits and must be considered wherever feasible. In selected patients, simultaneous kidney-pancreas transplantation may be offered with improved survival benefit.

References

1. American Diabetes Association. Standards of medical care in diabetes—2015 abridged for primary care providers. Clin Diabetes. 2015;33(2):97–111. https://doi.org/10.2337/diaclin.33.2.97.
2. Varughese S, John GT, Alexander S, et al. Pre-tertiary hospital care of patients with chronic kidney disease in India. Indian J Med Res. 2007;126(1):28–33.
3. Lok CE, Huber TS, Lee T, et al. KDOQI clinical practice guideline for vascular access: 2019 update. Am J Kidney Dis. 2020;75(4):S1–S164. https://doi.org/10.1053/j.ajkd.2019.12.001.
4. Dupuis MÈ, Laurin LP, Goupil R, et al. Arteriovenous fistula creation and estimated glomerular filtration rate decline in advanced CKD: a matched cohort study. Kidney360. 2021;2(1):42–9. https://doi.org/10.34067/KID.0005072020.
5. Termorshuizen F, Korevaar JC, Dekker FW, et al. Hemodialysis and peritoneal dialysis: comparison of adjusted mortality rates according to the duration of dialysis: analysis of The Netherlands Cooperative Study on the Adequacy of Dialysis 2. J Am Soc Nephrol JASN. 2003;14(11):2851–60. https://doi.org/10.1097/01.asn.0000091585.45723.9e.
6. Noordzij M, Jager KJ. Survival comparisons between haemodialysis and peritoneal dialysis. Nephrol Dial Transplant. 2012;27(9):3385–7. https://doi.org/10.1093/ndt/gfs031.
7. Mehrotra R, Chiu YW, Kalantar-Zadeh K, Bargman J, Vonesh E. Similar outcomes with hemodialysis and peritoneal dialysis in patients with end-stage renal disease. Arch Intern Med. 2011;171(2):110–8. https://doi.org/10.1001/archinternmed.2010.352.
8. Khan IH, Catto GR, Edward N, MacLeod AM. Death during the first 90 days of dialysis: a case control study. Am J Kidney Dis. 1995;25(2):276–80. https://doi.org/10.1016/0272-6386(95)90009-8.
9. Mendelssohn DC, Malmberg C, Hamandi B. An integrated review of "unplanned" dialysis initiation: reframing the terminology to "suboptimal" initiation. BMC Nephrol. 2009;10:22. https://doi.org/10.1186/1471-2369-10-22.

10. Ivarsen P, Povlsen JV. Can peritoneal dialysis be applied for unplanned initiation of chronic dialysis? Nephrol Dial Transplant. 2014;29(12):2201–6. https://doi.org/10.1093/ndt/gft487.
11. Bargman J, François K. Evaluating the benefits of home-based peritoneal dialysis. Int J Nephrol Renov Dis. Published online December. 2014;7:447. https://doi.org/10.2147/IJNRD.S50527.
12. Akmal M. Hemodialysis in diabetic patients. Am J Kidney Dis. 2001;38(4):S195–9. https://doi.org/10.1053/ajkd.2001.27443.
13. Santoro D, Benedetto F, Mondello P, et al. Vascular access for hemodialysis: current perspectives. Int J Nephrol Renov Dis. 2014;7:281. https://doi.org/10.2147/IJNRD.S46643.
14. Li Q, Mao Z, Hu P, Kang H, Zhou F. Analysis of the short-term prognosis and risk factors of elderly acute kidney injury patients in different KDIGO diagnostic windows. Aging Clin Exp Res. 2020;32(5):851–60. https://doi.org/10.1007/s40520-019-01261-z.
15. Dierkx RI, van de Hoek W, Hoekstra JB, Erkelens DW. Smoking and diabetes mellitus. Neth J Med. 1996;48(4):150–62.
16. Joki N, Hase H, Ishikawa H, et al. Coronary artery disease as a definitive risk factor of short-term outcome after starting hemodialysis in diabetic renal failure patients. Clin Nephrol. 2001;55(2):109–14.
17. Page MM, Watkins PJ. Cardiorespiratory arrest and diabetic autonomic neuropathy. Lancet. 1978;1(8054):14–6. https://doi.org/10.1016/s0140-6736(78)90360-4.
18. Ewing DJ, Campbell IW, Clarke BF. Assessment of cardiovascular effects in diabetic autonomic neuropathy and prognostic implications. Ann Intern Med. 1980;92(2 Pt 2):308–11. https://doi.org/10.7326/0003-4819-92-2-308.
19. Shideman JR, Buselmeier TJ, Kjellstrand CM. Hemodialysis in diabetics: complications in insulin-dependent patients accepted for renal transplantation. Arch Intern Med. 1976;136(10):1126–30. https://doi.org/10.1001/archinte.136.10.1126.
20. Ritz E, Strumpf C, Katz F, Wing AJ, Quellhorst E. Hypertension and cardiovascular risk factors in hemodialyzed diabetic patients. Hypertension. 1985;7(6 Pt 2):II118-124. https://doi.org/10.1161/01.hyp.7.6_pt_2.ii118.
21. Diabetes Control and Complications Trial Research Group, Nathan DM, Genuth S, et al. The effect of intensive treatment of diabetes on the development and progression of long-term complications in insulin-dependent diabetes mellitus. N Engl J Med. 1993;329(14):977–86. https://doi.org/10.1056/NEJM199309303291401.
22. Rhee CM, Leung AM, Kovesdy CP, Lynch KE, Brent GA, Kalantar-Zadeh K. Updates on the management of diabetes in dialysis patients. Semin Dial. 2014;27(2):135–45. https://doi.org/10.1111/sdi.12198.
23. Ghavamian M, Gutch CF, Kopp KF, Kolff WJ. The sad truth about hemodialysis in diabetic nephropathy. JAMA. 1972;222(11):1386–9.
24. Ritz E, Rychlík I, Locatelli F, Halimi S. End-stage renal failure in type 2 diabetes: a medical catastrophe of worldwide dimensions. Am J Kidney Dis. 1999;34(5):795–808. https://doi.org/10.1016/S0272-6386(99)70035-1.
25. Shapiro F, Compty C. Hemodialysis in diabetics—1981 update. In: Diabetic renal retinal syndrome. Grune & Stratton; 1981. p. 309–19.
26. Jaar BG, Hermann JA, Furth SL, Briggs W, Powe NR. Septicemia in diabetic hemodialysis patients: comparison of incidence, risk factors, and mortality with nondiabetic hemodialysis patients. Am J Kidney Dis. 2000;35(2):282–92. https://doi.org/10.1016/s0272-6386(00)70338-6.
27. Vanholder R, Ringoir S. Infectious morbidity and defects of phagocytic function in end-stage renal disease: a review. J Am Soc Nephrol. 1993;3(9):1541–54. https://doi.org/10.1681/ASN.V391541.
28. Vanholder R, Ringoir S, Dhondt A, Hakim R. Phagocytosis in uremic and hemodialysis patients: a prospective and cross sectional study. Kidney Int. 1991;39(2):320–7. https://doi.org/10.1038/ki.1991.40.
29. Descamps-Latscha B, Herbelin A. Long-term dialysis and cellular immunity: a critical survey. Kidney Int Suppl. 1993;41:S135–42.

30. Schömig M, Ritz E. Cardiovascular problems in diabetic patients on renal replacement therapy. Nephrol Dial Transplant. 2000;15(Suppl 5):111–6. https://doi.org/10.1093/ndt/15.suppl_5.111.
31. Foley RN, Culleton BF, Parfrey PS, et al. Cardiac disease in diabetic end-stage renal disease. Diabetologia. 1997;40(11):1307–12. https://doi.org/10.1007/s001250050825.
32. Blagg CR. Visual and vascular problems in dialyzed diabetic patients. Kidney Int Suppl. 1974;1:27–31.
33. Goldstein DA, Massry SG. Diabetic nephropathy: clinical course and effect of hemodialysis. Nephron. 1978;20(5):286–96. https://doi.org/10.1159/000181239.
34. Jacobs C, Rottembourg J, Frantz P, Slama G, Legrain M. Treatment of end-stage renal failure in the insulin-dependent diabetic patient. Adv Nephrol Necker Hosp. 1979;8:101–26.
35. Vijayan M, Radhakrishnan S, Abraham G, Mathew M, Sampathkumar K, Mancha NP. Diabetic kidney disease patients on hemodialysis: a retrospective survival analysis across different socioeconomic groups. Clin Kidney J. 2016;9(6):833–8. https://doi.org/10.1093/ckj/sfw069.
36. Murea M, Moossavi S, Garneata L, Kalantar-Zadeh K. Narrative review of incremental hemodialysis. Kidney Int Rep. 2020;5(2):135–48. https://doi.org/10.1016/j.ekir.2019.11.014.
37. George N, Alexander S, David VG, et al. Comparison of early mechanical and infective complications in first time blind, bedside, midline percutaneous Tenckhoff catheter insertion with ultra-short break-in period in diabetics and non-diabetics: setting new standards. Perit Dial Int. 2016;36(6):655–61. https://doi.org/10.3747/pdi.2015.00097.
38. Duong U, Mehrotra R, Molnar MZ, et al. Glycemic control and survival in peritoneal dialysis patients with diabetes mellitus. Clin J Am Soc Nephrol. 2011;6(5):1041–8. https://doi.org/10.2215/CJN.08921010.
39. Park J, Lertdumrongluk P, Molnar MZ, Kovesdy CP, Kalantar-Zadeh K. Glycemic control in diabetic dialysis patients and the burnt-out diabetes phenomenon. Curr Diab Rep. 2012;12(4):432–9. https://doi.org/10.1007/s11892-012-0286-3.
40. Kalantar-Zadeh K, Kopple JD, Regidor DL, et al. A1C and survival in maintenance hemodialysis patients. Diabetes Care. 2007;30(5):1049–55. https://doi.org/10.2337/dc06-2127.
41. National Kidney Foundation. KDOQI clinical practice guideline for diabetes and CKD: 2012 update. Am J Kidney Dis. 2012;60(5):850–86. https://doi.org/10.1053/j.ajkd.2012.07.005.
42. Rossing P, Caramori ML, Chan JCN, et al. KDIGO 2022 clinical practice guideline for diabetes management in chronic kidney disease. Kidney Int. 2022;102(5):S1–S127. https://doi.org/10.1016/j.kint.2022.06.008.
43. Grodstein GP, Blumenkrantz MJ, Kopple JD, Moran JK, Coburn JW. Glucose absorption during continuous ambulatory peritoneal dialysis. Kidney Int. 1981;19(4):564–7. https://doi.org/10.1038/ki.1981.53.
44. Meier-Kriesche HU, Kaplan B. Waiting time on dialysis as the strongest modifiable risk factor for renal transplant outcomes: a paired donor kidney analysis. Transplantation. 2002;74(10):1377–81. https://doi.org/10.1097/00007890-200211270-00005.
45. Wolfe RA, Ashby VB, Milford EL, et al. Comparison of mortality in all patients on dialysis, patients on dialysis awaiting transplantation, and recipients of a first cadaveric transplant. N Engl J Med. 1999;341(23):1725–30. https://doi.org/10.1056/NEJM199912023412303.
46. Lentine KL, Brennan DC, Schnitzler MA. Incidence and predictors of myocardial infarction after kidney transplantation. J Am Soc Nephrol. 2005;16(2):496–506. https://doi.org/10.1681/ASN.2004070580.
47. Lentine KL, Schnitzler MA, Abbott KC, et al. De novo congestive heart failure after kidney transplantation: a common condition with poor prognostic implications. Am J Kidney Dis. 2005;46(4):720–33. https://doi.org/10.1053/j.ajkd.2005.06.019.
48. Meier-Kriesche HU, Schold JD, Srinivas TR, Reed A, Kaplan B. Kidney transplantation halts cardiovascular disease progression in patients with end-stage renal disease. Am J Transplant. 2004;4(10):1662–8. https://doi.org/10.1111/j.1600-6143.2004.00573.x.
49. Lentine KL, Rocca Rey LA, Kolli S, et al. Variations in the risk for cerebrovascular events after kidney transplant compared with experience on the waiting list and after graft failure. Clin J Am Soc Nephrol. 2008;3(4):1090–101. https://doi.org/10.2215/CJN.03080707.

50. Meier-Kriesche HU, Port FK, Ojo AO, et al. Effect of waiting time on renal transplant outcome. Kidney Int. 2000;58(3):1311–7. https://doi.org/10.1046/j.1523-1755.2000.00287.x.
51. Mohamed Ali AA, Abraham G, Khanna P, et al. Renal transplantation in the elderly: south Indian experience. Int Urol Nephrol. 2011;43(1):265–71. https://doi.org/10.1007/s11255-010-9887-4.
52. Massie AB, Luo X, Chow EKH, Alejo JL, Desai NM, Segev DL. Survival benefit of primary deceased donor transplantation with high-KDPI kidneys. Am J Transplant. 2014;14(10):2310–6. https://doi.org/10.1111/ajt.12830.
53. Gruessner AC, Gruessner RWG. Long-term outcome after pancreas transplantation: a registry analysis. Curr Opin Organ Transplant. 2016;21(4):377–85. https://doi.org/10.1097/MOT.0000000000000331.
54. Weiss AS, Smits G, Wiseman AC. Twelve-month pancreas graft function significantly influences survival following simultaneous pancreas-kidney transplantation. Clin J Am Soc Nephrol. 2009;4(5):988–95. https://doi.org/10.2215/CJN.04940908.

18 Diabetes Mellitus and Cancer

Jovita M. Martin Daniel, Gopinathan Mathiazhagan, and Insara Jaffer Sathick

18.1 Introduction

Diabetes mellitus is one of the common chronic diseases, which is very closely associated with cancer because they have shared risk factors. These risk factors are dietary factors such as obesity, sedentary lifestyle, and smoking. Type 1 DM or Juvenile diabetes or insulin-dependent DM (IDDM) is characterized by pancreatic failure to produce insulin due to beta cell destruction. It is prevalent in children, adolescents, and young adults. Type 2 DM (T2DM) is adult-onset diabetes which is due to the inability of cells/tissues to respond properly to the action of insulin and is non-insulin dependent. There is increasing evidence suggesting abnormal glucose homeostasis is an independent risk factor for the development of specific cancers and affecting the outcome [1, 2].

In the USA, adults with Type II DM who also had a history of cancer is 11.5% according to the National Health Interview surveys 2009–2010 in comparison to adults with Type 1 DM which is 8.9% [1, 2].

There has been a huge rise in DM globally more so in developing economies like India, China, and other South Asian countries. This is due to the increasing prevalence of obesity and unhealthy lifestyles. The estimates in 2019 revealed that 77 million individuals had DM in India. The numbers are expected to rise to over 134

J. M. Martin Daniel (✉)
Medical Oncology, MGM Healthcare, Chennai, Tamil Nadu, India

G. Mathiazhagan
Hematology, MGM Cancer Institute, Chennai, Tamil Nadu, India

I. J. Sathick
Department of Medicine, Renal Service, Memorial Sloan Kettering Cancer Center, New York, NY, USA

Weill Cornell Medical College, New York, NY, USA

G. Abraham et al. (eds.), *Management of Diabetic Complications*, https://doi.org/10.1007/978-981-97-6406-8_18

million by 2045. About 57% of these individuals remain undiagnosed in their prediabetic state. Type II DM, which accounts for a majority of the cases, can lead to multiorgan (microvascular and macrovascular) complications. These complications lead to increased premature morbidity and mortality among individuals with DM. This contributes to reduced life expectancy, increasing financial and social burdens of DM leading to enormous economic stress on the Indian health care system. The risk for DM is largely influenced by ethnicity, age, physical inactivity, obesity, unhealthy diet, and behavioral habits in addition to genetics and family history. Optimal control of blood sugar blood pressure and blood lipid levels prevents and delay the onset of DM complications. Recent studies show DM is also being linked to complications such as mental health, cancer, disability, and liver disease [1, 2].

Meta-analysis of large observational studies shows the specific risk for cancer pancreas with a relative risk (RR) being 1.94; colon cancer RR 1.38; rectal cancer RR 1.20; hepatocellular cancer RR 2.20: renal cancer RR 1.42; urinary bladder cancer RR 1.29; breast cancer RR 1.27; and endometrial cancer RR 2.10.

DM also increases the risk of mortality from cancer. The American Society Cancer Prevention study reported increased mortality of colon cancer with DM with a RR of 1.20; pancreatic cancer RR 1.48 males and females 1.44; bladder cancer RR 1.43 males, females 2.00; breast cancer RR 1.27 [3, 4].

18.2 Cancer Incidence and Diabetes

Because of metabolic aberrations, DM is significantly interlinked with cancer risk across all types of cancer with HbA1c > 5.7% having an increased risk of cancer ratio of 1.30.

18.3 Prediabetes and the Risk of Cancer

Prediabetes defined as IFG (FPG in the range either 5.6–6.9 mmol/l (100.8–124.2 mg/dl) or 6.1–6.9 mmol/l, (110–125 mg/dl) depending on the study) and/or IGT (2 h plasma glucose 7.8–11.1 mmol/l (140.4–199.8 mg/dl) during an OGTT) was clearly associated with an increased risk of cancer (RR 1.15; 95% CI 1.06, 1.23) in a meta-analysis, the risk increased with fasting plasma glucose (FPG) as low as 5.6 mmol/l (100 mg/dl) [5].

In this meta-analysis of 16 prospective cohort studies comprising more than 890,000 individuals, prediabetes at baseline was significantly associated with increased risks of cancer in the general population, particularly for liver, stomach pancreas, breast, and endometrium or colorectal cancer. However, this cancer relationship was not observed with other cancers such as cancer of the bronchus/lung, prostate, ovary, kidney, or bladder. Prediabetes is associated with obesity which is a recognized risk factor for cancer.

18.4 Metabolic Changes in Hyperglycemia

(a) Chronic hyperglycemia leads to chronic oxidative stress and accumulation of advanced glycation end products (AGE) which are carcinogenic drivers. Further augmented production of reactive **oxygen species** leads to oxidative DNA damage and cytotoxicity, which is correlated with the level of HbA1c in prediabetic patients.
(b) Hyperglycaemia also leads to oxidative stress through inhibition of the antioxidant function of thioredoxin. **Thioredoxin** is a ubiquitous oxidoreductase with antioxidant activity which will lead to dysregulated angiogenesis DM [5].
(c) The AGEs are detrimental to protein structures and cause extracellular matrix modification directly, and also indirectly by binding with the receptor for advanced glycation end products (**RAGE**).
(d) For the development of DM, insulin resistance is the core defect in Type II DM. Insulin **Resistance leads to increased availability of IGF1** and compensatory hyperinsulinemia promotes cancer cell growth.
(e) There is also evidence for association of genetic interferences and cancer in prediabetic individuals -**deficiency of nuclear receptor activator 5** increases the susceptibility to both glucose intolerance and hepatocellular carcinoma partially by increasing the interleukin 6 levels.
(f) Men with DM are less likely to develop prostate cancer with genetic mechanisms linked to the **HNF 1 Beta gene** (also known as TCF 2 gene). This leads to the protection of DM population from prostate cancer [5].

Hyperglycemia → Chronic Hyperglycaemia and related conditions as carcinogenic factors → Augmented production of reactive **oxygen species** → Oxidative damage DNA damage and cytotoxicity → Cancer

Hyperglycemia → Oxidative stress through inhibition of the antioxidant function of thioredoxin by Thioredoxin-interacting protein (TXNIP) (glucose-inducible gene) → Impaired angiogenesis found in diabetes mellitus → Cancer

Hyperglycemia → High rates of protein glycation leading to glycation end products (**AGEs**) → The results of AGEs are to damage the protein structures and cause extracellular matrix modification directly. → Eventually indirectly binding with the receptor for advanced glycation end products (**RAGE**). → Cancer → Cancer

Hyperglycemia → **Resistance leads to increased availability of IGF1** → compensatory hyper insulinemia → Cancer

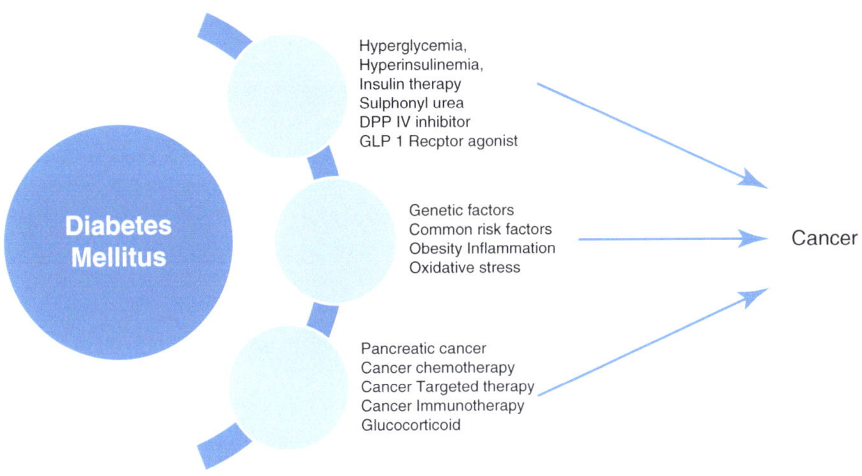

Fig. 18.1 Predisposing factors for cancer in DM

18.5 DM in Cancer Patients

A community-based cohort of 2481 adults who had cancer and DM showed increased case fatality with a hazard ratio of 1.34 compared to those without DM (Fig. 18.1) [6].

18.6 DM and Stage of Cancer Diagnosis

Women with a history of comorbidity of DM had a greater risk of developing early breast cancer in comparison to nondiabetic patients. Women also have increased tumor cell proliferation and metastasis in a pathophysiological environment of hyperglycemia and hypercholesterolemia [7, 8].

18.7 DM with Anticancer Therapy

The results of Dutch patients with breast cancer, colon cancer, ovarian cancer, or oesophageal cancer with a co-morbidity such as DM had a poor outcome, compared to those patients without DM [8, 9].

18.8 DM and Recurrence of Cancer or Second Malignancies

Patients with DM and cancer are less responsive to systemic therapy and radiotherapy therapeutic effects. Due to compromised therapies in view of increased adverse reactions and intolerance, the outcome is inferior leading to the recurrence of cancers or even developing second cancers. Clinical studies have alluded to the increase in the risk of recurrence with acute lymphocytic leukemia, colon cancer, and endometrial cancer [8, 9].

18.9 DM Complications in Cancer Patients on Treatment

DM is an established risk factor for infection and sepsis in the general population. Derr et al. have reported an association between pre-neutropenia glycemia and subsequent infection. An increase in the blood sugar level of 10 mg/dl or 0.56 mmol/l is associated with an increased risk ratio of 1.15, resulting in a rise in the mean pre-neutropenia and bloodstream infections. DM is also a chronic risk factor for multiple microvascular and macrovascular diseases such as atherosclerosis and coronary artery diseases [8, 10].

Some of the chemotherapeutic agents such as Oxaliplatin and Paclitaxel increase the risk of peripheral neuropathy adding to the pre-existing diabetic neuropathy complicates the treatment decisions.

18.10 Need for Multidisciplinary Approach

DM has a strong impact on over complete spectrum of cancers across the board on all stages and ages of cancer and in all subsites, in the development and progression of cancer until death. Therefore, there is a mandatory need for the involvement of a Multidisciplinary Team with Physicians, Surgeons, Oncologists, Endocrinologists, Primary Healthcare Physicians, Cancer care Nurses, Occupational and Physiotherapists in order to understand the biological mechanisms which are behind the metabolic aberrations of DM in the development of cancer and also with clinical outcomes. There is a mandatory requirement for recommendations on a healthy diet, increased physical activity proper weight management, psychotherapy, and lifestyle measures in order to mitigate the onset of DM and its control [8, 10].

18.11 Diabetic Medications and Cancer Risks

Several studies have alluded to the role of Metformin and Sulfonylurea having a protective role in cancer and others such as thiazolidinediones (TZD), insulin, AND incretin-based therapies are associated with cancer risk [11].

18.12 Sulfonylureas

Previous studies have indicated that patients treated with sulfonylureas (SUs) therapy have a high incidence of cancer and risk of cancer mortality, particularly in pancreatic and breast cancer. However, few randomized controlled trials show no statistically significant difference in the risk of cancer between the use of SUs and other treatments. SU has shown cytostatic effects on human breast cancer cell lines and anticancer activity against non-small cell lung carcinoma tissues and cell lines. However, there are contradictory statements on SU causing cancer and acting as anticancer drugs [11].

As an anti-cancer drug

1. SU is an inhibitor of ATP-binding cassette transporters. These transporters belong to a group of transmembrane proteins including multidrug-resistant proteins (MRPs). SU inhibits the MRP sensitizing cancer cells to chemotherapeutic agents.
2. SU through the mechanism of accumulation of calcein an MRP1 substrate, with overexpressed MRP1, the molecule glibenclamide might act as a sensitizer of cancer cells to chemotherapeutic agents. Glibenclamide suppresses cell growth, cell-cycle progression, epithelial-mesenchymal transition, and cell migration.
3. In addition, the glibenclamide down-regulates the expression of p70S6K and up-regulates the expression of Krüppel-like factor 4, a tumor suppressor.

18.13 Metformin

Metformin has shown potential mechanisms of inhibition of cancer development. It improves the increasing Insulin sensitivity and reduces the circulating Insulin. It activates the Adenosine monophosphate (AMP) Kinase with decreased protein synthesis and proliferation of cancer cells. In 2005, Ahmed et al. concluded that there is a reduction of cancer risk associated with Metformin usage to 23% alluding to a protective role of Metformin and cancer risk. 2012 meta-analysis open studies reported a significant decrease in cancer with Metformin usage in comparison to non-Metformin users [11].

18.14 Thiazolidinedione

The peroxisome proliferator-activated receptor-gamma (PPAR-γ)-activating TZD medications include pioglitazone and rosiglitazone, which are a class of drugs used to improve lipid and glucose metabolism in type II DM. However, preclinical studies have documented an increased risk of bladder cancer. The relative risk of bladder cancer with Pioglitazone usage after 100 days was 1.01 [11].

18.15 Insulin

Studies have shown increased cancer in type II DM with the use of **Insulin Glargine** is a long-acting Insulin monogenic. Studies have shown an increased risk of prostate and colorectal cancer and breast cancer to a relative risk of 1.3. The overall average ratio of Glargine Insulin compared to NPH insulin was 1.12. The outcome reduction within the initial Glargine intervention origin trial showed an incidence of cancer with a hazard ratio of 1. Hence the number of cancer cases was not sufficient to study associations with specific cancer types. MORE Registry which included 50,000 patients with an average of 1.2 years of follow-up reported that patients initiating insulin glargine rather than NPH were not at an increased risk for cancer [11].

18.16 Incretin-Based Therapies

Incretin-based therapies, including GLP-1 agonists and DPP-4 inhibitors, cause a significantly higher risk of pancreatic cancer, and thyroid cancer. Therefore, there is a requirement for continuous monitoring of cancer occurrence while augmenting the dosage [11].

18.17 Role of the Microbiome in Cancer and Diabetes

There is an evolving role of the gut microbiome in the development of diabetes and cancer. The human digestive tract carries 100 trillions of microbes including bacteria, viruses, yeast, protozoa, and fungi that interact with each other as well as the host and play a role in homeostasis and dysbiosis leads to the development of several diseases including cancer. Chronic inflammation leads to the production of carcinogenic byproducts along with impaired host immune function, and disruption of programmed cell death. In addition to these, there is emerging evidence that certain infection such as candidiasis, which is more common in patients with diabetes, has been associated with an increased risk of cancer [12].

18.18 Cancer and Solid Tumors

18.18.1 Pancreatic Cancer

Pancreatic cancer (Pac) or Ductal adenocarcinoma of the pancreas (DPAC) is the 13th most common type of cancer worldwide and is the fifth leading cause of death related to cancer in developed countries. Abnormal glucose homeostasis may be the underlying factor for pancreatic cancer with DM [2] (Table 18.1).

18.18.2 Gastric Cancer

Studies examining the relationship between DM and the risk of gastric cancer-related mortality have produced inconsistent results. However, 2 meta-analyses have alluded to a positive correlation [2] (Table 18.2).

18.18.3 Hepatic Cancer

Literature shows an association of DM with liver cancer. It has been suggested that low insulin and hyperglycemia in diabetes may account for increased virological response and impairment in HCV eradication leading to fibrosis which progresses to cirrhosis in patients with T2DM and HCV and HBV [2] (Table 18.3).

Table 18.1 Summary of included studies involving the association between diabetes and cancer risk

Cancer	References	Design	Characteristic findings
Pancreatic cancer	Gullo et al. (1994)	Cohort	DM in patients with pancreatic cancer is frequently of recent onset and is presumably caused by DM itself [13]
	Gupta et al. (2006)	Cohort	New-onset DM was associated with a significantly increased rate of pancreatic cancer diagnosis, particularly in the first 2 years after the diagnosis. Factors associated with pancreatic cancer diagnosis included younger age groups and the presence of gastrointestinal symptoms [14]
	Ogunleye et al. (2009)	Cohort	More studies are necessary to definitively identify DM as a risk factor for pancreatic cancer taking into consideration that approximately 10 years are needed to diagnose symptomatic pancreatic cancer [15]
	Batabyal et al. (2014)	Meta-analysis of 88 cohort	94% increase in the risk of pancreatic cancer in individuals with diabetes compared to nondiabetic individuals [16]
	Ben et al. (2011)	Meta-analysis	Diabetes duration <1 year was reported to carry the highest risk for DPAC [17]
	Pannala et al. (2008)	Case-control	The reported prevalence of DM in PaC varies from 4–64% [18]
	Chen et al. (2017)	Cohort [19]	According to recent reviews, patients with T2DM have three fold increase in developing pancreatic cancer Increased mortality risk for pancreatic cancer in diabetic subjects [19]

18.18.4 Colo-Rectal Cancer (CRC)

A systemic analysis of 8 studies showed a robust correlation of T2DM with the 1.21-fold; enhanced risk; and exhibited a greater risk of developing CRC than men [2] (Table 18.4).

18.18.5 Breast Cancer

There is a positive association between DM and the risk of breast cancer in females. Breast cancer has emerged as the most common cancer in females worldwide. Hyperinsulinemia alongside of hyperestrogenemia with low sex hormone-binding globulin (SHBG) levels are considered as etiological factors responsible for stimulating the proliferation of endometrial cells causing cancer [2] (Table 18.5).

Table 18.2 Summary of included studies involving the association between diabetes and cancer risk

Cancer	References	Design	Characteristic findings
Gastric cancer	**Chen et al. (2017)**	**Cohort** [19]	**A positive association between DM and gastric cancer** [19]
	Miao et al. (2017)	Meta-analysis	Meta-analysis of 22 studies and 13,538 incident gastric cancer found no association between DM and gastric cancer RR = 1.10 [20]
	Inoue et al. (2006)	Cohort	No association between diabetes history and gastric cancer risk [21]
	Kuruki et al. (2007)	Case-control	Inconsistent results [22]
	Ge et al. (2011)	**Meta-analysis**	**DM was significantly associated with GC with a RR of 1.41** [23]
	Xu et al.	Cohort	No significant association between DM and gastric cancer [24]
	Codick et al. (2015)	Cohort	No significant correlation between the incidence of gastric cancer and diabetes [25]
	Jee et al. (2005)	Cohort	Increased FBS and DM were considered as independent risk factors for gastric cancer, and the relative risk tends to increase accompanying an increased fasting serum glucose level [26]
	Lin et al. (2011)	Cohort	Hyperglycemia may account for the generation of imbalance in the energy/metabolism and impairment of the immune system that could progressively lead to gastric cancer [27]

Table 18.3 Summary of included studies involving the association between diabetes and cancer risk

Cancer	References	Design	Characteristic findings
Liver cancer	Davila et al. (2005)	Case-control	A 2.8-fold enhancement in the risk of hepatic cancer in diabetic individuals was reported. Positive correlation of diabetes with HCC [28]
	Lagiou et al. (2000)	Case-control	**Excess** risk of primary liver cancer in patients with DM [29]
	Ogunleye et al. (2009)	Cohort	A history of DM at baseline is highly associated with non-viral HCC [30]
	Li et al. (2017)	Case-control	The risk of HCC was found to double in diabetic individuals in China with chronic hepatitis [31]
	Wang et al. (2017)	Meta-analysis	The risk of hepatic cancer increased in diabetes associated with HBV, HCV, or alcoholic cirrhosis [32]
	Amano et al. (2014)	Cohort	HCC patients with HBV infection found T2DM to be significantly related to HCC [33]
	Gao et al. (2013)	Cohort	DM was found to be independent risk factor in HCC with cirrhotic patients with HBV infection [34]

HCV Hepatitis C virus, *HBV* Hepatitis B virus, *HCC* hepatocellular carcinoma

Table 18.4 Summary of included studies involving the association between diabetes and cancer risk

Cancer	References	Design	Characteristic findings
CRC	Zhu et al. (2017)	Meta-analysis 36 cohort studies with 2,299,012 participants	Patients with type II DM have a 5-year shorter survival (18%) in CRC compared to nondiabetic patients [35]
	Zelenko et al. (2014)	Meta-analysis	Increased risk of CRC in DM compared to nondiabetic patients [36]
	Guraya et al. (2015)	Meta-analysis of cohort studies	Diabetic females have a greater risk of developing CRC than men [37]

Table 18.5 Summary of included studies involving the association between diabetes and cancer risk

Cancer	References	Design	Characteristic findings
Breast cancer	Hardefeldt et al. (2012)	Meta-analysis [38]	Significantly increased risk of breast cancer in diabetic women compared to men and nondiabetic females [39]
	Larsson et al. (2007)	Meta-analysis	A 20% enhancement in the risk of breast cancer in type 2 DM [40]

Table 18.6 Summary of included studies involving the association between diabetes and cancer risk

Cancer	References	Design	Characteristic findings
Prostate cancer	Lee et al. (2016)	Meta-analysis	A 29% increase in prostate cancer-specific mortality was observed in preexisting diabetes [41]
	Bonvas et al. (2004)	Meta-analysis	People with diabetes have a significant decrease in risk of developing prostate cancer [42]

18.18.6 Prostate Cancer

Contrasting results were obtained for prostate cancer compared with other type of cancer. The presence of low levels of testosterone and Sex Hormone Binding Globulin (SHBG) in diabetic men could be responsible for these conflicting results [2] (Table 18.6).

18.19 DM and Haematological Cancers

The biological plausibility between DM and hematological malignancies is explained by immunosuppression, chronic inflammation, and lymphocyte dysfunction all of which are implicated in hematological malignancies [38, 43]. The immunosuppression, chronic inflammation, and lymphocyte (B and T cells) dysfunction may occur in the form of impaired neutrophil activity, suppression of cellular immunity, and alterations in serum immunoglobulin levels. Immune dysfunction is well known pathophysiologic mechanism in the development of lymphoproliferative disorders. Hyperinsulinemia, IGF overproduction, and upregulation of IGF-1 receptor are additional mechanisms contributing to malignancy. Given that obesity is a known major risk factor for development of diabetes, obesity may be an important mediator of the relationship between diabetes and malignancy [44]. Castillo JJ et al. has shown 22% overall increase in hematological malignancies in those patients having diabetes [45]. Population-based studies have shown that there is a 36% increase in all-cause mortality for patients of hematological malignancies with diabetes.

Apart from this, the drugs used in hematological malignancies that deregulate glycaemic control are steroids and L-asparaginase which are used in acute lymphoid leukemia. Cyclosporine commonly used as posttransplant immunosuppression in haematolymphoid malignancies can alter lipid profile and endothelial activation adding to end-organ complications of diabetes. Phosphatidyl kinase inhibitors like idelalisib used in the treat of Chronic lymphoid leukemia and low-grade lymphomas can induce hyperglycemia [46]. On the other hand, metformin the commonly used anti-diabetic improves glycemic profile and outcome in hematological malignancies. It also halts the progression from monoclonal protein of undetermined significance (MGUS) to multiple myeloma [47]. Pioglitazone a thiazolidone derivative used in DM leads to sustained molecular response when used in addition to imatinib for chronic myeloid leukaemia [48].

The above observations demand further studies to assess independent risk associated with DM beyond BMI, severity of diabetes, malignancy stage and glucose-lowering medications. Lifestyle modification not only reduces DM burden and its complications but may also potentially lower risk of malignancy and mortality.

18.20 Conclusion

- Adults with DM are more prone to develop cancer than their nondiabetic counterparts, particularly pancreatic cancer.
- Adults with DM are more prone to die of cancer than their nondiabetic counterparts.
- Adults with DM are associated with greater cancer-specific case fatality than adults with cancer, particularly with colorectal cancer.
- In patients with cancer, adults with DM had higher all-cause mortality than those without diabetes.
- Novel cancer biomarkers (CBs) are under study to evaluate the risk of cancer in both prediabetic and nondiabetic individuals.
- A plethora of cancer types has been documented to be remarkably linked to DM. Even though, an interesting phenomenon of "reverse causality" is also there, in which cancer leads to DM onset as in the case of pancreatic cancer.
- As opposed to the cancers of the endometrium, colorectal, breast, bladder, kidney, and non-Hodgkin lymphoma; prostate cancer is reported to be less likely in men with type 2 diabetes, which is seemingly attributed to the reduced levels of circulating testosterone in diabetic men [12].

References

1. Pradeepa R, Mohan V. Epidemiology of type 2 diabetes in India. Indian J Ophthalmol. 2021;69:2932–8.
2. Abudawood M. Diabetes and cancer: a comprehensive review. J Res Med Sci. 2019;24:94.
3. Yeh H-C, Golozar A, Brancati FL. Cancer and diabetes. 3rd ed. Diabetes in America.
4. Vigneri P, Frasca F. Diabetes and cancer. Endocr Relat Cancer. 2009;16:1103–23.
5. Huang Y, Cai X, Qiu M, Chen P, Tang H, Hu Y, Huang Y. A meta-analysis. Diabetologia. 2014;57:2261–9.
6. Zhu B, Shen Q. The relationship between diabetes mellitus and cancers and its underlying mechanisms. Front Endocrinol. 2022;13:800995. https://doi.org/10.3389/fendo.2022.800995.
7. Fleming ST, Pursley HG, Newman B, Pavlov D, Chen K. Comorbidity as a predictor of the stage of illness for patients with breast cancer. Med Care. 2005;43:132–40.
8. Yeh H-C, Golozar A, Brancati FL. Diabetes in America, 3rd edition. Chapter 29 Cancer and diabetes. 2022.
9. Van de Poll-Franse LV, Houterman S, Janssen-Heijnen ML, Dercksen MW, Coebergh JW, Haak HR. Less aggressive treatment and worse overall survival in cancer patients with diabetes: a large population-based analysis. Int J Cancer. 2007;120:1986–92.
10. Derr RL, Hsiao VC, Saudek CD. Antecedent hyperglycemia is associated with an increased risk of neutropenic infections during bone marrow transplantation. Diabetes Care. 2008;31:1972–7.
11. Olatunde A, Nigam M, Olatunde, et al. Cancer and diabetes: the interlinking metabolic pathways and repurposing actions of antidiabetic drugs. Cancer Cell Int. 2021;21:499.
12. Shahid RK. Diabetes and cancer: risk, challenges, management and outcomes cancers 2021, 13, 5735.
13. Gullo L, Pezzilli R, Morselli-Labate AM, Italian Pancreatic Cancer Study Group. Diabetes and the risk of pancreatic cancer. N Engl J Med. 1994;331:81–4.
14. Gupta S. New-onset diabetes and pancreatic cancer. Clin Gastroenterol Hepatol. 4(11):1366–72. quiz 1301
15. Ogunleye A, Ogston S, Morris A, et al. A cohort study of the risk of cancer associated with type 2 diabetes. Br J Cancer. 2009;101:1199–201.
16. Batabyal P, Vander Hoorn S, Christophi C, Nikfarjam M. Association of diabetes mellitus and pancreatic adenocarcinoma: a meta-analysis of 88 studies. Ann Surg Oncol. 2014;21:2453–62.
17. Ben Q, Xu M, Ning X, Liu J, Hong S, Huang W, et al. Diabetes mellitus and risk of pancreatic cancer: a meta-analysis of cohort studies. Eur J Cancer. 2011;47:1928–37.
18. Pannala R, Leirness JB, Bamlet WR, Basu A, Petersen GM, Chari ST. Prevalence and clinical profile of pancreatic cancer-associated diabetes mellitus. Gastroenterology. 2008;134(4):981–7. https://doi.org/10.1053/j.gastro.2008.01.039. Epub 2008 Jan 18. PMID: 18395079; PMCID: PMC2323514
19. Chen Y, Wu F, Saito E, Lin Y, Song M, Luu HN, et al. Association between type 2 diabetes and risk of cancer mortality: a pooled analysis of over 771,000 individuals in the Asia cohort consortium. Diabetologia. 2017;60:1022–32.
20. Miao ZF, Xu H, Xu YY, Wang ZN, Zhao TT, Song YX, et al. Diabetes mellitus and the risk of gastric cancer: a meta-analysis of cohort studies. Oncotarget. 2017;8:44881–92.
21. Inoue M, Iwasaki M, Otani T, Sasazuki S, Noda M, Tsugane S. Diabetes mellitus and the risk of cancer: results from a large-scale population-based cohort study in Japan. Arch Intern Med. 2006;166:1871–7.
22. Kuriki K, Hirose K, Tajima K. Diabetes and cancer risk for all and specific sites among Japanese men and women. Eur J Cancer Prev. 2007;16:83–9.
23. Ge Z, Ben Q, Qian J, Wang Y, Li Y. Diabetes mellitus and risk of gastric cancer: a systematic review and meta-analysis of observational studies. Eur J Gastroenterol Hepatol. 2011;23:1127–35.
24. Xu HL, Tan YT, Epplein M, Li HL, Gao J, Gao YT, et al. Population-based cohort studies of type 2 diabetes and stomach cancer risk in Chinese men and women. Cancer Sci. 2015;106:294–8.

25. Chodick G, Heymann AD, Rosenmann L, Green MS, Flash S, Porath A, et al. Diabetes and risk of incident cancer: a large population-based cohort study in Israel. Cancer Causes Control. 2010;21:879–87.
26. Jee SH, Ohrr H, Sull JW, Yun JE, Ji M, Samet JM. Fasting serum glucose level and cancer risk in Korean men and women. JAMA. 2005;293:194–202.
27. Lin SW, Freedman ND, Hollenbeck AR, Schatzkin A, Abnet CC. Prospective study of self-reported diabetes and risk of upper gastrointestinal cancers. Cancer Epidemiol Biomarkers Prev. 2011;20:954–61.
28. Davila JA, Morgan RO, Shaib Y, McGlynn KA, El-Serag HB. Diabetes increases the risk of hepatocellular carcinoma in the United States: a population-based case-control study. Gut. 2005;54:533–9.
29. Lagiou P, Kuper H, Stuver SO, Tzonou A, Trichopoulos D, Adami HO. Role of diabetes mellitus in the etiology of hepatocellular carcinoma. J Natl Cancer Inst. 2000;92:1096–9.
30. Ogunleye AA, Ogston SA, Morris AD, Evans JM. A cohort study of the risk of cancer associated with type 2 diabetes. Br J Cancer. 2009;101:1199–201.
31. Li X, Xu H, Gao Y, Pan M, Wang L, Gao P. Diabetes mellitus increases the risk of hepatocellular carcinoma in treatment-naïve chronic hepatitis C patients in China. Medicine (Baltimore). 2017;96:e6508.
32. Wang M, Yang Y, Liao Z. Diabetes and cancer: epidemiological and biological links. World J Diabetes. 2020;11(6):227–38. https://doi.org/10.4239/wjd.v11.i6.227. PMID: 32547697; PMCID: PMC7284016
33. Amano K, Kawaguchi T, Komatsu R, Kawaguchi A, Miyajima I, Ide T, Kakuma T, Sata M. Time trends of clinical characteristics in hepatocellular carcinoma patients with chronic hepatitis B virus infection: a field survey between 2000 and 2012. Mol Clin Oncol. 2014;2:927–34.
34. Gao C, Fang L, Zhao HC, Li JT, Yao SK. Potential role of diabetes mellitus in the progression of cirrhosis to hepatocellular carcinoma: a cross-sectional case-control study from Chinese patients with HBV infection. Hepatobiliary Pancreat Dis Int. 2013;12:385–93.
35. Zhu B, Wu X, Wu B, Pei D, Zhang L, Wei L. The relationship between diabetes and colorectal cancer prognosis: a meta-analysis based on the cohort studies. PLoS One. 2017;12:e0176068.
36. Zelenko Z, Gallagher EJ. Diabetes and cancer. Endocrinol Metab Clin N Am. 2014;43:167–85.
37. Guraya SY. Association of type 2 diabetes mellitus and the risk of colorectal cancer: a meta-analysis and systematic review. World J Gastroenterol. 2015;21(19):6026–31. https://doi.org/10.3748/wjg.v21.i19.6026. PMID: 26019469; PMCID: PMC4438039
38. Smedby KE, Hjalgrim H, Askling J, et al. Autoimmune and chronic inflammatory disorders and risk of non-Hodgkin lymphoma by subtype. J Natl Cancer Inst. 2006;98(1):51–60. https://doi.org/10.1093/jnci/djj004.
39. Hardefeldt PJ, Edirimanne S, Eslick GD. Diabetes increases the risk of breast cancer: a meta-analysis. Endocr Relat Cancer. 2012;19:793–803.
40. Larsson SC, Mantzoros CS, Wolk A. Diabetes mellitus and risk of breast cancer: a meta-analysis. Int J Cancer. 2007;121:856–62.
41. Lee J, Giovannucci E, Jeon JY. Diabetes and mortality in patients with prostate cancer: a meta-analysis. Springerplus. 2016;5:1548.
42. Bonovas S, Filioussi K, Tsantes A. Diabetes mellitus and risk of prostate cancer: a meta-analysis. Diabetologia. 2004;47:1071–8.
43. Engels EA, Cerhan JR, Linet MS, et al. Immune-related conditions and immune-modulating medications as risk factors for non-Hodgkin's lymphoma: a case-control study. Am J Epidemiol. 2005;162(12):1153–61. https://doi.org/10.1093/aje/kwi34110.
44. Birmann BM, Neuhouser ML, Rosner B, et al. Prediagnosis biomarkers of insulin-like growth factor-1, insulin, and interleukin6 dysregulation and multiple myeloma risk in the Multiple Myeloma Cohort Consortium. Blood. 2012;120(25):4929–37. https://doi.org/10.1182/blood-2012-03-417253.
45. Castillo JJ, Mull N, Reagan JL, Nemr S, Mitri J. Increased incidence of non-Hodgkin lymphoma, leukemia, and myeloma in patients with diabetes mellitus type 2: a meta-analysis of observational studies. Blood. 2012;119(21):4845–50. https://doi.org/10.1182/blood-2011-06-362830.

46. Cheah CY, Fowler NH. Idelalisib in the management of lymphoma. Blood. 2016;128(3):331–6. https://doi.org/10.1182/blood-2016-02-702761.
47. Chang S-H, Luo S, O'Brian KK, et al. Association between metformin use and progression of monoclonal gammopathy of undetermined significance to multiple myeloma in US veterans with diabetes mellitus: a population-based retrospective cohort study. Lancet Haematol. 2015;2(1):e30–6. https://doi.org/10.1016/s2352-3026(14)00037-4.
48. Rousselot P, Prost S, Guilhot J, et al. Pioglitazone together with imatinib in chronic myeloid leukemia: a proof of concept study. Cancer. 2017;123(10):1791–9.

Diabetes Mellitus and Hearing Loss 19

Ashish Varghese, Sunil Sam Varghese, and Jubbin Jagan Jacob

19.1 Introduction

Hearing loss is a very common problem worldwide, affecting one in three individuals above the age of 65 years. Hearing loss can have a significant impact on the quality of life of an individual. Bilateral hearing loss can result in social isolation of the affected individuals, which can affect their psychological wellbeing. This is known to reduce their cognitive capability leading to decreased physical activity. Hearing loss is known to be an independent risk factor in the development of dementia and depression. Hearing loss is also associated with an increased risk of fall in the elderly.

Diabetes mellitus is associated with higher odds (OR-2.12) of developing sensorineural hearing loss when compared with individuals without diabetes mellitus [1]. Hearing impairment is not dependent on the type of diabetes mellitus (type 1 or type 2) [2]. Hearing impairment is present across all the frequencies in diabetes mellitus, however at higher frequencies the hearing thresholds are affected to a greater extent [1, 3]. Microvascular angiopathy leads to retinopathy, nephropathy, neuropathy, and macrovascular complications to the development of cerebrovascular accidents,

A. Varghese (✉)
Endocrinology and Metabolism, Christian Medical College Hospital, Ludhiana, Ludhiana, Punjab, India

ENT- Thyroid Surgery Dept, Christian Medical College, Ludhiana, Punjab, India

S. S. Varghese
ENT- Thyroid Surgery Dept, Christian Medical College, Ludhiana, Punjab, India

J. J. Jacob
Endocrinology and Metabolism, Christian Medical College Hospital, Ludhiana, Ludhiana, Punjab, India

G. Abraham et al. (eds.), *Management of Diabetic Complications*,
https://doi.org/10.1007/978-981-97-6406-8_19

cardiovascular disease, and peripheral vascular disease, these are responsible for the morbidity associated with diabetes mellitus [1]. Thus, the physician actively screens their patients for these co-morbid conditions while treating diabetes mellitus, in order to detect them early and facilitate early intervention. There are many studies that conclude that there is an association between diabetes mellitus and hearing loss, but screening for hearing loss in patients with diabetes mellitus is not universally followed.

19.2 Ultrastructure and Function of THE Cochlea

The inner ear comprises the cochlea and the vestibule. The cochlea resembles a snail-like structure with approximately two and a half turns. It is housed in the petrous bone and is comprised scala vestibuli, scala media, and scala tympani. The scala media is filled with endolymph which has high concentration of potassium (140 mmol/l). The perilymph fluid occupies the scala vestibuli and scala tympani and is similar to the CSF fluid in its biochemical composition. The scala media is separated from the scala vestibuli and scala tympani by Reissner's membrane and the basilar membrane, respectively. The sensory epithelium of the cochlea is the organ of Corti, comprising narrow strip of hair cells called the inner hair cells placed over the basilar membrane. These hair cells have cilia projecting out of their apical cuticular plate called stereocilia. They are arranged such that the shortest cilia is at one end and the longest at the other. The tips of the cilia are connected to the shaft of the adjacent taller cilia by tip links, which activate mechanoelectrical transduction channels when there is relative movement between the stereocilia. Opening of these channels allows potassium to enter the haircells and depolarize them. The haircells are innervated by cochlear nerve through the spiral ganglions. The spiral ganglion cells are bipolar nerve cells that carry the electrical information from the haircells to the cochlear nucleus. There are outer hair cells also that are mainly supportive in function and play a role in modulating the movement of the basilar membrane. There is a highly vascular structure at the lateral wall of the scala media called the stria vascularis. The marginal cells of the stria vascularis separate it from the scala media, these cells are responsible for maintaining the integrity and volume of the endolymph. The relative high concentration of potassium in the endolymph, allows a positive potential difference of +80 mV between the scala media and scala tympani called the endocochlear potential. This potential difference is crucial for depolarization of the inner hair cells.

The scala vestibuli communicates with the saccule through the ductus reunion (Fig. 19.1).

The footplate of stapes lies over the oval window which opens into the saccule. Piston-like movements of the stapes will cause pressure changes in the endolymph of the saccule which will be transmitted to the cochlea. The difference in the pressure between the scala vestibuli and scala tympani will make the basilar membrane vibrate causing movement of the stereocilia and consequent depolarization of the inner haircells and the cochlear nerve.

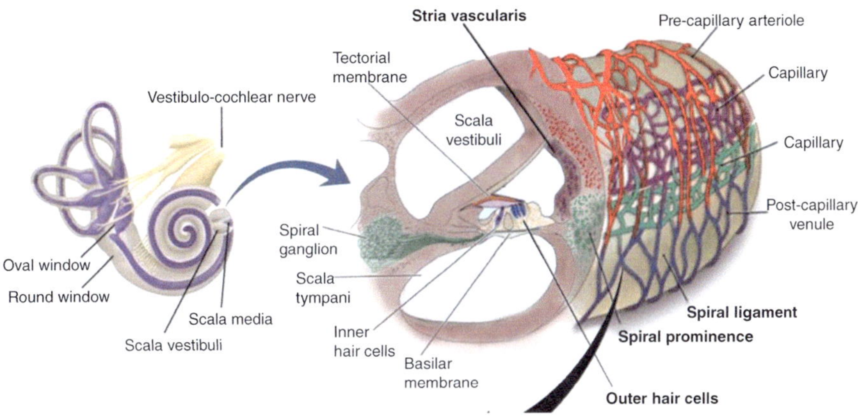

Fig. 19.1 Ultrastructure and function of the cochlea

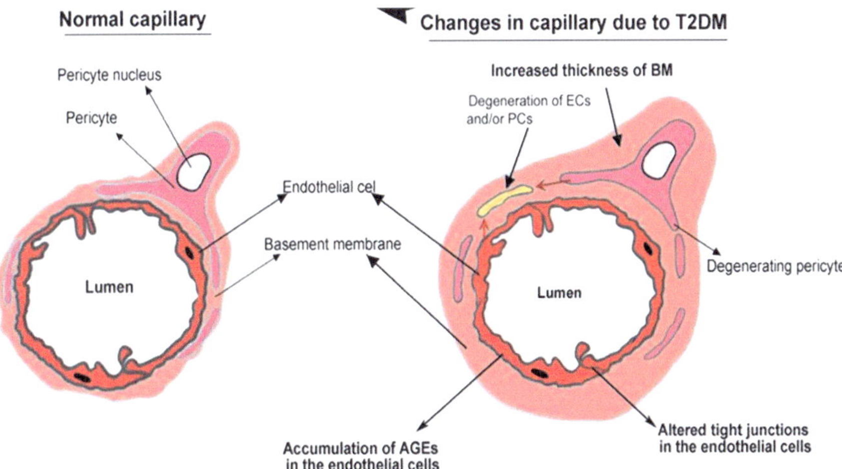

Fig. 19.2 Abnormalities were seen in the vessel wall of cochlea

19.2.1 Pathophysiology

19.2.1.1 Microangiopathy

Microvascular angiopathy occurs in diabetes mellitus due to the glycoprotein accumulation in the tunica intima and endothelial damage [1]. Cochlea being a microvascular-rich structure is extremely sensitivity to the blood supply and microangiopathy of the blood vessels in the cochlea can manifest as reduced hearing acuity (Fig. 19.2). Stria vascularis is a vascular-rich structure in the lateral wall of the cochlea and is responsible for maintaining the endo-cochlear potential. Atrophy of the stria vascularis and thickening of the vessel walls in the stria vascularis was seen more frequently in the cochlea of individuals treated for diabetes mellitus than in those without diabetes mellitus [4]. Reduction of spiral ganglion cells is seen in the cochlea of individuals with diabetes mellitus [5]. The vessel wall in the basilar membrane also showed significant thickening with outer hair cell damage [4]. The thickness of the capillary walls in the stria vascularis was found to be 10–20 times thicker in individuals with diabetes mellitus than in normal controls [5]. These changes are identical to vascular changes seen in other organs affected by diabetic microangiopathy [5]. These vessel changes can significantly reduce the blood flow to the haircells and the marginal cells of the stria vascularis violating the integrity and function of these cells.

Hyperglycemia induces an overproduction of superoxides through the mitochondrial electron transport chain and this plays a critical role in the pathogenesis of diabetes-related complications [6]. Thus oxidative stress and increased production of free radicals is another mechanism by which the vestibulo-cochlear nerve is damaged in diabetes mellitus leading to hearing loss, this was demonstrated by the increased latencies observed on auditory brainstem response tests [1]. High glucose levels can damage the mitochondrial DNA and alter oxidative phosphorylation, this can reduce ATP production affecting those organs that have high energy consumption such as the kidney and cochlea [1].

19.3 Risk Factors

Hearing loss is associated with increasing severity of diabetic neuropathy [7]. Incidence of hearing impairment of upto 33.3% was seen in individuals with moderate to severe diabetic nephropathy [3]. Increasing age is associated with an increased risk of developing hearing loss in individuals with diabetes mellitus [2, 8]. Males with diabetes mellitus are at an increased risk of developing sensorineural hearing loss when compared to females [8]. Presence and severity of neuropathy [3]. Hearing impairment was observed in early stages of chronic renal failure, with eGFR range of 60–89 ml/min/1.73m^2 [9]. Decreasing eGFR values was shown to increase hearing thresholds at 2000 Hz [3]. HbA1c levels of more than 12% were associated with hearing impairment in one study [8]. For every 10% increase in HbA1c, there is a 32% increase in speech perception and 19% increase in high-frequency hearing loss [10].

The ototoxic effects of the drugs used in the treatment of diabetes mellitus and its co-morbid conditions such as coronary artery disease, cerebrovascular accidents, pancreatic or liver cancer, and infection can be responsible for developing hearing impairment [2]. Aspirin is prescribed in low doses (75 mg/day) for many years which can potentially impair cochlear function. Anticancer medication such as cisplatin and antibiotics like aminoglycosides cause structural damage to the haircells leading to hearing impairment. Antidiabetic drugs such as biguanides, synthetic insulin, glucagon-like peptide -1 receptor agonists, and dipeptidyl-4 inhibitors are capable of causing hearing impairment [2].

19.4 Tools Used for Screening for Hearing Loss

- Single question screening—asking a single question—"Do you have difficulty with your hearing?" has specificity of 74% and a sensitivity of 80% in detecting moderate hearing impairment [1].
- Hearing Handicap Inventory for the Elderly Screening version (HHIE-S). This is a self-reported questionnaire comprising 10 questions. Each question is given a score of 4 if symptoms are present all the time, score of 2 if they are present sometimes and 0 if they are absent. A total score of 10 or more is suggestive of moderate hearing loss and the patient is referred to an audiologist for a formal hearing assessment [1]. The specificity of HHIE-S questionnaire is 75% and sensitivity of 89.1% [1].
- Hand-held audiometer.

19.5 Conclusion

This chapter gives a broad overview of the pathomechanism of hearing loss in diabetes mellitus and aims at creating awareness among physicians about this neglected complication of diabetes mellitus. Early detection of this entity will facilitate timely intervention in halting the progression of hearing loss and an opportunity to rehabilitate the patient with the use of hearing aids, this will further reduce the ill effects of hearing loss in the aged such as dementia, social isolation and depression.

References

1. Abraham AM, Jacob JJ, Varghese A. Should we screen patients with type 2 diabetes mellitus for hearing loss? Aging Med Healthc. 2023;14(3):102–13. https://doi.org/10.33879/AMH.143.2022.01008.
2. Samocha-Bonet D, Wu B, Ryugo DK. Diabetes mellitus and hearing loss: a review. Ageing Res Rev. 2021;71:101423.
3. Abraham AM, Jacob JJ, Varghese A. Prevalence of hearing loss in type 2 diabetes mellitus and its association with severity of diabetic neuropathy and glycemic control. J Assoc Physicians India. 2023;71(6):11–2.
4. Fukushima H, Cureoglu S, Schachern PA, Paparella MM, Harada T, Oktay MF. Effects of type 2 diabetes mellitus on cochlear structure in humans. Arch Otolaryngol Head Neck Surg. 2006;132(9):934–8.
5. Jorgensen MB. The inner ear in diabetes mellitus: histological studies. Arch Otolaryngol. 1961;74(4):373–81.
6. Ceriello A. Oxidative stress and diabetes-associated complications. Endocr Pract. 2006;12:60–2.
7. Sugimoto S, Teranishi M, Fukunaga Y, Yoshida T, Sugiura S, Uchida Y, Oiso Y, Nakashima T. Contributing factors to hearing of diabetic patients in an in-hospital education program. Acta Otolaryngol. 2013;133(11):1165–72.
8. Cruickshanks KJ, Nondahl DM, Dalton DS, Fischer ME, Klein BE, Klein R, Nieto FJ, Schubert CR, Tweed TS. Smoking, central adiposity, and poor glycemic control increase risk of hearing impairment. J Am Geriatr Soc. 2015;63(5):918–24.

9. Bainbridge KE, Cowie CC, Gonzalez F II, Hoffman HJ, Dinces E, Stamler J, Cruickshanks KJ. Risk factors for hearing impairment among adults with diabetes: the hispanic community health study/study of Latinos (HCHS/SOL). J Clin Transl Endocrinol. 2016;6:15–22.
10. Kalra S, Kaur N. Hear the ear: gear up, diabetes care. J Assoc Physicians India. 2023;71(6):11–2.

Diabetes Mellitus and Psychiatric Disorders

20

Anju Kuruvilla

20.1 Introduction

Diabetes Mellitus (DM) and psychiatric disorders are common comorbid conditions and both influence each other in many ways. While DM can increase the risk of developing certain mental disorders, the presence of a psychiatric disorder is associated with greater prevalence and incidence of DM.

The potential mediating mechanisms that may explain the association between DM and psychiatric disorders continue to be investigated. Some psychiatric presentations such as depression, anxiety, sleep problems, and substance use disorders can be a consequence of the burden of managing diabetes, a life-changing disease. Among persons with mental illness, a combination of biological factors such as genetic predisposition, lifestyle factors (lack of a balanced diet, physical inactivity, and smoking), comorbid conditions, and psychotropic medication contribute to metabolic problems and a greater risk of developing DM.

The detection of co-existing emotional disorders in persons with DM is often less than optimal resulting in greater morbidity and mortality. Given their high prevalence in general medical settings and the community, it is essential to be aware, recognize, and effectively manage these comorbid conditions.

20.2 Diabetes-Related Distress

The burden of living with diabetes, its daily management, and the threat of complications can lead to emotional distress; this is termed diabetes distress and is seen in up to 45% of people in community settings [1]. Early in the course of illness,

A. Kuruvilla (✉)
Department of Psychiatry, Christian Medical College, Vellore, Tamil Nadu, India
e-mail: sanju@cmcvellore.ac.in

G. Abraham et al. (eds.), *Management of Diabetic Complications*,
https://doi.org/10.1007/978-981-97-6406-8_20

patients are faced with challenges of accepting and adjusting to the diagnosis and the considerable lifestyle changes required to manage it. Individuals may experience a sense that the illness has taken over their lives. Anxiety and frustration may occur when sugars remain poorly controlled and medical complications occur despite all efforts to manage them [2]. The financial implications of the illness and its social impact—stigma, other people's lack of support and understanding—may also cause distress. These feelings can be overwhelming, causing discouragement and poor adherence to diabetes care regimens resulting in unhealthy habits, irregular monitoring of blood sugar, missing medication, and skipping doctor's appointments, leading to worse health outcomes [3].

20.3 Depressive Disorder

Major depressive disorder (MDD) is reported to be two to three times more common in people with type 2 and type 1 diabetes, respectively, than in the general population [4]. There is also an increased risk of persons with depression developing diabetes. Both conditions can worsen the outcome of the other. Depression in diabetes leads to suboptimal self-care and poorer glycaemic control, leading to an increased risk of complications and mortality; poor metabolic control can in turn worsen depression.

Patients with depression present with low mood and reduced interest in previously pleasurable activities. Other symptoms that are often present are feelings of guilt or worthlessness, fatigue, concentration problems, suicidal thoughts, psychomotor retardation or agitation, changes in sleep, appetite, and weight lasting for at least 2 weeks. Episodes may or may not be associated with psychotic features. A simple and quick method that can be used to screen for depression is to ask 2 questions: "During the past month, have you been bothered by having little interest or pleasure in doing things?" and "During the past month, have you been bothered by feeling down, depressed, or hopeless?" [5]. If the answer to either question is "yes," a detailed assessment needs to be carried out to elicit other symptoms of depression. Other useful screening instruments include scales such as the Beck Depression Inventory and Patient Health Questionnaire-9 (PHQ-9) [6].

Factors that are associated with an increased risk of depression in DM include female gender, lower educational level, early age of onset of illness, high body mass index (BMI), poor glycaemic control, and complications of diabetes [7]. Depressive disorder is less common than diabetes distress and is characterized by overall emotional distress, not only distress related to the burden of living with diabetes. Depressive symptoms can mimic symptoms of poorly managed diabetes—such as weight loss, fatigue, sleep disturbances, and difficulty concentrating. Both depression and diabetes are thought to be contributed to by biological factors such as hypothalamic-pituitary-adrenal axis activation and inflammation, as well as behavioral factors including a sedentary lifestyle, sleep disturbance, poor dietary habits, and other environmental factors which influence glucose transport, cortisol levels and insulin resistance factors [8].

20.4 Anxiety Disorders and Diabetes

There is a higher risk of anxiety disorders in patients with diabetes mellitus than among people without DM. The prevalence of anxiety among this population is reported to range from 14 to 55%, though there are several more who experience subclinical anxiety [9, 10]. The most common type of anxiety disorder reported in DM is generalized anxiety disorder (GAD) [11]. GAD is characterized by anxiety about a wide range of situations and issues, rather than about one specific event. Anxiety is experienced most of the time on most days, is difficult to control, and is associated with a feeling of restlessness, easy fatiguability, muscle tension, poor concentration, sleep disturbance, and irritability. Other less common anxiety disorders in DM are phobias and panic disorder. People with panic disorder have frequent and unexpected panic attacks characterized by sudden periods of intense fear, or sense of losing control even when there is no clear danger or trigger. During a panic attack, a person may experience a racing heart, sweating, tremulousness, and difficulty breathing. Patients worry about when the next attack will happen and actively try to avoid future attacks. People with a phobia experience an intense fear and avoidance of specific objects or situations, which are out of proportion to the actual danger caused by the situation or object. A phobia of needles in persons with diabetes can be a barrier to taking insulin as well as to regular blood monitoring.

Several factors may contribute to the development of anxiety disorders among patients with diabetes such as personality traits, stressful life events, substance use, and physical illness [12]. Seen more commonly among women, these disorders can result in poor adherence to treatment, inadequate glycaemic control, more medical complications, and poor functioning and quality of life. Mechanisms by which anxiety is postulated to influence diabetic control include activation of the hypothalamic–pituitary–adrenal axis, stimulation of the sympathetic nervous system-adrenal responses, increase in platelet aggregation and inflammation, decreased insulin sensitivity, and worsening glycaemic control complications [13].

20.5 Other Psychiatric Disorders

People with severe mental illness such as schizophrenia and bipolar affective disorder have a greater risk of developing diabetes, which in turn contributes to excess mortality [14]. When patients are acutely ill and behaviourally disturbed, it can be difficult to ensure adherence to treatment of DM. In persons with chronic illness, negative symptoms, poor adherence to treatment, a sedentary lifestyle, and poor dietary choices can contribute to impaired blood sugars. In addition, the use of antipsychotic medication can contribute to the onset of metabolic syndrome [15].

Patients with type 1 diabetes are known to have an increased risk of eating disorders compared with the general population, with the prevalence ranging from 6.4% to 10.1% [16]. Behaviors that are seen include deliberately taking inadequate amounts of insulin, restricting intake, self-induced vomiting, and binge eating. Eating disorders also occur in those with type 2 diabetes with binge eating disorder being the most common diagnosis; the prevalence of complications in type 2 is less than in type 1 DM [17].

Persons with comorbid alcohol use disorders are often found to have poor adherence to diabetes self-care behaviors. Heavy alcohol use could lead to excessive weight gain, elevated glucose levels, and may precipitate diabetic ketoacidosis. Alcohol can alter the metabolism of oral hypoglycaemic agents; concomitant use of chlorpropamide and alcohol could lead to disulfiram-ethanol type of reaction. Those using insulin are at risk of hypoglycemia. Smoking can affect glycemic control and increase the risk of diabetic complications. In view of the significant interactions, all patients with diabetes should be routinely screened for substance use [18].

Sleep disturbances such as insomnia, poor sleep quality, daytime sleepiness, and use of sedative drugs are common among persons with diabetes. These may be a direct effect of DM or may be due to associated complications such as peripheral neuropathy or polyuria. Conversely, poor sleep hygiene itself is associated with a greater risk of obesity, metabolic syndrome, and DM [19]. Maladaptive personality and coping styles have been recognized to contribute significantly to the "brittle" form of diabetes characterized by severe glycemic instability and recurrent hospital admissions [20].

20.6 Management

The first step to effective management of psychiatric conditions in patients with DM is to recognize them. Patients should be routinely screened for these conditions during their reviews with the clinician. Taking time to ask about the patient's well-being at every consultation is also necessary to build a therapeutic rapport. Regularly assessing how patients are coping with the demands of living with diabetes and addressing those stressors can help improve outcomes.

Psychological Management For patients who are distressed regarding the diagnosis of DM, provide opportunity for them to talk about their concerns about the different aspects of the disease. Acknowledge their distress and reassure them that such feelings are normal. Provide adequate health information regarding the nature of diabetes and its management and allow patients to clarify their doubts. A better understanding of the condition will improve the patient's ability and confidence to manage it [21]. Motivational interviewing is a useful tool to encourage patients who are ambivalent or reluctant to make changes in lifestyle; it involves pointing out the discrepancy between the patient's current behavior and his or her own health-related goals, and thus increase motivation for change [22]. Psychoeducation regarding the causes and symptoms of depression and anxiety help to improve the patient's understanding of his/her emotional difficulties, how these affect their quality of life, and how better to handle these problems.

Problem-solving techniques can be suggested to patients to deal with specific difficulties. This involves a series of steps: identify a problem to be addressed, list all possible solutions and the pros and cons of each, select the most suitable problem-solving method and execute it, then evaluate how successful the plan was and decide whether the problem needs to be reformulated or whether another solution needs to be implemented. These steps can help patients manage daily barriers to treatment adherence and to make appropriate adjustments to their self-care regimen [23].

Patients who are depressed, anxious, or distressed often have a variety of negative thoughts about themselves, their illness, and the world in general. They may see the diagnosis as a catastrophe, feel hopeless, helpless, and sad. Cognitive therapy can help the patient recognize how these negative thought patterns and distorted ways of thinking lead to feelings of depression and anxiety [3]. The patient needs to learn to identify such negative thoughts and then proceed to challenge them by asking themselves whether there is actual evidence to support such thoughts, or whether he/she is making assumptions. After successfully challenging the belief, it needs to be replaced with alternate beliefs that are realistic rather than negative. Thus, by reframing and restructuring their thoughts, patients can learn to improve their mood and feel better.

Deep breathing and muscular relaxation exercises help to reduce anxiety by creating a calming response within the body. These are helpful when confronting an anxiety-producing situation, as well as to reduce overall stress [10]. Patients need to understand that avoidance of anxiety-provoking situations worsens anxiety, while facing their fears helps to reduce it. Exposure therapy is useful as the patient is forced to confront the feared situation in a gradual and graded manner while using relaxation skills to manage their anxiety [2]. For example, for a person with needle phobia, the patient makes a hierarchy of feared situations: holding the insulin syringe, drawing up the correct dose of insulin, acting `as if" injecting, and actually injecting. The patient is then asked to practise the relaxation exercise and perform the first item on the list; he/she is asked to continue to practice it on a number of different occasions until it can be done with little or no fear. Then the patient moves onto the next step on the fear hierarchy and repeats the same process, and so on, till the completion of the items on the list. Additional techniques that can be used for patients with needle phobia include the use of premedication, topical anesthetic creams, and alternative injection devices without needles [24].

Lifestyle modification is a necessary and useful intervention for psychiatric conditions as well as diabetes. Regular physical exercise, diet modification, sleep hygiene, and avoidance of substance use improve both glycaemic control and depressive symptoms [25]. Incorporating lifestyle interventions as part of routine management of psychotic disorders helps to improve clinical outcomes [26]. Patients should also be encouraged to engage in social and leisure activities.

Medication Antidepressant medication is useful in the treatment of depressive and anxiety disorders though it is unlikely to benefit patients with diabetes distress. Since all antidepressants have similar efficacy in terms of depression outcome, the drug of choice depends largely on the side effect profile including effects on metabolic control, patient preference, and individual response [27]. Selective serotonin re-uptake inhibitors, such as sertraline, fluoxetine, and escitalopram, in addition to their antidepressant effects, have been reported to have a favorable effect on glycaemic control with improvement in HbA1c levels, weight loss, and enhanced insulin sensitivity [28]. In addition, they are less cardiotoxic than tricyclic antidepressants and are safer in overdose. The antidepressants that induce significant weight gain such as tricyclic antidepressants, paroxetine, and mirtazapine may be less suitable as they could increase insulin resistance and decrease glycaemic control [8].

Presence of psychotic symptoms requires the addition of antipsychotic medication. Since many second-generation antipsychotic agents such as clozapine, olanzapine, quetiapine, and risperidone are associated with a greater risk of metabolic syndrome, preferred drugs include high potency first-generation antipsychotics such as haloperidol and second-generation antipsychotics such as aripiprazole, amisulpride, cariprazine, and lurasidone in view of their low or minimal risk of diabetes and impaired glucose tolerance [28]. Once antidepressant and/or antipsychotic agents are started, blood glucose level and HbA1c must be carefully monitored.

20.7 Conclusion

Clinicians need to be aware that diabetes is a risk factor for different psychological disorders. Therefore, patients with DM should be routinely screened for psychiatric problems and those who screen positive must be evaluated in detail. Treatment should address both conditions simultaneously; the psychiatric condition should be treated with psychological interventions, appropriate weight-neutral pharmacological agents, and lifestyle modification.

References

1. Parsa S, Aghamohammadi M, Abazari M. Diabetes distress and its clinical determinants in patients with type II diabetes. Diabetes Metab Syndr. 2019;13:1275–9.
2. Doherty A. Psychiatric aspects of diabetes mellitus. BJPsych Adv. 2015;21(6):407–16.
3. Kreider KE. Diabetes distress or major depressive disorder? A practical approach to diagnosing and treating psychological comorbidities of diabetes. Diabetes Ther. 2017;8(1):1–7.
4. Roy T, Lloyd CE. Epidemiology of depression and diabetes: a systematic review. J Affect Disord. 2012;142(Suppl):S8–S21.
5. Kroenke K, Spitzer RL, Williams JB. The Patient Health Questionnaire-2: validity of a two-item depression screener. Med Care. 2003;41(11):1284–92.
6. Kroenke K, Spitzer RL, Williams JBW. The PHQ-9. J Gen Intern Med. 2001;16:606–13.
7. Chen F, Wei G, Wang Y, Liu T, Huang T, Wei Q, Ma G, Wang D. Risk factors for depression in elderly diabetic patients and the effect of metformin on the condition. BMC Public Health. 2019;19(1):1063.
8. Holt RI, de Groot M, Golden SH. Diabetes and depression. Curr Diab Rep. 2014;14(6):491.
9. Chaturvedi SK, Gowda SM, Ahmed HU, Alosaimi FD, Andreone N, Bobrov A, et al. More anxious than depressed: prevalence and correlates in a 15-nation study of anxiety disorders in people with type 2 diabetes mellitus. Gen Psychiatr. 2019;32(4):e100076.
10. Bickett A, Tapp H. Anxiety and diabetes: innovative approaches to management in primary care. Exp Biol Med (Maywood). 2016;241(15):1724–31.

11. Grigsby AB, Anderson RJ, Freedland KE, Clouse RE, Lustman PJ. Prevalence of anxiety in adults with diabetes: a systematic review. J Psychosom Res. 2002;53:1053–60.
12. Hendrieckx C, Halliday JA, Beeney LJ, Speight J. Diabetes and emotional health: a handbook for health professionals supporting adults with type 1 or type 2 diabetes. Canberra: National Diabetes Services Scheme; 2016.
13. dos Santos MAB, Ceretta LB, Réus GZ, Abelaira HM, Jornada LK, Schwalm MT, Neotti MV, Tomazzi CD, Gulbis KG, Ceretta RA, Quevedo J. Anxiety disorders are associated with quality of life impairment in patients with insulin-dependent type 2 diabetes: a case-control study. Braz J Psychiatry. 2014;36(4):298–304.
14. Schoepf D, Potluri R, Uppal H, Natalwala A, Narendran P, Heun R. Type-2 diabetes mellitus in schizophrenia: increased prevalence and major risk factor of excess mortality in a naturalistic 7-year follow-up. Eur Psychiatry. 2012;27:33–42.
15. Newcomer JW. Second-generation (atypical) antipsychotics and metabolic effects: a comprehensive literature review. CNS Drugs. 2005;19(suppl 1):1–93.
16. Young V, Eiser C, Johnson B, Brierley S, Epton T, Elliott J, Heller S. Eating problems in adolescents with type 1 diabetes: a systematic review with meta-analysis. Diabet Med. 2013;30:189–98.
17. Winston AP. Eating disorders and diabetes. Curr Diab Rep. 2020;20(8):32.
18. Balhara YP. Diabetes and psychiatric disorders. Indian J Endocrinol Metab. 2011;15(4):274–83.
19. Khandelwal D, Dutta D, Chittawar S, Kalra S. Sleep Disorders in Type 2 Diabetes. Indian J Endocrinol Metab. 2017;21(5):758–61.
20. Pelizza L, Bonazzi F, Scaltriti S, Milli B, Giuseppina C. Brittle diabetes: psycho-pathological aspects. Acta Biomed. 2014;85:18–29.
21. Fagherazzi G. Technologies will not make diabetes disappear: how to integrate the concept of diabetes distress into care. Diabet Epidemiol Manag. 2023;11:100140.
22. Welch G, Zagarins SE, Feinberg RG, Garb JL. Motivational interviewing delivered by diabetes educators: does it improve blood glucose control among poorly controlled type 2 diabetes patients? Diabetes Res Clin Pract. 2011;91(1):54–60.
23. Hill-Briggs F. Problem solving in diabetes self-management: a model of chronic illness self-management behavior. Ann Behav Med. 2003;25:182–93.
24. Duncanson E, Le Leu RK, Shanahan L, Macauley L, Bennett PN, Weichula R, McDonald S, Burke ALJ, Collins KL, Chur-Hansen A, Jesudason S. The prevalence and evidence-based management of needle fear in adults with chronic disease: a scoping review. PLoS One. 2021;16(6):e0253048.
25. Gregory JM, Rosenblat JD, McIntyre RS. Deconstructing diabetes and depression: clinical context, treatment strategies, and new directions. Focus (Am Psychiatr Publ). 2016;14(2):184–93.
26. Caemmerer J, Correll CU, Maayan L. Acute and maintenance effects of non-pharmacologic interventions for antipsychotic associated weight gain and metabolic abnormalities: a meta-analytic comparison of randomized controlled trials. Schizophr Res. 2012;140:159–68.
27. Fournier JC, DeRubeis RJ, Hollon SD, Dimidjian S, Amsterdam JD, Shelton RC, Fawcett J. Antidepressant drug effects and depression severity: a patient-level meta-analysis. JAMA. 2010;303(1):47–53.
28. Taylor DM, Barnes TRE, Young AH. The Maudsley prescribing guidelines in psychiatry. 14th ed. John Wiley & S; 2021.

21 Adverse Events Due to Oral Hypoglycemic Drugs

Nanditha Arun and Rebeccaa Eapen Vettath

21.1 Introduction

In the realm of type 2 diabetes mellitus management, an intricate interplay of patient characteristics, severity of hyperglycemia, and therapeutic options guides the course of treatment. Among the myriad factors contributing to the multifaceted landscape of T2DM, an "ominous octet" has been postulated as a crucial framework. This octet encompasses a collection of eight distinct pathophysiological mechanisms that, either individually or in combination, underlie the intricate web of hyperglycemia in T2DM (Fig. 21.1) [1]. These encompass a range of mechanisms, including reduced insulin secretion from pancreatic β-cells, heightened glucagon secretion from pancreatic α cells, increased hepatic glucose production, disrupted neurotransmitter function and insulin resistance within the brain, elevated lipolysis, augmented renal glucose reabsorption, diminished incretin effect in the small intestine, and impaired glucose uptake in peripheral tissues such as skeletal muscle, liver, and adipose tissue.

In response to these multifaceted challenges, contemporary glucose-lowering therapies are tailored to address one or more of these pivotal pathways. Effective glycemic control remains a cornerstone in the management of T2DM, playing a pivotal role in deterring or postponing the onset and progression of diabetic complications. Central to this approach is the recognition that treatment choices should be driven by a patient-centered paradigm, accounting for a spectrum of variables, including treatment efficacy, financial considerations, potential adverse effects, weight fluctuations, coexisting medical conditions, risk of hypoglycemia, and individual patient preferences.

N. Arun (✉)
Dr. A. Ramachandran's Diabetes Hospitals & India Diabetes Research Foundation, Chennai, Tamil Nadu, India
e-mail: research@ardiabetes.org

R. E. Vettath
Department of Nephrology, MGM Healthcare, Chennai, Tamil Nadu, India

G. Abraham et al. (eds.), *Management of Diabetic Complications*,
https://doi.org/10.1007/978-981-97-6406-8_21

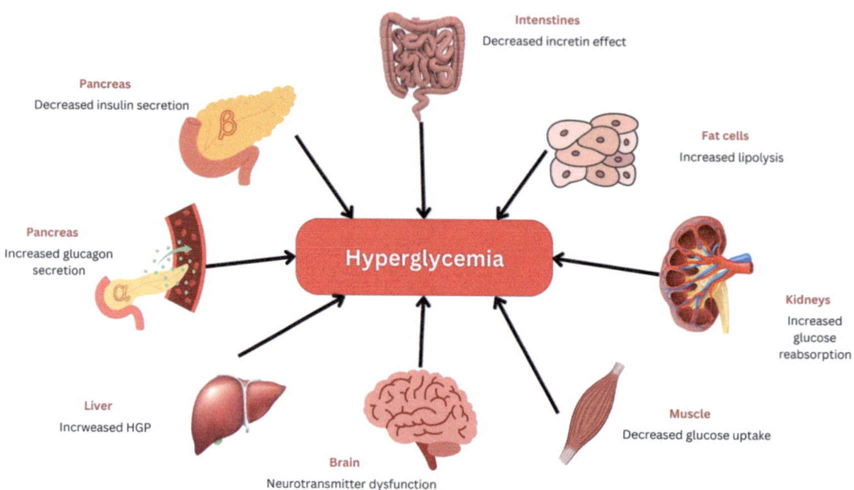

Fig. 21.1 Ominous octet

In the realm of oral antidiabetic medications, a range of classes are available, each addressing distinct facets of T2DM management. From biguanides to sulfonylureas, meglitinides to thiazolidinediones, dipeptidyl peptidase 4 inhibitors, sodium-glucose cotransporter 2 inhibitors, and α-glucosidase inhibitors, these agents target a spectrum of physiological pathways to restore glycemic equilibrium.

This chapter delves into the array of adverse effects associated with oral hypoglycemic drugs, shedding light on their implications for patient care and management (Table 21.1). With a primary focus on agents like SGLT2 inhibitors and DPP-4 inhibitors, we also address the safety profile of metformin, SUs, TZDs, and AGIs, which have weathered the test of time in clinical practice. In a landscape marked by evolving guidelines, global considerations, and individual patient needs, this exploration will navigate the nuances of adverse effects to equip clinicians with a comprehensive understanding of informed decision-making (Fig. 21.1).

Table 21.1 Oral hypoglycemic drugs and their adverse events

Class of drug	Drugs	Mechanism of action	Adverse events
Biguanide	Metformin	• Insulin sensitizer • Inhibition of hepatic glucose production	• Gastrointestinal intolerance • Vitamin B12 deficiency • Anemia • Neuropathy (risk in the elderly) • Low risk of lactic acidosis • Stop metformin if creatinine >1.5 mg/dL in males and > 1.4 mg/dL in females

(continued)

Table 21.1 (continued)

Class of drug	Drugs	Mechanism of action	Adverse events
Sulfonylureas	Glimepiride Exenatide Glyburide	• Insulin secretion	• High risk of hypoglycemia • Weight gain • Cardiovascular uncertainties
Thiazolidinediones	Rosiglitazone Pioglitazone	• True insulin sensitizer	• Weight gain • Fluid retention • Heart failure • Cardiovascular risks • Small risk of bone fractures • Small risk of bladder cancer • Macular edema • Worsening lipid profile
DPP-4 inhibitors	Sitagliptin Saxagliptin Vildagliptin Linagliptin Alogliptin	• Inhibition of degradation of GLP	• Small risk of pancreatitis • Upper RTI infection • Gastrointestinal intolerance • Heart failure • Rare cases of bullous pemphigoid • Arthralgias
Oral GLP-1 receptor agonist	Semaglutide	• Increased insulin secretion • Decreased glucagon • Delayed gastric • Emptying • Increased satiety	• Nausea • Vomiting • Pancreatitis • Gastrointestinal disorders
Alpha-glucosidase inhibitors	Acarbose Miglitol Voglibose	• Inhibit the absorption of carbohydrates from the small intestine	• Gastrointestinal intolerance • Rare cases of ileus
SGLT2 inhibitors	Canagliflozin' Dapagliflozin Empagliflozin	• Blocking of glucose reabsorption in renal PCT; insulin-independent mechanism of action	• Genital mycotic infection • Ketoacidosis (rare) • Acute kidney injury • Risk of orthostatic hypotension (falls) • Risk of dehydration (AKI) • Bone fractures

21.2 Metformin

Metformin, one of the oldest oral agents in the management of T2DM, is renowned for its remarkable efficacy in insulin resistance. However, alongside its undeniable therapeutic advantages, metformin is not without its share of adverse effects, warranting vigilant consideration in clinical practice.

Gastrointestinal Intolerance One of the most commonly encountered side effects of metformin is gastrointestinal intolerance, affecting approximately 10–20% of individuals with T2DM [2]. This can manifest as an array of symptoms, including nausea, anorexia, abdominal discomfort, and a metallic taste in the mouth. Perhaps the most vexing of these symptoms is diarrhea, a bothersome complication [2]. For older, frail patients, the reduction in appetite caused by metformin can be particularly problematic, further emphasizing the need for a tailored approach to medication selection [2]. Most notably, its propensity for gastrointestinal disturbances, including diarrhea, nausea, and dyspepsia, tends to affect less than 30% of individuals initiated on the medication [3].

Lactic Acidosis The specter of lactic acidosis looms over metformin therapy, representing a rare but potentially life-threatening complication [4, 5]. The historical association between biguanide compounds like phenformin and lactic acidosis in the 1980s led to their withdrawal from the pharmaceutical landscape. Although the risk of metformin-induced lactic acidosis is often overstated, it remains a concern, particularly in populations vulnerable to renal impairment and cardiovascular disease, including heart failure and organ hypoperfusion [5, 6].

In contrast to the notorious association between phenformin and lactic acidosis, metformin-associated lactic acidosis is exceedingly rare, with an estimated incidence ranging from 0 to 0.08 cases per 1000 patient years and a low mortality risk [7]. The risk associated with phenformin, on the other hand, was substantially higher, contributing to its discontinuation in numerous countries [8].

Vitamin B12 Deficiency Metformin's influence isn't confined to glucose metabolism; it can also impact vitamin B12 levels, with a higher risk observed in elderly residents [9]. Longer durations of metformin therapy (>2 years) and daily doses exceeding 1500 mg appear to escalate this risk. A potential association with peripheral neuropathy has also been suggested in older individuals receiving metformin for extended periods [10]. The exact causal relationship between metformin and vitamin B12 deficiency warrants further investigation. Concerns about vitamin B12 and folic acid deficiency, while present, have limited clinical significance [11, 12].

21.3 Sulfonylurea

Sulfonylureas (SUs), a class of oral hypoglycemic drugs with a long history of use, have demonstrated efficacy in managing type 2 diabetes by stimulating insulin secretion independently of plasma glucose levels. However, their utilization comes with notable concerns and potential adverse effects, which need careful consideration.

Risk of Hypoglycemia Sulfonylureas have a high propensity to induce hypoglycemia, which is a serious concern, particularly in the elderly population. This risk has been recognized for almost three decades [13]. A population-based cohort study conducted in England, which encompassed a significant proportion of elderly patients, reported a 2.5-fold increase in the risk of hypoglycemia in current users of SUs compared to those on metformin [14]. This risk was even more pronounced in patients with reduced kidney function (eGFR <30 mL/min/1.73 m^2), those taking high doses of SUs, and individuals using glibenclamide (glyburide). The second-generation SUs, gliclazide and glimepride are considered to have a relatively lower risk of hypoglycemia as compared to first generation SUs [14].

Weight Gain Another commonly observed side effect of SUs is weight gain. This is a consequence of their insulin-stimulating action, which promotes anabolic effects in the body. The weight gain associated with SUs can be particularly problematic for patients with obesity, as it exacerbates tissue insulin resistance [15].

Other Adverse Effects SUs can also lead to various other adverse effects. These include skin rashes, such as erythema multiforme, although they are relatively uncommon [16] and often drug-specific and reversible [16, 17]. Blood dyscrasias [18] and cholestatic jaundice [19] associated with SUs are very rare.

Cardiovascular Concerns The use of SUs has raised concerns about their impact on cardiovascular outcomes. Some studies have suggested an increased risk of cardiovascular events and mortality in patients treated with SUs, especially high doses of glibenclamide (glyburide) [20–22]. However, the relationship between SU-induced hypoglycemia and cardiovascular events is complex [23] and debated, with some studies suggesting no significant increase in cardiovascular risk [24]. During the cardiovascular outcome trial CAROLINA, out of the 6033 participants, 35.3% were aged between 65 and 74 years, and 14.0% were aged 75 years or older. Over the 6.3-year median follow-up period, there were no discernible differences in cardiovascular and mortality outcomes between glimepiride and linagliptin, both overall and across all age groups [25].

21.4 Thiazolidinediones

Thiazolidinediones (TZDs) are a class of oral hypoglycemic drugs used for the management of T2DM. Pioglitazone, an insulin sensitizer, PPAR 8 agonist is an effective agent in managing T2DM. However, due to some of its adverse effects, patient selection is key.

Cardiovascular Risks TZDs have been associated with certain cardiovascular risks. Specifically, rosiglitazone has been linked to increased levels of triglycerides (TG) and LDL particle concentrations, as well as a rise in LDL cholesterol levels [26]. Additionally, there have been concerns about an elevated risk of myocardial infarction associated with rosiglitazone, leading to its withdrawal from the market

[27]. Due to the risk of fluid retention, these drugs must be avoided in Congestive Cardiac Failure.

Risk of Bone Fractures Older patients with T2DM may be particularly susceptible to the adverse effects of TZDs. A meta-analysis of 18 trials found that TZD treatment resulted in modest bone loss, which was not reversed even one year after treatment cessation [28]. Women appear to be more affected by TZD-induced bone loss than men, and an increased incidence of fractures has been observed in women using TZDs [29]. However, the differences in fracture risk between TZDs and other treatments like metformin or sulfonylureas have not always reached statistical significance [30].

Fluid Retention and Heart Failure TZDs have been associated with fluid retention and congestive heart failure. This side effect is not limited to the elderly population, with some studies showing a doubling of the risk of congestive heart failure in patients with T2DM [31]. Several studies have suggested that rosiglitazone may have a worse cardiovascular risk profile compared to pioglitazone, especially in the elderly [32]. In a population-based study among older T2DM patients, TZD treatment, primarily with rosiglitazone, was linked to an increased risk of heart failure, acute myocardial infarction, and mortality [33]. Similar findings were reported in a large population-based cohort of elderly individuals [34].

Bladder Cancer Risk Pioglitazone has been associated with an increased risk of bladder cancer. Several systematic reviews and meta-analyses have reported a modest but significant increase in the risk of bladder cancer with pioglitazone, which seems to be related to cumulative dose and duration of exposure [35]. However, some studies have found conflicting results, and the risk appears to decrease after discontinuing pioglitazone [36].

Macular Edema Macular edema, a condition characterized by swelling in the macula of the eye, has been reported after initiating TZD treatment. As a result, the American Diabetes Association recommends using TZDs cautiously in T2DM patients with or at risk of macular edema [37].

21.5 DPP-4 Inhibitors

Dipeptidyl peptidase-4 inhibitors, commonly referred to as DPP-4 inhibitors or gliptins, are a class of oral hypoglycemic drugs used in the management of T2DM. These agents provide good glycemic efficacy with a low risk of hypoglycemia, due to their glucose-dependent action. They are generally well-tolerated agent. However, a few adverse effects are worth noting.

Nonsignificant Adverse Events In clinical studies, certain adverse events have been reported at a higher but not statistically significant rate in individuals treated with DPP-4 inhibitors. These events include constipation, nasopharyngitis, myalgias, arthralgias, headache, and dizziness [38–42]. However, it is worth noting that these adverse effects are fairly uncommon.

Gastrointestinal Side Effects DPP-4 inhibitor may rarely cause mild to moderate gastrointestinal side effects like belching, nausea and diarrhea. In some instances, a transient elevation of pancreatic enzymes may be found [43].

Pancreatitis Case reports of pancreatitis, including a notable number of post-marketing cases between 2006 and 2009, led to the Food and Drug Administration (FDA) requiring a warning statement on all DPP-4 inhibitor product labels. While rare, the risk of acute pancreatitis has been associated with DPP-4 inhibitor use. Some meta-analyses have reported a slight but significant increase in the incidence of acute pancreatitis compared to placebo [44, 45]. The risk appears to be small, and for most patients, the benefits of DPP-4 inhibitors outweigh this risk [46].

Heart Failure Large cardiovascular trials involving different DPP-4 inhibitors have yielded mixed results regarding cardiovascular outcomes [47, 48]. The risk of heart failure hospitalization was particularly associated with saxagliptin use [47], but this unfavorable signal was not consistently observed with other DPP-4 inhibitors such as sitagliptin, vildagliptin, linagliptin, and alogliptin [49–54]. The FDA issued a safety warning in 2016 regarding the association of heart failure with saxagliptin and alogliptin, highlighting preexisting cardiovascular disease, prior heart failure, and chronic kidney disease as risk factors [55].

Joint Pain and Arthralgia In 2015, the FDA issued a warning that sitagliptin, saxagliptin, linagliptin, and alogliptin may cause significant joint pain. Symptoms were relieved upon discontinuation of the DPP-4 inhibitor. Joint pain has recurred in some patients even after switching to a different DPP-4 inhibitor [56]. Some studies have reported a small but significant increase in non-severe arthralgia in individuals on DPP-4 inhibitors, with long-standing T2DM or using DPP-4 inhibitors as add-on therapy potentially being risk factors [57]. Immunologic or genetic mechanisms have also been suggested as possible associations between arthralgias and DPP-4 inhibitors [58].

Bullous Pemphigoid An observed association exists between bullous pemphigoid, an autoimmune blistering disorder, and the use of DPP-4 inhibitors, particularly vildagliptin and linagliptin. This association appears to be more prevalent in younger male individuals [59, 60]. Discontinuation of DPP-4 inhibitor treatment has resulted in improved clinical outcomes.

21.6 GLP-1 Analogues

The Glucagon Like Peptide-1 Receptor Agonist (GLP-1 RA) are agents that have enriched the landscape of T2DM management. As a class, these agents provide glycemic control, alongside pleiotropic benefits including, weight loss and cardiovascular benefits. Recently oral semaglutide is available for the management of T2DM.

Gastrointestinal Effects Mild to moderate gastrointestinal side effects are the most common adverse effects associated with GLP-1 RAs. These effects can include nausea, vomiting, diarrhea, and occasionally, gallstone disease. These adverse events tend to be dose-dependent and transient, often diminishing as treatment continues [61].

Acute Pancreatitis Reports of acute pancreatitis have been associated with the use of GLP-1 RAs. However, a definitive causal relationship has not been established yet [62]. Both the FDA and the European Medicines Agency have agreed to monitor and report potential pancreatic side effects [63]. Patients should be informed about the signs and symptoms of pancreatitis, and healthcare providers should remain vigilant. Easow and colleagues documented two cases involving patients on long-term liraglutide treatment: one concerned a male patient who experienced recurrent gallstone diseases accompanied by cholestatic jaundice and acute pancreatitis (Fig. 21.2), and the other involved a female kidney transplant patient who, despite no prior history of gallstone disease, developed an asymptomatic large gallstone [64] (Fig. 21.2).

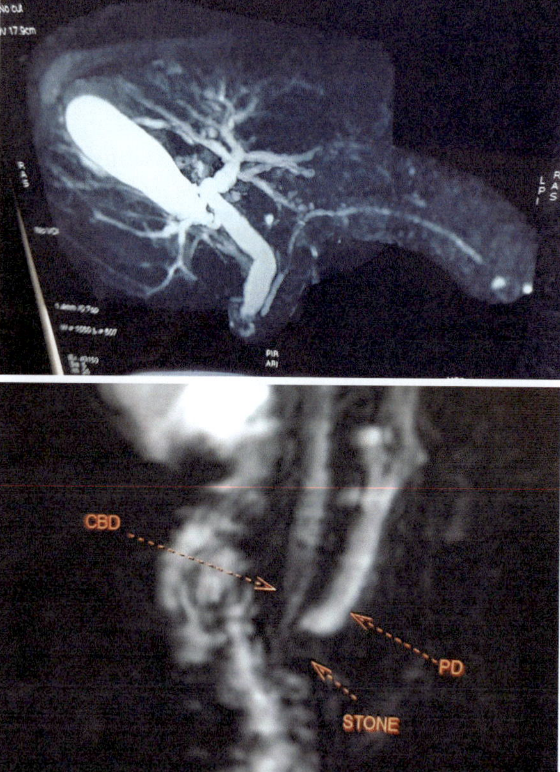

Fig. 21.2 Recurrent gallstone disease following use of liraglutide in individual with type 2 diabetes

Immunogenic Response Some individuals using GLP-1 RAs have mounted an immunogenic response, leading to the development of antibodies against these agents. The clinical significance of this immune response remains unclear [61]. However, it's an aspect that healthcare providers should be aware of and monitor.

Retinopathy In the SUSTAIN-6 trial, participants in the injectable, once-weekly semaglutide arm reported higher rates of retinopathy-associated complications. It's postulated that the worsening of these symptoms may be associated with poor glycemic control at baseline, advanced diabetic retinopathy, and rapid achievement of euglycemia [65]. However, this finding may also reflect an incidental occurrence, as higher retinopathy-associated complication rates have not been consistently detected in other randomized trials, PIONEER trails, with oral semaglutide [66].

21.7 Alpha Glucosidase Inhibitors

Alpha-glucosidase inhibitors, such as acarbose and voglibose, are oral hypoglycemic drugs used in the management of T2DM that specifically help to target postprandial blood glucose. While they have shown effectiveness in controlling blood sugar levels, they are associated with some adverse effects that should be considered when prescribing them.

Gastrointestinal Side Effects The most commonly reported adverse effects of alpha-glucosidase inhibitors are gastrointestinal. These include flatulence (excessive gas production) and diarrhea. These side effects can be quite bothersome and have led to a high rate of noncompliance among patients. In some studies, the incidence of flatulence was reported to be as high as 30%, compared to 12% in the placebo group, and diarrhea was reported in 16% of patients compared to 8% in the placebo group [67, 68].

Gastrointestinal symptoms, including abdominal pain, bloating, flatulence, and diarrhea, have been reported by up to 80% of patients during the initial weeks of therapy. However, it's worth noting that these symptoms tend to decrease over time [69].

Rare Adverse Effects While alpha-glucosidase inhibitors are not associated with serious or life-threatening adverse effects, there have been rare reports of more serious issues. For instance, there have been a few case reports of paralytic ileus, a condition where the intestines become paralyzed, reported in elderly and middle-aged diabetic patients treated with acarbose and voglibose [70].

Liver transaminase elevation has been observed in rare cases, primarily in patients receiving higher doses of acarbose [71]. However, these adverse effects are very rare.

21.8 SGLT2 Inhibitors

Sodium-glucose cotransporter 2 (SGLT2) inhibitors are a class of oral hypoglycemic drugs used in the management of T2DM. SGLT2 inhibitors provide insulin-independent glucose lowering by blocking glucose reabsorption in the proximal renal tubule by inhibiting SGLT2 [72]. While these medications have proven effective in lowering blood glucose levels, it's essential to be aware of their potential adverse effects when prescribing them to patients.

Genital and Urinary Tract Infections Reports of signs and symptoms suggestive of urinary tract and genital infections have been noted more frequently in individuals receiving SGLT-2 inhibitors, with dapagliflozin demonstrating a notable association [73]. Genital infections, particularly mycotic, are a common occurrence in patients treated with SGLT-2 inhibitors [74]. While these infections are generally mild, they can be a source of discomfort. Despite this, the rates of urinary tract infections (UTI), complicated UTIs, or pyelonephritis do not significantly differ from placebo in most trials [73, 75, 76]. However, caution should be exercised in patients with a history of similar infections.

Euglycemic Ketoacidosis A recent warning from the FDA highlights the potential for euglycemic ketoacidosis associated with SGLT-2 inhibitor use [77]. Based on 20 case reports, this alarm underscores the need for vigilance in monitoring and identifying this rare but serious complication. The exact mechanisms contributing to euglycemic ketoacidosis remain under investigation but may involve increased glucagon levels and reduced insulin secretion, culminating in a shift toward free fatty acid oxidation and ketosis [77].

Acute Kidney Injury Perhaps one of the most concerning adverse effects associated with SGLT-2 inhibitors is acute kidney injury, with canagliflozin and dapagliflozin implicated in 101 confirmable cases [78]. In approximately 50% of these cases, the adverse outcome materialized within 1 month of initiating SGLT-2 inhibitor therapy and demonstrated improvement upon discontinuation [78]. The FDA has responded by issuing and strengthening warnings, particularly for individuals with co-morbid factors such as chronic kidney insufficiency [78]. Notably, the risk of acute kidney injury escalates when SGLT-2 inhibitors are co-administered with certain medications, including diuretics, angiotensin-converting enzyme inhibitors, angiotensin II receptor blockers, and nonsteroidal anti-inflammatory drugs [78].

Dehydration and Hypotension Due to the osmotic diuretic effect of SGLT2 inhibitors, patients may experience polyuria, leading to dehydration and postural hypotension, especially in elderly individuals and those on diuretics. It's important to monitor patients for signs of dehydration, especially during hot weather.

Falls and Fractures The volume depletion caused by SGLT2 inhibitors, which can lead to orthostatic hypotension, may contribute to an increased risk of falls, particularly in older adults. This, in turn, may lead to an elevated risk of fractures.

21.9 Conclusion

In conclusion, the management of T2DM requires careful consideration of various factors, including patient characteristics, comorbidities, and the potential adverse effects associated with oral hypoglycemic drugs. Each class of these medications offers unique benefits and drawbacks, and the choice of therapy should be individualized to best suit the patient's needs.

Sulfonylureas remain a viable option for T2DM treatment, especially when considering them as an add-on therapy to metformin or in situations where metformin is contraindicated. However, their use can be challenging in patients who are elderly, overweight, have impaired renal function, or are at risk of cardiovascular complications. The potential for hypoglycemia and weight gain must be carefully balanced against their efficacy.

Thiazolidinediones have faced concerns related to cardiovascular and cancer risks, leading to a decreased preference for this class of drugs. Their use is now limited and should be approached cautiously until further clarification of these risks.

Dipeptidyl peptidase-4 inhibitors offer an excellent alternative, especially when metformin is limited due to gastrointestinal side effects or when SUs pose a risk of hypoglycemia or weight gain. They can be considered as add-on therapy when maximal doses of other oral medications have not achieved glycemic control. Adjusting the dosage based on renal function makes them suitable for patients with various stages of chronic kidney disease.

Alpha-glucosidase inhibitors act on the gut and are equally effective as DPP-4 inhibitors but are often poorly tolerated due to gastrointestinal side effects. They may be an option for patients already taking multiple daily medications and experiencing constipation.

When initiating DPP-4 inhibitors, it is essential to discuss the potential risks of pancreatitis and joint pain with the patient. Similarly, the introduction of sodium-glucose cotransporter 2 inhibitors should involve a discussion regarding the risks of ketoacidosis, amputation, and genital infections.

In summary, the choice of oral hypoglycemic drugs for managing T2DM should be based on a comprehensive assessment of the patient's clinical profile, preferences, and risk factors. It is essential to engage in open and informed discussions with patients to ensure that the selected therapy aligns with their individual needs while minimizing the potential for adverse effects. Additionally, ongoing monitoring and evaluation are crucial to optimize glycemic control and minimize risks throughout treatment.

References

1. Defronzo RA. From the triumvirate to the ominous octet: a new paradigm for the treatment of type 2 diabetes mellitus. 2009; Available from: http://diabetes.diabetesjournals.org/
2. Bonnet F, Scheen A. Understanding and overcoming metformin gastrointestinal intolerance. Diabetes Obes Metab. 2017;19(4):473–81. Available from: https://pubmed.ncbi.nlm.nih.gov/27987248/ [cited 2023 Oct 22]
3. Hermann LS. Metformin: a review of its pharmacological properties and therapeutic use. Diabete Metab. 1979;5(3):233–45. Available from: https://pubmed.ncbi.nlm.nih.gov/387488/ [cited 2023 Oct 22]
4. Bicsak TA, Walsh B, Fineman M. Metformin-associated lactic acidosis: moving towards a new paradigm? Diabetes Obes Metab. 2017;19(11):1499. Available from: /pmc/articles/PMC5655765/ [cited 2023 Oct 22]
5. Defronzo R, Fleming GA, Chen K, Bicsak TA. Metformin-associated lactic acidosis: current perspectives on causes and risk. Metabolism. 2016;65(2):20–9. Available from: https://pubmed.ncbi.nlm.nih.gov/26773926/ [cited 2023 Oct 22]
6. Scheen AJ, Paquot N. Metformin revisited: a critical review of the benefit-risk balance in at-risk patients with type 2 diabetes. Diabetes Metab. 2013;39(3):179–90. Available from: https://pubmed.ncbi.nlm.nih.gov/23528671/ [cited 2023 Oct 22]
7. Bailey CJ, Nattrass M. 11 treatment—metformin. Bailliere Clin Endocrinol Metab. 1988;2(2):455–76.
8. Kreisberg RA. Lactate homeostasis and lactic acidosis. Ann Intern Med. 1980;92(2 Pt 1):227–37. Available from: https://pubmed.ncbi.nlm.nih.gov/6766289/ [cited 2023 Oct 22]
9. Wong CW, Leung CS, Leung CP, Cheng JN. Association of metformin use with vitamin B12 deficiency in the institutionalized elderly. Arch Gerontol Geriatr. 2018;79:57–62. Available from: https://pubmed.ncbi.nlm.nih.gov/30114554/ [cited 2023 Oct 22]
10. Serra MC, Kancherla V, Khakharia A, Allen LL, Phillips LS, Rhee MK, et al. Long-term metformin treatment and risk of peripheral neuropathy in older veterans. Diabetes Res Clin Pract. 2020;170. Available from: https://pubmed.ncbi.nlm.nih.gov/33035597/ [cited 2023 Oct 22]
11. Tomkin GH. Malabsorption of vitamin B12 in diabetic patients treated with phenformin: a comparison with metformin. Br Med J. 1973;3(5882):673. Available from: https://pubmed.ncbi.nlm.nih.gov/4742454/ [cited 2023 Oct 22]
12. Boman G, Wiholm BE. Epidemiology of adverse drug reactions to phenformin and metformin. Br Med J. 1978;2(6135):464–6. Available from: https://pubmed.ncbi.nlm.nih.gov/678924/ [cited 2023 Oct 22]
13. Robertson DA, Home PD. Problems and pitfalls of sulphonylurea therapy in older patients. Drugs Aging. 1993;3(6):510–24. Available from: https://pubmed.ncbi.nlm.nih.gov/8312676/ [cited 2023 Oct 22]
14. Van Dalem J, Brouwers MCGJ, Stehouwer CDA, Krings A, Leufkens HGM, Driessen JHM, et al. Risk of hypoglycaemia in users of sulphonylureas compared with metformin in relation to renal function and sulphonylurea metabolite group: population based cohort study. BMJ. 2016;354. Available from: https://pubmed.ncbi.nlm.nih.gov/27413017/ [cited 2023 Oct 22]
15. Stout RW. Insulin and atheroma. 20-yr perspective. Diabetes Care. 1990;13(6):631–54. Available from: https://pubmed.ncbi.nlm.nih.gov/2192848/ [cited 2023 Oct 22]
16. Undesired effects of the sulphonylurea drugs—PubMed [Internet]. Available from: https://pubmed.ncbi.nlm.nih.gov/3890480/ [cited 2023 Oct 22].
17. Jackson JE, Bressler R. Clinical pharmacology of sulphonylurea hypoglycaemic agents: part 1. Drugs. 1981;22(3):211–45. Available from: https://pubmed.ncbi.nlm.nih.gov/7021124/ [cited 2023 Oct 22]
18. Malacarne P, Castaldi G, Bertusi M, Zavagli G. Tolbutamide-induced hemolytic anemia. Diabetes. 1977;26(2):156–8. Available from: https://pubmed.ncbi.nlm.nih.gov/838166/ [cited 2023 Oct 22]

19. Clarke BF, Campbell IW, Ewing DJ, Beveridge GW, MacDonald MK. Generalized hypersensitivity reaction and visceral arteritis with fatal outcome during glibenclamide therapy. Diabetes. 1974;23(9):739–42. Available from: https://pubmed.ncbi.nlm.nih.gov/4213123/ [cited 2023 Oct 22]
20. Evans JMM, Ogston SA, Emslie-Smith A, Morris AD. Risk of mortality and adverse cardiovascular outcomes in type 2 diabetes: a comparison of patients treated with sulfonylureas and metformin. Diabetologia. 2006;49(5):930–6. Available from: https://pubmed.ncbi.nlm.nih.gov/16525843/ [cited 2023 Oct 22]
21. Roumie CL, Hung AM, Greevy RA, Grijalva CG, Liu X, Murff HJ, et al. Comparative effectiveness of sulfonylurea and metformin monotherapy on cardiovascular events in type 2 diabetes mellitus: a cohort study. Ann Intern Med. 2012;157(9):601–10. Available from: https://pubmed.ncbi.nlm.nih.gov/23128859/ [cited 2023 Oct 22]
22. Simpson SH, Majumdar SR, Tsuyuki RT, Eurich DT, Johnson JA. Dose-response relation between sulfonylurea drugs and mortality in type 2 diabetes mellitus: a population-based cohort study. CMAJ. 2006;174(2):169–74. Available from: https://pubmed.ncbi.nlm.nih.gov/16415461/ [cited 2023 Oct 22]
23. Abdelmoneim AS, Eurich DT, Light PE, Senior PA, Seubert JM, Makowsky MJ, et al. Cardiovascular safety of sulphonylureas: over 40 years of continuous controversy without an answer. Diabetes Obes Metab. 2015;17(6):523. Available from: https://pubmed.ncbi.nlm.nih.gov/25711240/ [cited 2023 Oct 22]
24. Gangji AS, Cukierman T, Gerstein HC, Goldsmith CH, Clase CM. A systematic review and meta-analysis of hypoglycemia and cardiovascular events: a comparison of glyburide with other secretagogues and with insulin. Diabetes Care. 2007;30(2):389–94. Available from: https://pubmed.ncbi.nlm.nih.gov/17259518/ [cited 2023 Oct 22]
25. Espeland MA, Pratley RE, Rosenstock J, Kadowaki T, Seino Y, Zinman B, et al. Cardiovascular outcomes and safety with linagliptin, a dipeptidyl peptidase-4 inhibitor, compared with the sulphonylurea glimepiride in older people with type 2 diabetes: a subgroup analysis of the randomized CAROLINA trial. Diabetes Obes Metab. 2021;23(2):569–80. Available from: https://onlinelibrary.wiley.com/doi/full/10.1111/dom.14254 [cited 2023 Oct 22]
26. Goldberg RB, Kendall DM, Deeg MA, Buse JB, Zagar AJ, Pinaire JA, et al. A comparison of lipid and glycemic effects of pioglitazone and rosiglitazone in patients with type 2 diabetes and dyslipidemia. Diabetes Care. 2005;28(7):1547–54. Available from: https://pubmed.ncbi.nlm.nih.gov/15983299/ [cited 2023 Oct 22]
27. Nissen SE, Wolski K. Effect of rosiglitazone on the risk of myocardial infarction and death from cardiovascular causes. N Engl J Med. 2007;356(24):2457–71. Available from: https://pubmed.ncbi.nlm.nih.gov/17517853/ [cited 2023 Oct 22]
28. Billington EO, Grey A, Bolland MJ. The effect of thiazolidinediones on bone mineral density and bone turnover: systematic review and meta-analysis. Diabetologia. 2015;58(10):2238–46. Available from: https://pubmed.ncbi.nlm.nih.gov/26109213/ [cited 2023 Oct 22]
29. Zhu ZN, Jiang YF, Ding T. Risk of fracture with thiazolidinediones: an updated meta-analysis of randomized clinical trials. Bone. 2014;68:115–23. Available from: https://pubmed.ncbi.nlm.nih.gov/25173606/ [cited 2023 Oct 22]
30. Solomon DH, Cadarette SM, Choudhry NK, Canning C, Levin R, Stürmer T. A cohort study of thiazolidinediones and fractures in older adults with diabetes. J Clin Endocrinol Metab. 2009;94(8):2792–8. Available from: https://pubmed.ncbi.nlm.nih.gov/19470635/ [cited 2023 Oct 22]
31. Singh S, Loke YK, Furberg CD. Thiazolidinediones and heart failure: a teleo-analysis. Diabetes Care. 2007;30(8):2148–53. Available from: https://pubmed.ncbi.nlm.nih.gov/17536074/ [cited 2023 Oct 22]
32. Viljoen A, Sinclair A. Safety and efficacy of rosiglitazone in the elderly diabetic patient. Vasc Health Risk Manag. 2009;5:389. Available from: /pmc/articles/PMC2686257/ [cited 2023 Oct 22]

33. Lipscombe LL, Gomes T, Lévesque LE, Hux JE, Juurlink DN, Alter DA. Thiazolidinediones and cardiovascular outcomes in older patients with diabetes. JAMA. 2007;298(22):2634–43. Available from: https://pubmed.ncbi.nlm.nih.gov/18073359/ [cited 2023 Oct 22]
34. Winkelmayer WC, Setoguchi S, Levin R, Solomon DH. Comparison of cardiovascular outcomes in elderly patients with diabetes who initiated rosiglitazone vs pioglitazone therapy. Arch Intern Med. 2008;168(21):2368–75. Available from: https://pubmed.ncbi.nlm.nih.gov/19029503/ [cited 2023 Oct 22]
35. Turner RM, Kwok CS, Chen-Turner C, Maduakor CA, Singh S, Loke YK. Thiazolidinediones and associated risk of bladder cancer: a systematic review and meta-analysis. Br J Clin Pharmacol. 2014;78(2):258–73. Available from: https://pubmed.ncbi.nlm.nih.gov/24325197/ [cited 2023 Oct 22]
36. Garry EM, Buse JB, Gokhale M, Lund JL, Nielsen ME, Pate V, et al. Study design choices for evaluating comparative safety of diabetic medications: an evaluation of pioglitazone and bladder cancer risk among older US adults with Type-2 diabetes. Diabetes Obes Metab. 2019;21(9):2096. Available from: /pmc/articles/PMC7025290/ [cited 2023 Oct 22]
37. Association AD. 12. Older adults: standards of medical Care in Diabetes—2021. Diabetes Care. 2021;44(Supplement_1):S168–S79. https://doi.org/10.2337/dc21-S012. [cited 2023 Oct 22]
38. Aschner P, Kipnes MS, Lunceford JK, Sanchez M, Mickel C, Williams-Herman DE. Effect of the dipeptidyl peptidase-4 inhibitor sitagliptin as monotherapy on glycemic control in patients with type 2 diabetes. Diabetes Care. 2006;29(12):2632–7. Available from: https://pubmed.ncbi.nlm.nih.gov/17130196/ [cited 2023 Oct 22]
39. Raz I, Hanefeld M, Xu L, Caria C, Williams-Herman D, Khatami H. Efficacy and safety of the dipeptidyl peptidase-4 inhibitor sitagliptin as monotherapy in patients with type 2 diabetes mellitus. Diabetologia. 2006;49(11):2564–71. Available from: https://pubmed.ncbi.nlm.nih.gov/17001471/ [cited 2023 Oct 22]
40. Pi-Sunyer FX, Schweizer A, Mills D, Dejager S. Efficacy and tolerability of vildagliptin monotherapy in drug-naïve patients with type 2 diabetes. Diabetes Res Clin Pract. 2007;76(1):132–8. Available from: https://pubmed.ncbi.nlm.nih.gov/17223217/ [cited 2023 Oct 22]
41. Nauck MA, Meininger G, Sheng D, Terranella L, Stein PP, Tesone P, et al. Efficacy and safety of the dipeptidyl peptidase-4 inhibitor, sitagliptin, compared with the sulfonylurea, glipizide, in patients with type 2 diabetes inadequately controlled on metformin alone: a randomized, double-blind, non-inferiority trial. Diabetes Obes Metab. 2007;9(2):194–205. Available from: https://pubmed.ncbi.nlm.nih.gov/17300595/ [cited 2023 Oct 22]
42. Rosenstock J, Brazg R, Andryuk PJ, Lu K, Stein P. Efficacy and safety of the dipeptidyl peptidase-4 inhibitor sitagliptin added to ongoing pioglitazone therapy in patients with type 2 diabetes: a 24-week, multicenter, randomized, double-blind, placebo-controlled, parallel-group study. Clin Ther. 2006;28(10):1556–68. Available from: https://pubmed.ncbi.nlm.nih.gov/17157112/ [cited 2023 Oct 22]
43. Galvus 50 mg Tablets—Summary of Product Characteristics (SmPC)—(emc). Available from: https://www.medicines.org.uk/emc/medicine/20734#POSOLOGY [cited 2023 Oct 22].
44. Buse JB, Bethel MA, Green JB, Stevens SR, Lokhnygina Y, Aschner P, et al. Pancreatic safety of Sitagliptin in the TECOS study. Diabetes Care. 2017;40(2):164–70. Available from: https://pubmed.ncbi.nlm.nih.gov/27630212/ [cited 2023 Oct 22]
45. Tkáč I, Raz I. Combined analysis of three large interventional trials with gliptins indicates increased incidence of acute pancreatitis in patients with type 2 diabetes. Diabetes Care. 2017;40(2):284–6. Available from: https://pubmed.ncbi.nlm.nih.gov/27659407/ [cited 2023 Oct 22]
46. Deacon CF. Dipeptidyl peptidase 4 inhibitors in the treatment of type 2 diabetes mellitus. Nat Rev Endocrinol. 2020;16(11):642–53. Available from: https://pubmed.ncbi.nlm.nih.gov/32929230/ [cited 2023 Oct 22]
47. Scirica BM, Bhatt DL, Braunwald E, Steg PG, Davidson J, Hirshberg B, et al. Saxagliptin and cardiovascular outcomes in patients with type 2 diabetes mellitus. N Engl J Med. 2013;369(14):1317–26. Available from: https://pubmed.ncbi.nlm.nih.gov/23992601/ [cited 2023 Oct 22]

48. White WB, Kupfer S, Zannad F, Mehta CR, Wilson CA, Lei L, et al. Cardiovascular mortality in patients with type 2 diabetes and recent acute coronary syndromes from the EXAMINE trial. Diabetes Care. 2016;39(7):1267–73. Available from: https://pubmed.ncbi.nlm.nih.gov/27289121/ [cited 2023 Oct 22]
49. Schweizer A, Dejager S, Foley JE, Couturier A, Ligueros-Saylan M, Kothny W. Assessing the cardio-cerebrovascular safety of vildagliptin: meta-analysis of adjudicated events from a large phase III type 2 diabetes population. Diabetes Obes Metab. 2010;12(6):485–94. Available from: https://pubmed.ncbi.nlm.nih.gov/20518804/ [cited 2023 Oct 22]
50. Rosenstock J, Perkovic V, Johansen OE, Cooper ME, Kahn SE, Marx N, et al. Effect of Linagliptin vs placebo on major cardiovascular events in adults with type 2 diabetes and high cardiovascular and renal risk: the CARMELINA randomized clinical trial. JAMA. 2019;321(1):69–79. Available from: https://pubmed.ncbi.nlm.nih.gov/30418475/ [cited 2023 Oct 22]
51. Johansen OE, Neubacher D, von Eynatten M, Patel S, Woerle HJ. Cardiovascular safety with linagliptin in patients with type 2 diabetes mellitus: a pre-specified, prospective, and adjudicated meta-analysis of a phase 3 programme. Cardiovasc Diabetol. 2012;11. Available from: https://pubmed.ncbi.nlm.nih.gov/22234149/ [cited 2023 Oct 22]
52. McGuire DK, Alexander JH, Johansen OE, Perkovic V, Rosenstock J, Cooper ME, et al. Linagliptin effects on heart failure and related outcomes in individuals with type 2 diabetes mellitus at high cardiovascular and renal risk in CARMELINA. Circulation. 2019;139(3):351–61. https://doi.org/10.1161/CIRCULATIONAHA.118.038352. [cited 2023 Oct 22]
53. Green JB, Bethel MA, Armstrong PW, Buse JB, Engel SS, Garg J, et al. Effect of sitagliptin on cardiovascular outcomes in type 2 diabetes. N Engl J Med. 2015;373(3):232–42. Available from: https://pubmed.ncbi.nlm.nih.gov/26052984/ [cited 2023 Oct 22]
54. Zannad F, Cannon CP, Cushman WC, Bakris GL, Menon V, Perez AT, et al. Heart failure and mortality outcomes in patients with type 2 diabetes taking alogliptin versus placebo in EXAMINE: a multicentre, randomised, double-blind trial. Lancet. 2015;385(9982):2067–76. Available from: https://pubmed.ncbi.nlm.nih.gov/25765696/ [cited 2023 Oct 22]
55. FDA Drug Safety Communication: FDA adds warnings about heart failure risk to labels of type 2 diabetes medicines containing saxagliptin and alogliptin | FDA. Available from: https://www.fda.gov/drugs/drug-safety-and-availability/fda-drug-safety-communication-fda-adds-warnings-about-heart-failure-risk-labels-type-2-diabetes [cited 2023 Oct 22].
56. FDA Drug Safety Communication: FDA warns that DPP-4 inhibitors for type 2 diabetes may cause severe joint pain | FDA. Available from: https://www.fda.gov/drugs/drug-safety-and-availability/fda-drug-safety-communication-fda-warns-dpp-4-inhibitors-type-2-diabetes-may-cause-severe-joint-pain [cited 2023 Oct 22].
57. Men P, He N, Song C, Zhai S. Dipeptidyl peptidase-4 inhibitors and risk of arthralgia: a systematic review and meta-analysis. Diabetes Metab. 2017;43(6):493–500. Available from: https://pubmed.ncbi.nlm.nih.gov/28778563/ [cited 2023 Oct 22]
58. Mascolo A, Rafaniello C, Sportiello L, Sessa M, Cimmaruta D, Rossi F, et al. Dipeptidyl peptidase (DPP)-4 inhibitor-induced arthritis/arthralgia: a review of clinical cases. Drug Saf. 2016;39(5):401–7. Available from: https://pubmed.ncbi.nlm.nih.gov/26873369/ [cited 2023 Oct 22]
59. Kridin K, Bergman R. Association of Bullous Pemphigoid with dipeptidyl-peptidase 4 inhibitors in patients with diabetes: estimating the risk of the new agents and characterizing the patients. JAMA Dermatol. 2018;154(10):1152–8. Available from: https://pubmed.ncbi.nlm.nih.gov/30090931/ [cited 2023 Oct 22]
60. Lee SG, Lee HJ, Yoon MS, Kim DH. Association of dipeptidyl peptidase 4 inhibitor use with risk of bullous pemphigoid in patients with diabetes. JAMA Dermatol. 2019;155(2):172–7. Available from: https://pubmed.ncbi.nlm.nih.gov/30624566/ [cited 2023 Oct 22]
61. Fineman MS, Shen LZ, Taylor K, Kim DD, Baron AD. Effectiveness of progressive dose-escalation of exenatide (exendin-4) in reducing dose-limiting side effects in subjects with type 2 diabetes. Diabetes Metab Res Rev. 2004;20(5):411–7. Available from: https://pubmed.ncbi.nlm.nih.gov/15343588/ [cited 2023 Oct 22]

62. Li L, Shen J, Bala MM, Busse JW, Ebrahim S, Vandvik PO, et al. Incretin treatment and risk of pancreatitis in patients with type 2 diabetes mellitus: systematic review and meta-analysis of randomised and non-randomised studies. BMJ. 2014;348. Available from: https://www.bmj.com/content/348/bmj.g2366 [cited 2023 Oct 22]
63. Egan AG, Blind E, Dunder K, de Graeff PA, Hummer BT, Bourcier T, et al. Pancreatic safety of incretin-based drugs—FDA and EMA assessment. N Engl J Med. 2014;370(9):794–7. Available from: https://pubmed.ncbi.nlm.nih.gov/24571751/ [cited 2023 Oct 22]
64. Easow B, Mathew M, Rajagopalan U, Nagarajan P, Abraham G. Serious adverse effects following use of liraglutide in individuals with type 2 diabetes. J Diabetol. 2022;13(3):314. Available from: https://journals.lww.com/jodb/fulltext/2022/13030/serious_adverse_effects_following_use_of.18.aspx [cited 2023 Oct 31]
65. Marso SP, Bain SC, Consoli A, Eliaschewitz FG, Jódar E, Leiter LA, et al. Semaglutide and cardiovascular outcomes in patients with type 2 diabetes. N Engl J Med. 2016;375(19):1834–44. Available from: https://www.nejm.org/doi/full/10.1056/nejmoa1607141 [cited 2023 Oct 22]
66. Husain M, Birkenfeld AL, Donsmark M, Dungan K, Eliaschewitz FG, Franco DR, et al. Oral Semaglutide and cardiovascular outcomes in patients with type 2 diabetes. N Engl J Med. 2019;381(9):841–51. Available from: https://pubmed.ncbi.nlm.nih.gov/31185157/ [cited 2023 Oct 22]
67. Holman RR, Cull CA, Turner RC. A randomized double-blind trial of acarbose in type 2 diabetes shows improved glycemic control over 3 years (U.K. Prospective Diabetes Study 44). Diabetes Care. 1999;22(6):960–4. Available from: https://pubmed.ncbi.nlm.nih.gov/10372249/ [cited 2023 Oct 22]
68. Long-term efficacy and safety of acarbose in the treatment of obese subjects with non-insulin-dependent diabetes mellitus. PubMed. Available from: https://pubmed.ncbi.nlm.nih.gov/7979840/ [cited 2023 Oct 22].
69. Hollander P. Safety profile of acarbose, an alpha-glucosidase inhibitor. Drugs. 1992;44(Suppl 3):47–53. Available from: https://pubmed.ncbi.nlm.nih.gov/1280577/ [cited 2023 Oct 22]
70. Oba K, Suzuki K, Ouchi M, Matsumura N, Suzuki T, Nakano H. Repeated episodes of paralytic ileus in an elderly diabetic patient treated with voglibose. J Am Geriatr Soc. 2006;54(1):182–3. Available from: https://pubmed.ncbi.nlm.nih.gov/16420230/ [cited 2023 Oct 22]
71. https://www.accessdata.fda.gov/drugsatfda_docs/label/2009/021773s9s11s18s22s25lbl.pdf.
72. Taylor SR, Harris KB. The clinical efficacy and safety of sodium glucose cotransporter-2 inhibitors in adults with type 2 diabetes mellitus. Pharmacotherapy. 2013;33(9):984–99. Available from: https://pubmed.ncbi.nlm.nih.gov/23744749/ [cited 2023 Oct 22]
73. Steiner S. Empagliflozin, cardiovascular outcomes, and mortality in type 2 diabetes. Zeitschrift fur Gefassmedizin. 2016;13(1):17–8. https://doi.org/10.1056/nejmoa1504720. [cited 2023 Oct 22]
74. Scheen AJ. An update on the safety of SGLT2 inhibitors. Expert Opin Drug Saf. 2019;18(4):295–311. Available from: https://pubmed.ncbi.nlm.nih.gov/30933547/ [cited 2023 Oct 22]
75. Rajagopalan S, Brook R. Canagliflozin and cardiovascular and renal events in type 2 diabetes. N Engl J Med. 2017;377(21):2098–9. Available from: http://www.ncbi.nlm.nih.gov/pubmed/29182250 [cited 2023 Oct 22]
76. Wiviott SD, Raz I, Bonaca MP, Mosenzon O, Kato ET, Cahn A, et al. Dapagliflozin and cardiovascular outcomes in type 2 diabetes. N Engl J Med. 2019;380(4):347–57. Available from: https://pubmed.ncbi.nlm.nih.gov/30415602/ [cited 2023 Oct 22]
77. FDA revises labels of SGLT2 inhibitors for diabetes to include warnings about too much acid in the blood and serious urinary tract infections | FDA. Available from: https://www.fda.gov/drugs/drug-safety-and-availability/fda-revises-labels-sglt2-inhibitors-diabetes-include-warnings-about-too-much-acid-blood-and-serious [cited 2023 Oct 22].
78. FDA Drug Safety Communication: FDA strengthens kidney warnings for diabetes medicines canagliflozin (Invokana, Invokamet) and dapagliflozin (Farxiga, Xigduo XR) | FDA. Available from: https://www.fda.gov/drugs/drug-safety-and-availability/fda-drug-safety-communication-fda-strengthens-kidney-warnings-diabetes-medicines-canagliflozin [cited 2023 Oct 22].

Diabetic Foot Complications and Challenges

22

Vijay Viswanathan, Siva shankari, and Gordon Sloan

22.1 Introduction

Diabetes mellitus is considered a chronic debilitating metabolic disease, which is also one of the most common noncommunicable diseases in the world. It is associated with significant morbidity, mortality, and healthcare expenses and also affects the quality of life of innumerable patients. According to a study by the Indian Council of Medical Research-India Diabetes (ICMR-INDIAB), around 101 million people in India are found to be affected by diabetes [1]. These numbers are expected to increase with the rampantly expanding population and also with lifestyle modifications as well as the increasing prevalence of obesity [2]. This creates tremendous pressure and burden on the healthcare providers to prevent dangerous and devastating complications of the disease.

22.2 The Diabetic Foot

There are various micro as well as macrovascular complications associated with the disease because it affects the kidneys, heart, eyes as well as feet. Diabetic foot infection (DFI) is considered a major complication which is also one of the most common reasons for hospitalization in India. It can also result in dreadful complications like amputation and sometimes even death, if not treated properly. Thus appropriate diagnosis and treatment play a crucial role in the management of DFI.

V. Viswanathan (✉) · S. shankari
MV Hospital for Diabetes, Royapuram, Chennai, Tamil Nadu, India
e-mail: clinicalresearch@mvdiabetes.com

G. Sloan
Division of Clinical Medicine, University of Sheffield, Sheffield, UK
e-mail: gordon.sloan@nhs.net

G. Abraham et al. (eds.), *Management of Diabetic Complications*,
https://doi.org/10.1007/978-981-97-6406-8_22

22.3 Epidemiology and Burden of DFI

It is quite alarming to understand that every 20 s a limb is lost somewhere in this world, and the lifetime risk of developing DFI is approximately between 19% and 34% [3]. The worldwide prevalence of diabetic foot ulcers (DFU) is found to be around 6.3% [4]. In India, around 25% of people living with diabetes are found to be affected by DFU with nearly 50% of them requiring hospitalization and around 20% of them requiring amputation [5]. It has been estimated that an Indian spends approximately 5.7 years of his income on his expenses toward DFU expenditure which is in concordance with two other studies (Satyavani et al. and Shobana et al.) in which it was stated that an individual with DFU spends approximately four times more than a person without the ulcer [6, 7]. Vijay V et al. (2005) projected the prevalence of DFI in India to be between 6% and 11% with neuropathy considered a major risk factor for DFI. Infection was also a major risk factor for major amputations in another multicentric study by Vijay V et al. (2011) in which the prevalence of neuropathy and peripheral vascular disease (PVD) was estimated to be around 82% and 35%, respectively [8]. The enormous burden and the gigantic magnitude of the problem in India could be attributed to the low socio-economic status, insufficient foot care facilities, and the inadvertent practice of barefoot walking [2]. Table 22.1 shows the steps in physical examination of diabetic foot.

22.4 The Vicious Triad

The pathophysiology of DFI could be attributed to the vicious triad of neuropathy, PVD, and repetitive trauma (Fig. 22.1).

Table 22.1 Key components of the diabetic foot examination

Key components of the diabetic foot examination	
Dermatology: – Skin status, color, thickness, dryness, cracking – Sweating – Infection: Check between toes for fungal infection – Ulceration – Calluses/blistering: Hemorrhage into callus?	**Neurological assessment:** 10-g monofilament + 1 of the following 4 – Vibration using 128-Hz tuning fork – Pinprick sensation – Ankle reflexes – VPT
Musculoskeletal: – Deformity; e.g., claw toes, prominent metatarsal heads, Charcot joint – Muscle wasting (guttering between metatarsals)	**Vascular assessment:** – Foot pulses – ABI, if indicated

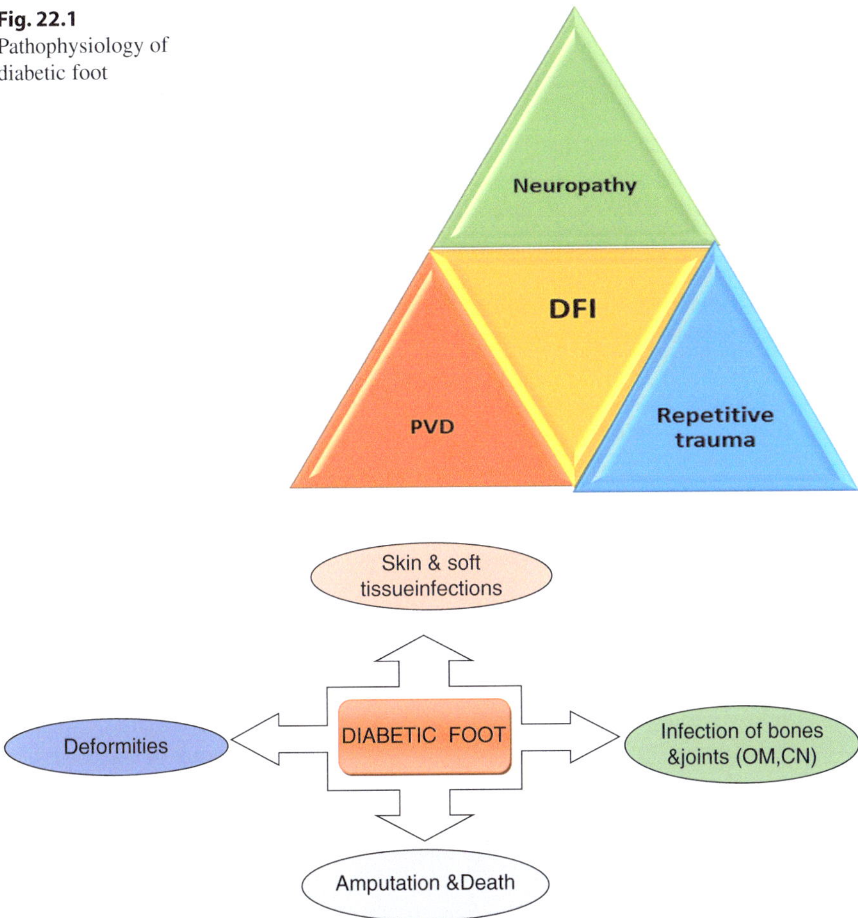

Fig. 22.1 Pathophysiology of diabetic foot

Fig. 22.2 Natural course of diabetic foot

22.5 Complications of Diabetic Foot

There are innumerable complications of diabetic foot encountered in clinical practice which require the most appropriate management. Some of the most common ones are depicted in the figure below (Fig. 22.2).

22.6 Skin and Soft Tissue Infections (STI)

The various foot infections ranging from superficial infections involving the nails to deep infections involving the bone are quite challenging in the management of DFI. Cellulitis, abscess, myositis, necrotizing fasciitis, and gangrene are some of the common skins and STIs. The microbes can spread through the skin ulcerations or sinus tracts and can cause soft tissue infections like cellulitis which affects deeper layers of skin. There can be swelling, partial or complete loss of facial planes, and sometimes even accumulation of gas which are evident from plain X-rays and computed tomography (CT) [9]. MRI findings like subcutaneous edema and increased thickness of skin are suggestive of Cellulitis [10]. Sometimes, prolonged foot infection can also result in abscess formation. Necrotizing fasciitis involves superficial and deep layers of skin which can be life-threatening. Foreign bodies can also pose a serious threat in people with insensate feet due to neuropathy and decreased protective reflexes. These impacted foreign bodies make the diabetic foot further susceptible to infections. Plain X-rays or probes in ultrasound can be used to remove these foreign bodies. Hyperglycemia causes impaired blood supply to the tissues which can decrease the blood supply to the feet, ultimately resulting in the formation of gangrene. Treatment depends upon the severity of the infection. Mild cases might require oral antibiotics whereas severe cases might require hospitalization and intravenous administration of antibiotics.

22.7 Infections of the Bone

The two potential life-threatening complications of diabetic foot affecting the bones are Osteomyelitis (OM) and Charcot neuroarthropathy (CN). A positive probe-to-bone (PTB) test can help in the clinical differentiation of STI from osteomyelitis. Plain radiographs and MRI are imaging modalities employed to diagnose OM and CN more accurately. Peripheral sensory and autonomic neuropathy in insensate feet along with repetitive trauma can result in an increase in osteoclastic activity and severe deformity contributing to the pathogenesis of CN. In the case of Acute CN, the foot appears red, hot, and swollen but in the case of Chronic CN, the local inflammatory changes are decreased with more pronounced bony changes finally resulting in deformities of the foot. The midfoot is usually affected and in some cases, there can be even collapse of the arch resulting in a rocker bottom deformity. This in turn can create high pressures making the foot more prone to the risk of ulceration [11].

An important diagnostic challenge can arise from the differentiation of acute CN and osteomyelitis which requires the usage of appropriate imaging modalities like plain radiographs and MRI. MRIs are usually highly sensitive as well as specific in the diagnosis of OM as well as the early stage of acute CN. However, plain radiographs are more affordable and easily available to distinguish between them though detection of CN at early stages might be difficult only with plain radiographs. Clinical classification of infections is given in Fig. 22.3.

Clinical classification of infection, definitions	IWGDF/IDSA classification
No systemic or local symptoms or signs of infection	1 / Uninfected
Infected: At least two of these items are present: • Local swelling or induration • Erythema > 0.5 but < 2 cm[b] around the wound • Local tenderness or pain • Local increased warmth • Purulent discharge And, no other cause of an inflammatory response of the skin (e.g., trauma, gout, acute Charcot neuro-arthropathy, fracture, thrombosis, or venous stasis)	2 / Mild
Infection with no systemic manifestations and involving: • erythema extending ≥ 2 cmb from the wound margin, and/or • tissue deeper than skin and subcutaneous tissues (e.g., tendon, muscle, joint, and bone)	3 / Moderate
Infection involving bone (osteomyelitis)	Add "(O)"
Any foot infection with associated systemic manifestations (of the systemic inflammatory response syndrome [SIRS]), as manifested by ≥ 2 of the following: • temperature, > 38°C or < 36°C • heart rate, > 90 beats/min • respiratory rate, >20 breaths/min, or PaCO2 < 4.3 kPa (32 mmHg) • white blood cell count >12,000/mm³, or < 4G/L, or > 10% immature (band) forms	4 / Severe
Infection involving bone (osteomyelitis)	Add "(O)"

Fig. 22.3 Classification system for the presence and severity of an infection of a DFU [26]. (1) refers to infection in any part of the foot not just a DFU; (2) if in any direction from the rim of the wound; (3) if osteomyelitis presents the foot can be classified as 3O (if <2 SIRS criteria) or 4O (if 2 or more SIRS criteria)

22.8 Deformities

Some of the common skeletal deformities seen among people with diabetic foot are Hallux vagus, pes planus, hammer/ claw toes, and rocker bottom deformities which can be detected in plain radiographs and CT. Hammer toes are usually caused by atrophy of intrinsic muscles due to hypertension of the metatarsophalangeal joint is also considered responsible for ulceration of plantar skin [12].

22.9 Amputation and Death

Lower extremity amputations and increased mortality rates due to complications of diabetic foot are two dreadful situations that are sometimes comparable to cancer. In a study by Armstrong et al., he estimated the five-year mortality rates of CN, DFU, minor, and major amputations to be 29, 30.5, 46.2, and 56.6, respectively [13]. Sometimes, the fear of amputation among patients is considered worse than even death. This also remains one of the major challenges encountered by diabetic foot specialists.

22.10 Potential Challenges Encountered in Resource-Constrained Setting for the Management of Diabetic Foot

Patients hesitate to approach diabetologists or podiatric surgeons in the early stages of DFI and adopt certain unconventional and nonvalidated home remedies which can have precarious consequences. This along with the irrational use of over-the-counter antibiotics are considered reasons for delay in the appropriate treatment required.

A longstanding 53-year-old male, diabetes mellitus since 19 years with ESKD for 6 months, foot ulcer with plain X-ray showing no arterial calcification and Doppler showing normal arterial flow (Fig. 22.4a, b).

Figure 22.4c shows 60-year-old male, with longstanding diabetes mellitus on hemodialysis and infected ulcer with severe calcified atherosclerotic arterial disease of the popliteal artery and branches. Now the ulcer has healed with angioplasty and infection control. He has also longstanding ESRD. 15 years smoker with 10 cigarettes/day.

22.11 Lack of Appropriate Footwear

In India, the usage of inappropriate footwear and improper foot care hygiene can increase the potential risk for ulceration. The choice of footwear is very important especially both indoors and outdoors, and it should pertain to the altered biomechanics or deformities of the foot, if any. The use of customized footwear and insole must be encouraged especially among patients who are identified to be at a higher risk due to insensate feet as in diabetic neuropathy. In a study by Vijay et al., it was concluded that around 65% of the study population lacked appropriate footcare practices which were also recognized as one of the chief reasons for the higher prevalence of DFI [14].

22.12 Lack of Adequate Training Programs for Healthcare Personnel

There is a definite need to develop systematic and integrated training programs for healthcare personnel across the globe especially in developing nations like India. The step-by-step program as well as Train the Foot Trainer programs are excellent examples of providing foot care education to healthcare professionals.

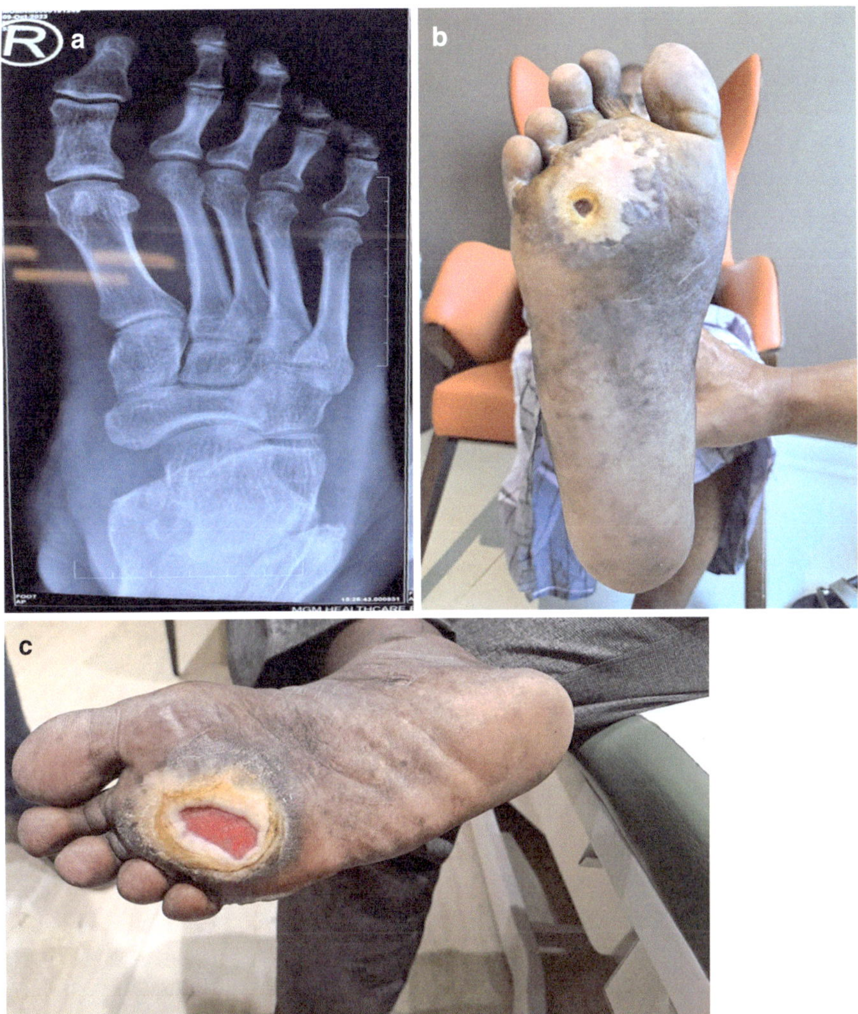

Fig. 22.4 (**a**, **b**, **c**) Showing foot ulcer with normal X-ray of foot

22.13 Inadequate Surveillance and Follow-Up

There is a desperate need for the development of a good surveillance system to assess the complications of diabetic foot [15]. The classification of diabetic foot by Meggitt–Wagner is given in Fig. 22.5. It becomes very difficult to receive patients for follow-up regularly to monitor them over foot care practices and thereby prevent complications. Patients living in rural areas are at a higher risk of developing DFI due to the practice of walking barefoot in the fields. They will have to travel long distances to obtain facilities from a well-equipped hospital for their treatment which is also considered as a potential barrier [2].

Fig. 22.5 Meggitt–Wagner classification of diabetic foot ulcers [15]

Grade	Description of the ulcer
0	Pre- or postulcerative lesion completely epithelialized
1	Superficial, full-thickness ulcer limited to the dermis, not extending to the subcutis
2	Ulcer of the skin extending through the subcutis with exposed tendon or bone and without osteomyelitis or abscess formation
3	Deep ulcers with osteomyelitis or abscess formation
4	Localized gangrene of the toes or the forefoot
5	Foot with extensive gangrene

22.14 Selection and Choice of Appropriate Antibiotics

An initial regimen of antibiotics has to be chosen based on the severity of DFI and resort to a more definitive therapy based on microbiology culture reports. In India, it is important to choose appropriate as well as affordable drugs because it can affect compliance [16]. IWGDF 2023 guidelines on infection suggest that the choice of antibiotics must depend on the causative pathogen and its susceptibility, clinical severity, cost, and potential risk of adverse events [17].

22.15 Strategies to Prevent Complications and Overcome the Challenges

An integrated approach is thus required to adequately manage the various complications associated with diabetic foot. A multidisciplinary team that comprises diabetologists, vascular, orthopedic and general surgeons, orthotists, podiatrists, nurses, radiologists, microbiologists, and psychologists is considered imperative and quintessential for the appropriate management of DFI.

The IWGDF guidelines 2023 recommends the following key principal components in the effective prevention as well as management of DFI [18] (Fig. 22.6).

22.15.1 Management of Diabetic Foot Ulcers

There are many considerations in the management of a patient with a DFU, which are often complex and require highly trained experts. In order to promote wound healing, the following factors need to be addressed: glucose control, ischemia,

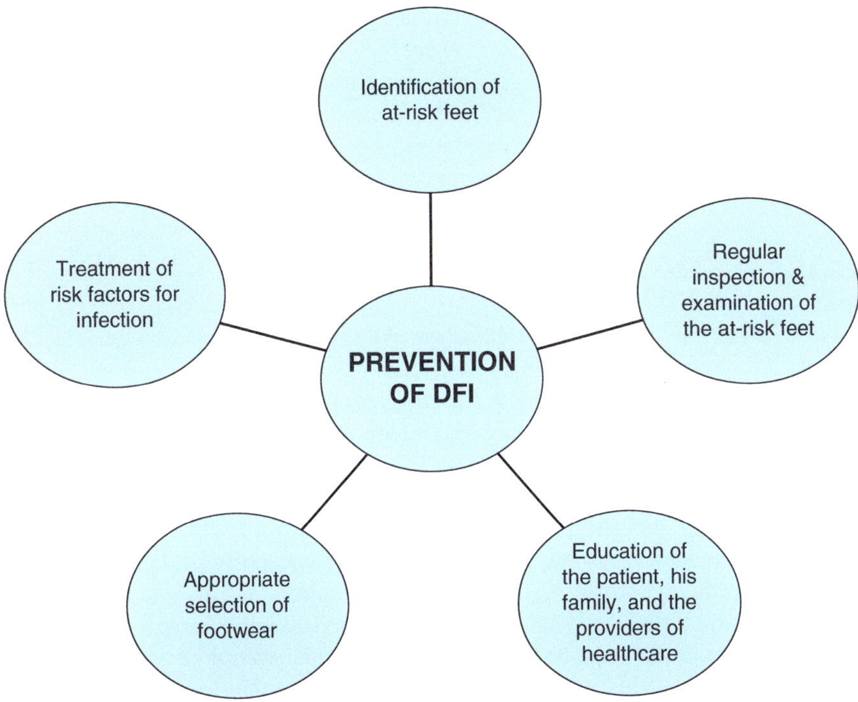

Fig. 22.6 Prevention of diabetic foot infection

infection, peri-wound tissue management (debridement), pressure, and edema. If any one of these factors is not addressed, then the wound may not heal. Thus, in order to effectively manage DFUs patients should be seen in specialist clinics with availability to multidisciplinary care teams, including diabetologists, diabetes specialist nurses, podiatrists, orthotics, orthopedic surgeons, vascular surgeons, and microbiology. Highly specialized, multidisciplinary teams with care algorithms and referral pathways are essential for the modern care of diabetic foot disease and have been shown to reduce amputations [19] with new diabetic foot disease should ideally be seen in 24–48 h within these outpatient services, unless they require immediate admission to hospital (e.g., limb/life-threatening conditions such as ischemia and infection).

22.15.2 Acute Management of the Limb/Life-Threatening DFU

The first, and most important distinction in a patient with a DFU is to determine whether the patient requires immediate (same day/within 24 h) treatment to avoid limb/life loss. Patients requiring such urgent care include those with bacteremia and sepsis, rapidly spreading infection, suspected (or confirmed) abscesses, and severe ischemia (e.g., gangrene, necrotizing infection, and ischemic rest pain). Most often, these patients would require an acute admission to receive such care. If patients have sepsis or severe cellulitis, then patients will require intravenous antibiotics tailored to microbiology samples. A DFU complicated by abscesses or severe ischemia will need to be evaluated by specialist surgeons for evaluate the need for surgical intervention [18]. DFU may deteriorate at any time, and it is important to educate patients on signs of deterioration (e.g., fever or unexplained hyperglycemia).

22.15.3 Treatment of Infection in DFU

Prompt treatment of superficial infection within the ulcer or deeper infection (abscess/osteomyelitis) is essential. The choice of antibiotics depends upon numerous factors; first, the first antibiotic of choice depends upon the likely causative bacterium, which is dependent upon the region, but most often are gram-positive cocci (e.g., staphylococci and streptococci) [20]. Patient factors must also be considered, such as the severity/depth of the infection, allergy status, and past microbiological history, including previous culture samples and antibiotic use. For mild infections, patients can usually be started on a cephalosporin/penicillin agent (or alternative if allergy) whilst awaiting swab/tissue culture results. It is important to review the patient frequently (at least weekly) to ensure improvement of the infection. The antibiotic can then be tailored to the individual according to microbiological culture results. This may require discussions with microbiology experts, as DFUs can be polymicrobial.

Generally, oral antibiotics for mild infections are sufficient; however, intravenous antibiotics may be necessary initially for moderate/severe infections or bacteremia for a few days before switching to oral antibiotics [21]. Source control of infection may also be necessary, such as debridement of infected/necrotic tissue and abscess drainage, as discussed above. It is recommended that 1–2 weeks of antibiotic therapy should be sufficient to treat infection, and patients should be re-assessed with careful consideration of reasons for lack of improvement (e.g., incorrect antibiotic treatment, misdiagnosis of infection, or deep infection). However, in the presence of osteomyelitis then at least 6-week antibiotic therapy will be necessary. Again, if there is no improvement with 6-week treatment of osteomyelitis then the patient should be re-assessed, and also bone sampling for culture where possible. If there continues to be no improvement, then bone resection, often in the presence of amputation (but ideally avoided), can be considered. Treatment of osteomyelitis is difficult, and bone infections often recur; therefore, surgical resection is commonly required to achieve a "cure" [22].

Traditionally, intravenous antibiotics had been recommended for osteomyelitis, but the OVIVA (Oral versus Intravenous Antibiotics for Bone and Joint Infection) study found oral antibiotics noninferior to intravenous antibiotics [23].

22.15.4 Treatment of Ischemia

Revascularization therapy may be necessary either to aid wound healing or prevent a new/recurrent DFU. Close collaboration with the vascular surgical team is essential to decide on the appropriateness and timing of vascular intervention. Some patients may not be deemed suitable for vascular intervention, such as those who are frail or felt to be very high risk (e.g., severe ischemic heart disease). The timing of revascularization therapy depends on the individual case, urgent intervention should be considered in purely ischemic ulcers and if there is severe ischemia on the basis of clinical signs/symptoms (e.g., necrosis or rest-pain) or on vascular assessment (e.g., impalpable pulses of ABPI <0.4). There is evidence that early intervention improves wound healing rates [24]. Thus, early vascular assessment should be considered in all patients [25]. Moreover, vascular status carefully reviewed in all patients with slowly/nonhealing DFU. The aim of revascularization is to restore in-line flow to arteries supplying the wound and can either be endovascular (e.g., stenting) or surgical (e.g., bypass surgery).

22.15.5 Off-Loading the Diabetic Foot Wound

Off-loading refers to the use of devices, surgeries, or lifestyle changes that reduce pressure, or the "load," at the site of a DFU, in order to improve healing [22]. Due to the presence of sensory neuropathy, people with DPN feel no pain at the site of DFUs, which would otherwise be enormously painful to walk on in the presence of normal sensation. When a person with DPN continues to walk on a DFU, each step prevents effective wound healing. Off-loading devices work by reducing pressure (often by spreading pressure over a larger area), reducing motion at the joint of the foot, and are often associated with reduced activity. The devices range from nonremovable devices (e.g., total-contact cast [TCC]), to customized shoes or inserts which can be put into normal or therapeutic footwear. Often, the most effective treatment (e.g., TCC) may not be the most suitable for the patient, for example, if they are frail, prone to falls, or have an ulcer that is at risk in a nonremovable device (e.g., in moderate-severe infection or moderate-severe ischemia). Moreover, the most intensive device might not be tolerable to the patient [26]. Thus, selection of an off-loading device requires tailoring to the individual.

Much of the evidence based on off-loading is for the treatment of uncomplicated neuropathic plantar foot ulcers [27]. The most efficacious off-loading devices for plantar foot ulcers are knee-high nonremovable devices, i.e., TCC or a knee-high walker which is nonremovable [24]. A TCC is a cast boot applied with minimal padding, whereas a knee-high walker is a prefabricated boot generally applied with straps/velcro. An important reason why these devices are so effective is the fact they cannot be removed, thereby ensuring compliance with treatment. TCCs may have higher initial treatment costs, but due to their efficacy over other treatment options, they are cost-effective over full duration of treatment. There is a small increase in risk with new lesions in nonremovable devices, and infection/ischemia may need to be managed before using a nonremovable device [26].

Removable knee-high offloading devices should be used if nonremovable devices are contraindicated/not tolerated, followed by ankle-high offloading devices. Unfortunately, there is scant evidence for the efficacy of these devices, in part this may be because they can be removed. A study demonstrated that patients used their prescribed removable devices for an average of only 29% of their daily steps, and the most adherent subset of patients still wore their device for 60% of their total daily activity [28].

Surgical off-loading treatments are adjuncts to nonsurgical offloading. Flexor tendon tenotomy can be used as a first-line treatment for DFU on the apex of the toes (except the great/first toe) [24].

Achilles tendon lengthening can also be performed if off-loading has failed for plantar forefoot ulcers. Other more complex orthopedic interventions can be considered in consultation with orthopedics with a specialist interest for ulcers that fail to heal with nonsurgical interventions (e.g., osteotomy, joint arthroplasty, or resection of bone at pressure points) [18].

22.15.6 Wound Debridement

Debridement involves the removal of nonviable tissues (e.g., callus or necrotic and/or infected tissue) that may be inhibiting wound healing at the bed or margin of the DFU. In addition, debridement makes it possible to accurately determine the size of wounds (e.g., DFU "hidden" beneath callus) and can allow drainage from a wound [29].

Similar to other treatments for DFU, there are numerous different debridement options, and many patients factors to be considered before choosing the best therapy [29]. The most used debridement method is sharp debridement, which involves the dissection of nonviable tissue from healthy tissues using a range of devices, such as curettes and scalpels. This technique requires well-trained and experienced members of the diabetic foot team, such as podiatrists or surgeons and can be performed either in operating rooms or in an outpatient clinic setting. Superficial and limited debridement, such as removing callus build up around neuropathic ulcers, can be performed in an outpatient clinic, whereas removal of infected and/or necrotic deeper tissues would need to be done in the operating theatre. In experienced hands, sharp debridement is safe and effective, although DFUs complicated with significant ischemia may require revascularization before debridement. Another factor to consider is the frequency of debridement, which is also dependent upon the availability of the service. However, in general it is recommended that debridement should occur 1–2 weekly. Other forms of mechanical debridement may nonselectively remove granulation tissue as well as nonviable tissue. These methods include high-pressure saline irrigation, wet-to-dry saline dressings, and ultrasound.

Biological debridement or Maggot Debridement Therapy (MDT), involves the application of medicinal maggots grown in a sterile environment which are introduced to a wound bed and contained with an overlying adherent dressing [22, 29]. The maggots then selectively feed on necrotic and nonviable tissue, without injuring living tissue. This method is effective if the wound has large quantities of slough tissue. The ability to employ this treatment is dependent upon the appropriate healthcare facilities able to develop medicinal larvae. Patients may have an aversion to the idea of the therapy, but in the correct circumstances it can be effective. Other forms of nonmechanical debridement involve application of chemical agents (enzymatic debridement) or using the body's own enzymatic processes (autolytic debridement), the latter by keeping the wound moist and thus facilitating endogenous enzymes to auto-digest nonviable tissue [29].

22.15.7 Dressings

There is little evidence to support the use of one dressing type. The IWGDF recommends the use of a dressing that absorbs exudate and maintains a moist wound environment but does not recommend the use of antimicrobial dressings [18]. One randomized controlled trial found sucrose octasulfate dressings to be more effective than control in neuroischemic DFUs [30].

22.15.8 Postoperative Wound Management

DFUs can require extensive surgical debridement and/or amputation at the level of the foot. It is important that these wounds are monitored by the operating surgeons, and appropriate off-loading footwear and dressings are applied. In addition, large post-surgical wounds may benefit from negative pressure therapy to reduce healing times [18].

22.15.9 Adjunctive Therapies

Adjunctive treatments for nonhealing ulcers have been developed. In general, these adjunctive treatments are not widely used, due to the limited efficacy, expense and availability. The 2023 IWGDF guidelines suggest that the following interventions can be considered in the noninfected DFU which fails to heal after 4–6 weeks:

- A multi-layered patch of autologous leucocytes, platelets and fibrin in ulcers with or without moderate ischemia.
- Placental membrane allografts in ulcers with or without moderate ischemia.
- Topical oxygen therapy.
- Systemic hyperbaric oxygen therapy as an adjunctive treatment for ischemic ulcers.

22.15.10 Charcot Neuroarthropathy

Charcot neuroarthropathy is a rarer but potentially devastating complication of DPN [31]. It is an inflammatory syndrome characterized by varying degrees of bone and joint disorganization secondary to underlying neuropathy, trauma, and perturbations of bone metabolism [32]. In the acute presentation, the foot is often swollen, warm, and erythematous with varying degrees of pain. If the condition is not rapidly recognized and joint immobilization instituted, chronic deformities can develop that subsequently put the foot at very high risk of ulceration. Pathways to Charcot neuroarthropathy and to foot ulceration and/or amputation are shown in Fig. 22.7.

In the presence of suspected Charcot neuroarthropathy, the foot should be immobilized in a non-weight-bearing cast at the earliest possible time (ideally same day). The first investigation is a weight-bearing plain X-ray, which can identify subtle and early signs of Charcot neuroarthropathy, but often further investigations are required such as an MRI scan, or serial X-rays if this is unavailable. The treatment involves off-loading using a TCC. Determining when the Charcot foot has become "inactive" is challenging and involves clinical assessment (reduction of foot swelling/temperature), but serial imaging can be useful too. Patients with Charcot Neuroarthropathy may need surgical intervention. In general, surgery is avoided early in the presentation, but it may be necessary in the presence of severe instability/deformity. Reconstructive surgery may also be required once the Charcot neuroarthropathy is quiet, to repair deformity and reduce the risk of future plantar foot ulceration.

22.15.11 Prevention of DFU Recurrence

The rate of DFU recurrence is very high, 40% may have a recurrence within 1 year of ulcer healing [3]. Despite treatment of a DFU, the precipitating factors for the ulcer in the first place (DPN, PVD, deformity, etc.) generally remain. Patients with a previous foot ulcer should be seen by foot care professionals on a regular basis, to identify new ulcers or "pre-ulcerative" lesions and provide ongoing education about foot care. Most patients will also require therapeutic footwear. Furthermore, vascular, and orthopedic interventions may be considered to treat PVD and biomechanical protection, respectively. Early recognition and treatment of new lesions is key, and patients with a previous DFU should have a clear pathway to rapidly access foot services. The prevention and treatment of diabetic foot complications in an at-risk patient are shown in Fig. 22.8.

22.16 Conclusion

Diabetic foot complications are already extremely common, and their prevalence is only going to increase with the increasing worldwide rates of type 2 diabetes. These complications are enormously expensive and lead to considerable patient morbidity, and limb and life loss. The key tenets of diabetic foot complications management

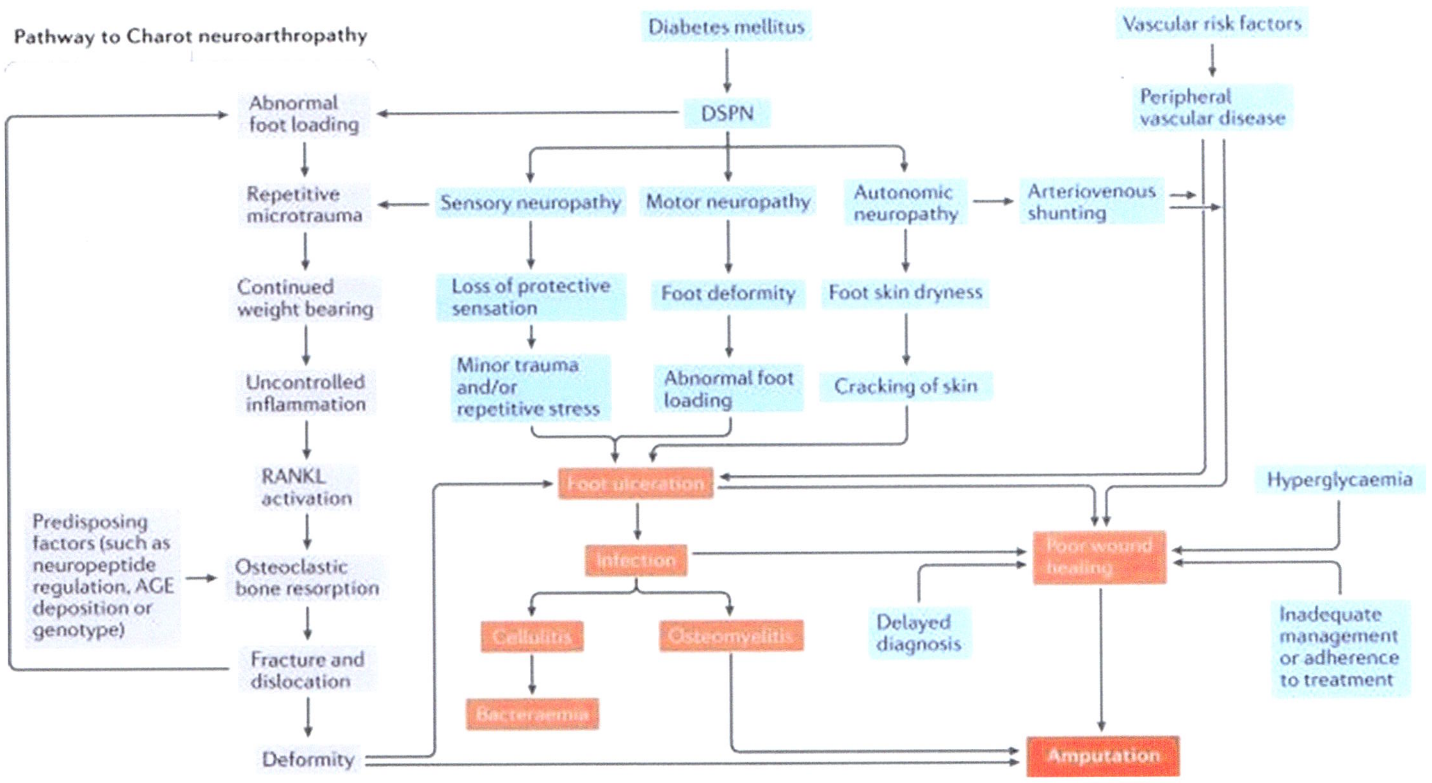

Fig. 22.7 The causal pathway of diabetic foot disease. Blue boxes signify risk factors to foot ulceration and poor wound healing. Grey boxes indicate the pathway to Charcot Neuroarthropathy. Orange boxes represent the pathway to amputation of the ulcerated foot [31]

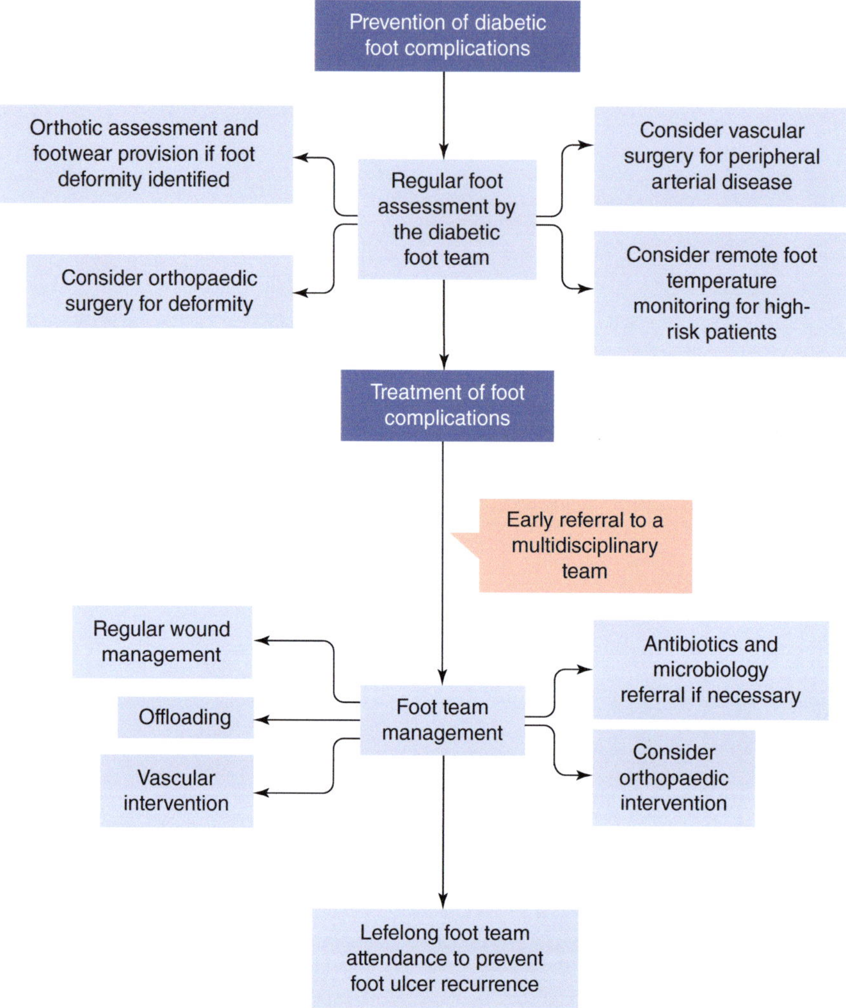

Fig. 22.8 Prevention and treatment of diabetic foot complications in an at-risk patient [13]

are early recognition and treatment, clear referral pathways, and multidisciplinary foot care teams with diabetic foot care experts.

It is imperative to be more pragmatic in dealing with diabetic foot complications and the potential challenges encountered especially in a resource-constrained setting like India. A multidisciplinary team is thus required for the comprehensive and integrated management of DFI. Thus, early screening and recognition of high-risk feet are considered key preventive strategies to prevent complications and overcome prospective challenges that may arise.

References

1. Anjana RM, Unnikrishnan R, Deepa M, Pradeepa R, Tandon N, Das AK, Joshi S, Bajaj S, Jabbar PK, Das HK, Kumar A, Dhandhania VK, Bhansali A, Rao PV, Desai A, Kalra S, Gupta A, Lakshmy R, Madhu SV, Elangovan N, Chowdhury S, Venkatesan U, Subashini R, Kaur T, Dhaliwal RS, Mohan V, ICMR-INDIAB Collaborative Study Group. Metabolic non-communicable disease health report of India: the ICMR-INDIAB national cross-sectional study (ICMR-INDIAB-17). Lancet Diabetes Endocrinol. 2023;11(7):474–89. https://doi.org/10.1016/S2213-8587(23)00119-5. Epub 2023 Jun 7
2. Viswanathan V. Epidemiology of diabetic foot and management of foot problems in India. Int J Low Extrem Wounds. 2010;9(3):122–6. https://doi.org/10.1177/1534734610380026.
3. Armstrong DG, Boulton AJM, Bus SA. Diabetic foot ulcers and their recurrence. N Engl J Med. 2017;376:2367–75.
4. Jodheea-Jutton A, Hindocha S, Bhaw-Luximon A. Health economics of diabetic foot ulcer and recent trends to accelerate treatment. Foot (Edinb). 2022;52:101909. https://doi.org/10.1016/j.foot.2022.101909. Epub 2022 Feb 4
5. Shankar EM, Mohan V, Premalatha G, Srinivasan RS, UshaAR. Bacterial etiology of diabetic foot infections in SouthIndia. Eur J Int Med. 2005;16:567–70.
6. Kumpatla S, Kothandan H, Tharkar S, Viswanathan V. The costs of treating long-term diabetic complications in a developing country: a study from India. J Assoc Physicians India. 2013;61(2):102–9.
7. Shobhana R, Rao PR, Lavanya A, Vijay V, Ramachandran A. Cost burden to diabetic patients with foot complications—a study from southern India. J Assoc Physicians India. 2000;48(12):1147–50. PMID: 11280217
8. Viswanathan V, Kumpatla S. Pattern and causes of amputation in diabetic patients—a multicentric study from India. J Assoc Phys India. 2011;59:148–51.
9. Wilson DJ, Berendt AR. Bone and soft tissue infection. In: Adam A, Dixon AK, editors. Grainger and Allison's diagnostic radiology. Edimburgh, UK: Churchill Livingstone; 2008. p. 1153–69.
10. Russell JM, Peterson JJ, Bancroft LW. MR imaging of the diabetic foot. Magn Reson Imaging Clin N Am. 2008;16:59–70., vi. https://doi.org/10.1016/j.mric.2008.02.004.
11. Ertugrul BM, Lipsky BA, Savk O. Osteomyelitis or Charcot neuro-osteoarthropathy? Differentiating these disorders in diabetic patients with a foot problem. Diabet Foot Ankle. 2013;5:4. https://doi.org/10.3402/dfa.v4i0.21855. PMID: 24205433; PMCID: PMC3819473
12. Naidoo P, Liu VJ, Mautone M, Bergin S. Lower limb complications of diabetes mellitus: a comprehensive review with clinicopathological insights from a dedicated high-risk diabetic foot multidisciplinary team. Br J Radiol. 2015;88(1053):20150135. https://doi.org/10.1259/bjr.20150135. Epub 2015 Jun 25. PMID: 26111070; PMCID: PMC4743571
13. Armstrong DG, Swerdlow MA, Armstrong AA, et al. Five year mortality and direct costs of care for people with diabetic foot complications are comparable to cancer. J Foot Ankle Res. 2020;13:16. https://doi.org/10.1186/s13047-020-00383-2.
14. Viswanathan V, Thomas N, Tandon N, Asirvatham A, Rajasekar S, Ramachandran A, Senthilvasan K, Murugan VS, Muthulakshmi. Profile of diabetic foot complications and its associated complications—a multicentric study from India. J Assoc Physicians India. 2005;53:933–6.
15. Abbas ZG, Archibald LK. Challenges for management of the diabetic foot in Africa: doing more with less. Int Wound J. 2007;4(4):305–13. https://doi.org/10.1111/j.1742-481X.2007.00376.x. Epub 2007 Oct 24. PMID: 17961157; PMCID: PMC7951481
16. Rastogi A, Bhansali A. Diabetic foot infection: an Indian scenario. J Foot Ankle Surg Asia-Pacific. 2016;3(2):71–9.
17. Available from www.iwgdfguidelines.org, Last accessed online 30 August 2023.

18. Schaper NC, van Netten JJ, Apelqvist J, et al. Practical guidelines on the prevention and management of diabetes-related foot disease (IWGDF 2023 update). Diabetes Metab Res Rev. 2023:e3657. https://doi.org/10.1002/dmrr.3657.
19. Musuuza J, Sutherland BL, Kurter S, Balasubramanian P, Bartels CM, Brennan MB. A systematic review of multidisciplinary teams to reduce major amputations for patients with diabetic foot ulcers. J Vasc Surg. 2020;71(4):1433–46.e1433. https://doi.org/10.1016/j.jvs.2019.08.244.
20. Lipsky BA, Senneville É, Abbas ZG, et al. Guidelines on the diagnosis and treatment of foot infection in persons with diabetes (IWGDF 2019 update). Diabetes Metab Res Rev. 2020;36(Suppl 1):e3280. https://doi.org/10.1002/dmrr.3280.
21. Nelson KA, Park KM, Robinovitz E, Tsigos C, Max MB. High-dose oral dextromethorphan versus placebo in painful diabetic neuropathy and postherpetic neuralgia 1997. PMID: 9153445 https://doi.org/10.1212/wnl.48.5.1212.
22. Boulton AJM, Armstrong DG, Kirsner RS, et al. Diagnosis and management of diabetic foot complications 2018 ID: NBK538977PMID: 30958663. https://doi.org/10.2337/db20182-1.
23. Li HK, Rombach I, Zambellas R, et al. Oral versus intravenous antibiotics for bone and joint infection. N Engl J Med. 2019;380(5):425–36. https://doi.org/10.1056/NEJMoa1710926.
24. Armstrong DG, Tan TW, Boulton AJM, Bus SA. Diabetic foot ulcers: a review. JAMA. 2023;330(1):62–75. https://doi.org/10.1001/jama.2023.10578.
25. Fitridge R, Chuter V, Mills J, et al. The intersocietal IWGDF, ESVS, SVS guidelines on peripheral artery disease in people with diabetes and a foot ulcer. Diabetes Metab Res Rev. 2023;e3686 https://doi.org/10.1002/dmrr.3686.
26. Bus SA, Armstrong DG, Crews RT, et al. Guidelines on offloading foot ulcers in persons with diabetes (IWGDF 2023 update). Diabetes Metab Res Rev. 2023;e3647 https://doi.org/10.1002/dmrr.3647.
27. Cavanagh PR, Bus SA. Off-loading the diabetic foot for ulcer prevention and healing. J Vasc Surg. 2010;52(3 Suppl):37S–43S. https://doi.org/10.1016/j.jvs.2010.06.007.
28. Armstrong DG, Lavery LA, Kimbriel HR, Nixon BP, Boulton AJ. Activity patterns of patients with diabetic foot ulceration: patients with active ulceration may not adhere to a standard pressure off-loading regimen. Diabetes Care. 2003;26(9):2595–7. https://doi.org/10.2337/diacare.26.9.2595.
29. Dayya D, O'Neill OJ, Huedo-Medina TB, Habib N, Moore J, Iyer K. Debridement of diabetic foot ulcers. Adv Wound Care (New Rochelle). 2022;11(12):666–86. https://doi.org/10.1089/wound.2021.0016.
30. Edmonds M, Lázaro-Martínez JL, Alfayate-García JM, et al. Sucrose octasulfate dressing versus control dressing in patients with neuroischaemic diabetic foot ulcers (explorer): an international, multicentre, double-blind, randomised, controlled trial. Lancet Diabetes Endocrinol. 2018;6(3):186–96. https://doi.org/10.1016/S2213-8587(17)30438-2.
31. Sloan G, Selvarajah D, Tesfaye S. Pathogenesis, diagnosis and clinical management of diabetic sensorimotor peripheral neuropathy. Nat Rev Endocrinol. 2021; https://doi.org/10.1038/s41574-021-00496-z.
32. Rogers LC, Frykberg RG, Armstrong DG, et al. The Charcot foot in diabetes. Diabetes Care. 2011;34(9):2123–9. https://doi.org/10.2337/dc11-0844.

Diabetic Ketoacidosis 23

Aisha Elamin and Suneeta Teckchandani

23.1 Introduction

Diabetic ketoacidosis (DKA) is a severe and occasionally fatal medical condition that impacts individuals with diabetes mellitus (DM), especially those with type 1 diabetes mellitus (T1DM). DKA may herald the onset of a new diagnosis of T1DM or may present in patients with known diabetes due to poor compliance or intercurrent illness. DKA is characterised by a profound blood glucose disruption in the body, resulting in metabolic acidosis. The hallmarks of DKA are hyperglycaemia, acidosis, and ketonaemia. The accumulation of ketones in the blood can result in life-threatening complications.

DKA is a medical emergency that necessitates immediate management. In the absence of immediate intervention, the condition can swiftly advance and result in a coma or even fatality. Gaining knowledge on the aetiology, manifestations, and appropriate treatment of DKA is essential for individuals with diabetes, healthcare practitioners, and anybody engaged in providing care for individuals afflicted by this ailment.

A. Elamin
Sheffield Teaching Hospitals NHS Foundation Trust, Sheffield, UK
e-mail: aisha.elamin@nhs.net

S. Teckchandani (✉)
Chesterfield Royal Hospital NHS Foundation Trust, Chesterfield, UK
e-mail: suneeta.teckchandani@nhs.net

G. Abraham et al. (eds.), *Management of Diabetic Complications*,
https://doi.org/10.1007/978-981-97-6406-8_23

23.2 Aetiology and Precipitating Factors

There are two main causes of DKA: inadequate insulin therapy and infection. Other causal factors include myocardial infarction, cerebrovascular accidents, pulmonary embolism, pancreatitis, alcohol, and illicit drug use. Some medications can cause massive volume depletion by induction of counter-regulatory hormone release or impairment of water access and can be the culprit drugs in some cases. Some noteworthy examples of such medications are corticosteroids, thiazide diuretics, sympathomimetic agents such as dobutamine and terbutaline, and second-generation antipsychotic agents.

A large systematic literature review identified patient characteristics that were significantly associated with increased risk of DKA, higher HbA1c, lower socioeconomic status, female sex, and depression or psychiatry history. It should, however, also be noted that the overall picture shows a decreasing incidence of DKA with increasing patient age [1].

It should be emphasised that DKA, regardless of its origins, can be avoided and its complications mitigated with proper education, prompt treatment, and avoidance of precipitating situations. Sick-day protocols for type 1 diabetes have been used to help prevent DKA in type 1 diabetes by providing precise guidance regarding extra bolus insulin or carbohydrates as needed, depending on blood glucose and ketone levels.

Though the absolute risk of DKA in patients treated with SGLT-2 inhibitors is small, this class of medications raises DKA risk by two- to four-fold in patients with type 2 diabetes mellitus T2DM, and its incidence can be up to 5% in patients with T1DM. In people with T2DM, low-carbohydrate diet, excessive alcohol intake, presence of autoimmunity, and exposure to stress situations such as infection, surgery, trauma, and dehydration are now identified as DKA risk factors in those treated with SGLT-2 inhibitors [2].

Anti-cancer medications that belong to classes of immune checkpoint inhibitors can cause new-onset diabetes mellitus in up to 1% of the patients receiving immune checkpoint inhibitors, with about half of these patients presenting with DKA as the initial presentation of diabetes, particularly in those individuals who may have underlying beta-cell autoimmunity.

In younger patients, non-adherence to insulin treatment due to fear of hypoglycaemia or weight gain and eating disorders can cause DKA. Mechanical problems with continuous subcutaneous insulin infusion (CSII) devices can precipitate DKA.

23.3 Pathophysiology

The pathogenesis of DKA is marked by a complex interaction of metabolic abnormalities, particularly a lack of insulin and increased release of counter-regulatory hormones. Insufficient insulin leads to poor glucose absorption by peripheral tissues, causing hyperglycaemia [3]. Hyperglycaemia results in an osmotic diuresis, which leads to the increased excretion of water and electrolytes, especially potassium, through urine. The subsequent reduction in volume and electrolyte abnormalities lead to the clinical symptoms of diabetic ketoacidosis (DKA). Concurrently, the body reacts to the apparent lack of energy by metabolising fatty acids through lipolysis to provide energy. This process leads to the generation of free fatty acids, which will be degraded into ketone bodies, which include β-hydroxybutyrate (β-OHB), acetoacetate, and acetone. The build-up of these ketone molecules in the circulation decreases blood pH, causing metabolic acidosis. The increased production of ketone bodies contributes to the distinctive fruity odour often associated with DKA. Together, these pathophysiological processes underlie the clinical presentation of DKA, including hyperglycaemia, dehydration, electrolyte imbalances, and metabolic acidosis (Fig. 23.1).

The underlying defects in DKA are (1) reduced net effective action of circulating insulin, (2) elevated levels of counter-regulatory hormones: glucagon,

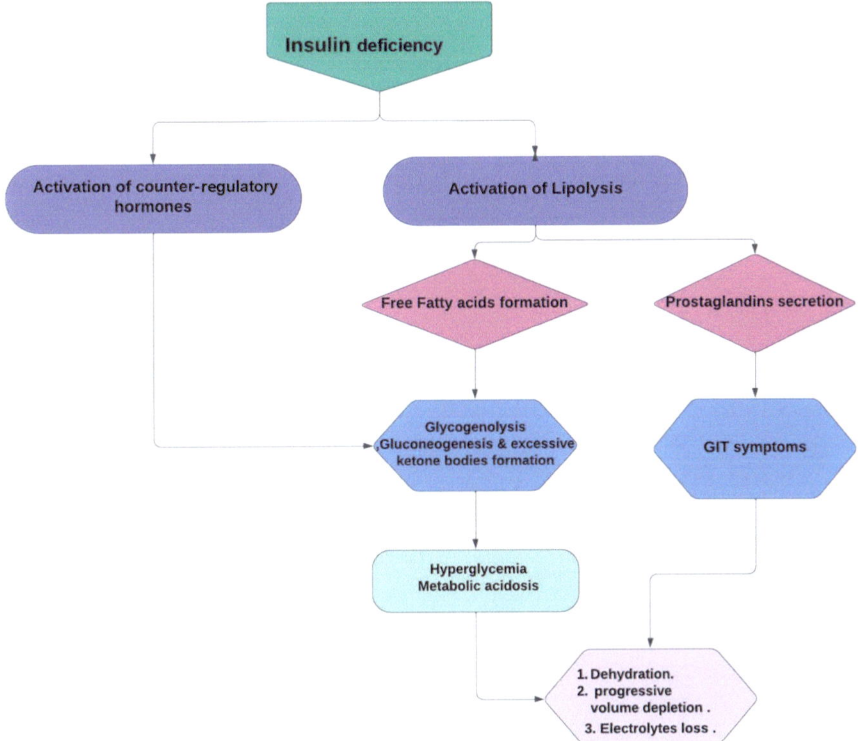

Fig. 23.1 Schematic framework of the pathophysiology of diabetic ketoacidosis. In DKA, insulin insufficiency sets off a cascade of maladaptive physiologic responses involving activation of lipase, increased free fatty acids that trigger excessive ketone bodies, leading to metabolic acidosis. The hyperglycaemia and ketoacidosis cause osmotic diuresis, dehydration, and electrolyte imbalance. Activation of counter-regulatory hormones drives hyperglycaemia via various mechanisms including increased glycogenolysis and gluconeogenesis, resulting in progressive volume depletion and electrolyte loss [4]. *GIT* gastrointestinal tract

catecholamines, cortisol, and growth hormone, resulting in increased hepatic glucose production and impaired glucose utilisation in peripheral tissues, and (3) dehydration and electrolyte abnormalities, mainly due to osmotic diuresis caused by glycosuria.

23.4 Diagnosis

The onset of DKA can vary from several hours to days, with progressive polyuria, polydipsia, and other symptoms of hyperglycaemia. Patients can present with generalised symptoms like weakness, lethargy, nausea, vomiting, and a few nonspecific symptoms like upper abdominal pain. Neurological symptoms may emerge, reflecting underlying acidosis.

Clinical examination reveals mainly findings secondary to dehydration, hyperglycaemia, and acidosis, which include dry skin and mucous membranes, reduced jugular venous pressure, tachycardia, orthostatic hypotension, depressed conscious level with or without coma, and deep, rapid respirations (Kussmaul breathing) [5].

DKA consists of the biochemical triad of hyperglycaemia, ketonaemia, and high anion gap metabolic acidosis (Fig. 23.2).

The American Diabetes Association diagnostic criteria for DKA include elevated serum glucose level above 250 mg/dL, arterial pH of ≤7.30, bicarbonate level of ≤18 mEq/L, an elevated serum ketone level, a pH less than 7.3, a serum bicarbonate level less than 18 mEq per L (18 mmol/L), and an adjusted albumin anion gap of >10–12.3. Conversely, The Joint British Diabetes Societies (JBDS) has a lower threshold for bicarbonate levels to diagnose DKA, not higher.

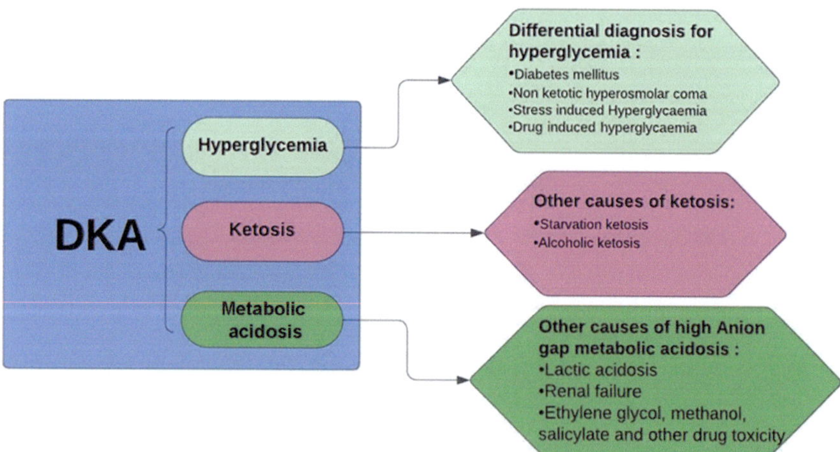

Fig. 23.2 The triad of DKA (hyperglycaemia, acidemia, and ketonaemia) and other conditions with which the individual components are associated [6]

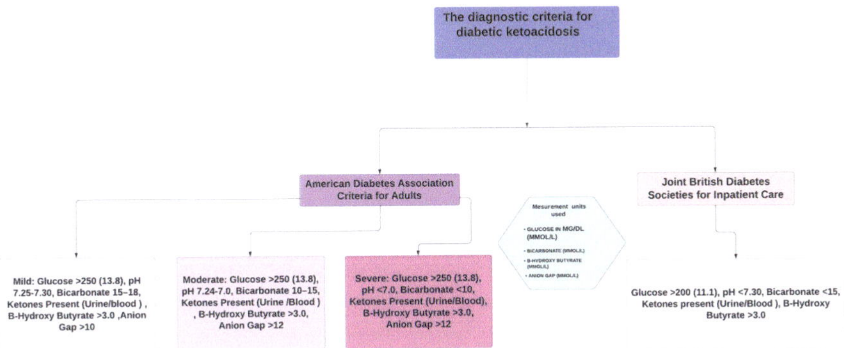

Fig. 23.3 The diagnostic criteria for diabetic ketoacidosis [7]

Figure 23.3 shows detailed flow chart of the diagnostic criteria for various stages of DKA based on the degree of acidosis. This reference work allows greater insight into the relationship between diagnostic parameters and the level of acidosis during DKA.

23.5 Evaluation of the Degree of Severity as per JBDS

Severe DKA may be indicated by the presence of one or more of the following, which may necessitate an extensive intervention and admission to a higher care unit:

- Blood ketones >6.0 mmol/L (34.86 mEq/L)
- HCO_3 level <5.0 mmol/L or mEq/L
- Venous/arterial pH <7.0
- Serum potassium levels at admission <3.5 mmol/L
- Glasgow Coma Scale (GCS) score <12 or an abnormal (AVPU) scale
- Oxygen saturation below 92% while breathing normal air (assuming normal baseline respiratory function)
- Systolic blood pressure (SBP) less than 90 mmHg
- Heart rate >100 or <60 beats per minute
- Anion gap exceeding 16 [Anion Gap = (Sodium + Potassium) − (Chloride + Bicarbonate)]

In three studies, serum osmolality was also the most important determinant of mental status changes [6]. A retrospective study showed that acidosis was independently associated with altered sensorium, but hyperosmolarity and serum "ketone" levels were not. In this study, a combination of acidosis and hyperosmolarity at presentation may identify a subset of patients with severe DKA (7% in this study) who may benefit from more aggressive treatment and monitoring [8].

Based on the 2009 publication of the American Diabetes Association, a condition called "euglycemic DKA" exhibits the characteristics of metabolic acidosis, ketosis, and blood glucose levels less than 250. Such syndrome occurs in about 10%

of DKA. It mainly occurs in patients who have little glycogen reserves or high glucosuria rates, such as in pregnancy, liver disorders, alcohol intake, and type 2 diabetes mellitus treatment using SGLT inhibitors.

23.6 Other Initial Investigations

Apart from measuring blood glucose (BG) levels, blood and/or urine ketone, and blood gases (arterial blood gas (ABG)/venous blood gas (VBG)), the initial laboratory analysis of a patient with diabetic ketoacidosis (DKA) should encompass kidney function (urea and creatinine), serum electrolyte levels (sodium, potassium, calcium, magnesium, phosphate, chloride), serum osmolality, complete blood count (CBC) with differential, and urine analysis. The evaluation for sepsis should include taking blood and urine culture samples and performing a chest X-ray if it is clinically necessary. Further examinations comprise an electrocardiogram (ECG) and the haemoglobin A1c level evaluation. The latter determines the extent and chronicity of hyperglycaemia. Consider pregnancy tests in female patients of reproductive age.

23.7 Differential Diagnosis

Distinguishing DKA from other conditions with similar clinical presentations is paramount. Differential diagnoses should consider hyperosmolar hyperglycaemic state (HHS), starvation ketosis, alcohol ketoacidosis, and other high anion gap metabolic acidosis.

HHS can gradually develop over a long period, such as days and sometimes weeks; it has a predominance of neurological symptoms. Patients with HHS typically have pH >7.30, bicarbonate level >20 mEq/L, and negative ketone bodies in plasma and urine.

In alcoholic ketoacidosis (AKA), total ketone bodies are much greater than in DKA, with a higher β-OHB to acetoacetate ratio of 7:1 versus a ratio of 3:1 in DKA. The AKA patients seldom present with hyperglycaemia. In starvation ketosis, serum bicarbonate concentration of less than 18 or hyperglycaemia will rarely be present.

23.8 Treatment Strategies

Effective DKA management necessitates meticulous attention to fluid and electrolyte balance, correcting the hyperglycaemia with insulin therapy and identifying and treating precipitating factors. The treatment protocol can be summarised as follows:

1. **Fluid Replacement**: Hyperglycaemia in DKA leads to osmotic diuresis and severe dehydration; therefore, the mainstay treatment herein is rehydration. It is

the most crucial initial therapeutic measure in DKA management. It mainly aims to correct fluid deficit, metabolic acidosis, and electrolyte imbalance [9]. Since DKA patients experience fluid loss of approximately 6–9 L, the goal of fluid resuscitation aims to replete that volume within 24–36 h with 50% of resuscitation fluid administered within the first 8–12 h of presentation. If renal function is not significantly altered, fluid resuscitation will decrease hyperglycaemia by stimulating osmotic diuresis and restoring the peripheral action of insulin.

Crystalloid solutions, such as 0.9% sodium chloride (normal saline), are preferred for fluid resuscitation. The first infusion rate commonly consists of 0.9% saline solution at a rate of 15–20 mL/kg/h or 1–1.5 L in the first hour, with adjustments made according to the patient's clinical response, urine output, and blood pressure.

The table below shows the typical fluid and electrolyte imbalances in DKA. However, if the systolic blood pressure (SBP) is less than 90 mmHg, it is recommended to give a bolus of 500 mL of normal saline 0.9% and consult a senior if SBP remains <90 mmHg. Fluid replacement may require modification in patients with renal failure, heart failure, advanced age, pregnant women, complex patients with multiple comorbidities, and adolescents [9].

A 10% dextrose infusion should be administered to avoid hypoglycaemia when blood glucose drops below 14.0 mmol/L (<250 mg/dL). 0.9% sodium chloride and 10% dextrose must often be infused together, or 0.45% saline with dextrose can be used.

Typical deficits in ketoacidosis in adults [9]

Water	100 mL/kg
Sodium	7–10 mmol/kg
Chloride	3–5 mmol/kg
Potassium	3–5 mmol/kg

2. **Insulin Therapy**: Insulin therapy is effective regardless of the route of administration, whether insulin is delivered via continuous intravenous infusion or by frequent subcutaneous or intramuscular injections in DKA patients, as evidenced by randomised controlled trials [10].

   However, IV continuous infusion with regular insulin remains the mainstay of treatment due to its short half-life and easy titration in comparison to other modes of administration. Studies have shown insulin infusion with or without bolus doses to be effective [4].

   The most important effects of insulin are suppression of ketogenesis, reduction of blood glucose, and correction of electrolyte disturbances. According to JBDS guidelines, it is advised to initiate insulin therapy with a continuous fixed rate intravenous insulin infusion (FRIII), monitor glucose levels regularly, and target euglycaemia, which should be the goals for treatment.

   Regular insulin (short-acting) is the preferred choice, typically started at a rate of 0.1 unit/kg/h; an estimated weight can be used if the weight is not known [9]. Serum glucose should be monitored frequently (hourly), and the insulin infusion rate should be adjusted to lower blood glucose by 3 mmol/L/h. It is crucial to avoid excessively aggressive insulin therapy, as it can result in cerebral oedema. Consideration should be given to lowering the rate of intravenous insulin infusion to 0.05 units/kg/h if the pace of decline is fast or the glucose decreases to less than 14.0 mmol/L (<250 mg/dL) in addition to adding dextrose to the infusion fluid.

The recommended targets are reduction of the blood ketone concentration by 0.5 mmol/L/h, increase the venous bicarbonate by 3.0 mmol/L/h, lowering capillary blood glucose by 3.0 mmol/L/h (54 mg/dL/h), and maintain potassium between 4.0 and 5.5 mmol/L. If these goals are not accomplished, it is essential to reevaluate the FRIII delivery rate for better results.

Maintaining the previous long-acting basal subcutaneous (S/C) insulin injections at the regular dosages while also using the insulin infusion is important. In those newly diagnosed, long-acting basal insulin should be commenced at a dose of 0.25 units/kg subcutaneously once daily.

3. **Potassium Replacement**: DKA is often associated with total body potassium depletion despite normal or elevated serum potassium (K) levels due to the K shifts from intracellular to extracellular due to hyperglycaemia, lack of insulin, and metabolic acidosis. As insulin therapy corrects hyperglycaemia, K transfers back to intracellular space, increasing the risk of hypokalaemia. Therefore, potassium supplementation should be started early and continued while serum levels are strictly monitored. In hypokalaemia patients, potassium replacement should begin with fluid therapy. However, it should be noted that insulin administration must be delayed until potassium concentration exceeds 3.3 mmol (mEq)/L. This is done to ensure the treatment is safe and effective. The patient's potassium levels should be monitored regularly upon arrival until the FRII is discontinued. These checks should be done at 2–4-h intervals for the first 12–24 h. Then, two potassium checks daily are required for FRIII till the fluids are no longer needed. If K was 3.5 mmol/L or less at presentation, an extensive intravascular replacement through a central venous line in a high dependency or critical care unit may be required; as stated previously, K is anticipated to decrease further after initiating FRIII. Therefore, the patient's blood potassium should be regularly tracked to avoid deficient levels.

   Potassium management in DKA can be highly individualised based on a patient's specific clinical condition and laboratory results, and local protocols and guidelines may vary. This paragraph offers a comprehensive overview of potassium management in DKA; however, it should be used with clinical judgement and any institution-specific protocols or guidelines.
4. **Identification and Treatment of Precipitating Factors**: It is essential to identify and address the underlying causes of DKA, which frequently involve infections, failure to comply with insulin therapy, and other medical disorders that heighten the body's stress response, such as myocardial infarction (MI).
5. **Bicarbonate Therapy**: Bicarbonate therapy for correcting acidosis remains controversial, as the observed acidosis serves as an adaptive response, shifting the oxygen dissociation curve rightward, thereby improving tissue oxygen delivery. Excessive bicarbonate in the circulation can raise the CO_2 partial pressure in

cerebrospinal fluid (CSF), which worsens CSF acidosis [9]. It is generally reserved for severe cases with a pH below 6.9 in the intensive care unit (ICU) and when the pH remains low despite requiring adequate medical treatment and inotropes.

23.9 Management Considerations

Several factors require careful consideration during DKA management. These include checking the patient's hydration level and taking care of it, avoiding complications like cerebral oedema, keeping an eye on electrolyte imbalances, spotting signs of worsening quickly, and calling the intensive care team as soon as necessary [9].

23.10 Resolution of DKA and Transition to Subcutaneous Insulin

As the patient stabilises clinically and biochemically (blood ketones <0.6 mmol/L, pH > 7.3), the transition from intravenous to subcutaneous insulin can be considered, along with addressing the patient's long-term diabetic management [9]. A variable rate insulin infusion might be needed for a short transition period if the patient cannot eat or drink or remains critically ill.

It is crucial to recognise that HCO_3 levels may remain low even after the resolution of DKA due to a non-gap acidosis caused by the aggressive intravenous infusion of crystalloid fluids, which is why it is not a reliable parameter for resolution [9].

23.11 Complications

Among the complications of DKA are cerebral oedema, acute respiratory distress syndrome (ARDS), renal impairment, and electrolyte imbalances.

Although cerebral oedema is uncommon, it remains a major cause of altered consciousness in DKA, especially in paediatric patients [8]. It is a feared complication, often necessitating treatment with mannitol or hypertonic saline [11].

Respiratory failure in DKA worsens prognosis but is preventable. Factors like electrolyte deficiencies and pulmonary oedema contribute to it. Respiratory infections, pre-existing conditions, and other recognisable factors can also lead to it. Early recognition and management of these conditions can prevent respiratory failure and improve DKA mortality. Early intervention is crucial for better DKA outcomes [12].

Due to hypovolemia and dehydration, renal impairment can manifest as acute kidney injury.

DKA frequently results in electrolyte disturbances, including hypokalaemia, which can lead to muscle weakness, cardiac arrhythmias, and even cardiac arrest if left untreated [13]. Identifying and effectively managing these complications are essential components of DKA treatment for optimal patient outcomes.

In summary, managing DKA necessitates a systematic approach encompassing fluid resuscitation, insulin therapy, potassium replacement, identification of precipitating factors, and vigilant monitoring. The key to successful DKA management is prompt diagnosis, close monitoring, and a thorough understanding of the underlying pathophysiology. Timely and comprehensive management can significantly improve patient outcomes and minimise the risk of complications associated with this life-threatening condition.

References

1. Fazeli Farsani S, Brodovicz K, Soleymanlou N, et al. Incidence and prevalence of diabetic ketoacidosis (DKA) among adults with type 1 diabetes mellitus (T1D): a systematic literature review. BMJ Open. 2017;7:e016587. https://doi.org/10.1136/bmjopen-2017-016587.
2. Fadini GP, Bonora BM, Avogaro A. SGLT2 inhibitors and diabetic ketoacidosis: data from the FDA adverse event reporting system. Diabetologia. 2017;60(8):1385–9.
3. Eledrisi MS, Alshanti MS, Shah MF, et al. Overview of the diagnosis and management of diabetic ketoacidosis. Am J Med Sci. 2006;331:243–51.
4. El-Remessy AB. Diabetic ketoacidosis management: updates and challenges for specific patient population. Endocrine. 2022;3:801–12. https://doi.org/10.3390/endocrines3040066.
5. Kitabchi AE, Umpierrez GE, Miles JM, Fisher JN. Hyperglycemic crises in adult patients with diabetes. Diabetes Care. 2009;32(7):1335–43. https://doi.org/10.2337/dc09-9032.
6. Gosmanov AR, Gosmanova EO, Kitabchi AE. Hyperglycemic crises: diabetic ketoacidosis and hyperglycemic hyperosmolar state. [Updated 9 May 2021]. In: Feingold KR, Anawalt B, Blackman MR, et al., editors. Endotext. South Dartmouth (MA): MDText.com, Inc.; 2000. https://www.ncbi.nlm.nih.gov/books/NBK279052/.
7. Dhatariya KK, Glaser NS, Codner E, Umpierrez GE. Diabetic ketoacidosis. Nat Rev Dis Primers. 2020;6(1):40. https://doi.org/10.1038/s41572-020-0165-1. PMID: 32409703.
8. Nyenwe EA, Razavi LN, Kitabchi AE, Khan AN, Wan JY. Acidosis: the prime determinant of depressed sensorium in diabetic ketoacidosis. Diabetes Care. 2010;33(8):1837–9.
9. Dhatariya KK, The Joint British Diabetes Societies for Inpatient Care. The management of diabetic ketoacidosis in adults—an updated guideline from the Joint British Diabetes Society for Inpatient Care. Diabet Med. 2022;39:e14788. https://doi.org/10.1111/dme.14788.
10. Fisher JN, Shahshahani MN, Kitabchi AE. Diabetic ketoacidosis: low-dose insulin therapy by various routes. N Engl J Med. 1977;297:238–41.
11. Glaser NS, Wootton-Gorges SL, Buonocore MH, et al. Frequency of sub-clinical cerebral edema in children with diabetic ketoacidosis. Pediatr Diabetes. 2006;7(2):75–80.
12. Konstantinov NK, et al. Respiratory failure in diabetic ketoacidosis. World J Diabetes. 2015;6(8):1009–23. https://doi.org/10.4239/wjd.v6.i8.1009.
13. Lizzo JM, Goyal A, Gupta V. Adult diabetic ketoacidosis. [Updated 10 Jul 2023]. In: StatPearls. Treasure Island (FL): StatPearls Publishing; 2024. https://www.ncbi.nlm.nih.gov/books/NBK560723/.

Hypoglycemia

24

Aisha Elamin and Suneeta Teckchandani

24.1 Introduction

The risk of hypoglycemia, which is defined as dangerously low blood glucose levels, is a serious problem with diabetes treatment, particularly when administering insulin or medications that stimulate insulin secretion (such as meglitinides and sulfonylureas). Because glucose targets in diabetes are being lowered to prevent microvascular and macrovascular effects, hypoglycemia has become increasingly prevalent. Numerous studies have shown that individuals undertaking intensive treatment to achieve a strict HbA1C are more likely to have hypoglycemic episodes [1–3].

Those with type 1 diabetes often have two bouts of moderate hypoglycemia each week. Even though it happens less often in type 2 diabetics on insulin, severe hypoglycemia is still a significant therapeutic problem in (T2DM). Severe hypoglycemia affects between 30 and 40 percent of unselected populations annually. Hypoglycemia is linked to a death rate of 6–10% in cases of type 1 diabetes; its effects on type 2 diabetes are less well-documented. To enhance the quality of therapy, healthcare professionals need to become proficient in this intricate subject [4–6]. Hypoglycemia is more common in patients with chronic kidney disease (CKD), pancreatic insufficiency, and advanced age.

It might be challenging to pinpoint a particular plasma glucose value that is indicative of hypoglycemia in diabetic individuals due to variations in the onset of symptoms. This threshold drops in patients with recurrent episodes of hypoglycemia and is slightly higher in individuals with uncontrolled diabetes.

A. Elamin
Sheffield Teaching Hospitals NHS Foundation Trust, Sheffield, UK

S. Teckchandani (✉)
Department of Acute Medicine, Chesterfield Royal Hospital, Calow, Derbyshire, UK
e-mail: suneeta.teckchandani@nhs.net

G. Abraham et al. (eds.), *Management of Diabetic Complications*,
https://doi.org/10.1007/978-981-97-6406-8_24

Measuring blood glucose levels using venous, arterial, or capillary samples is possible. Most conventional measurements are venous blood glucose levels. The interstitial fluid compartment is a good approximation of the steady-state plasma glucose concentration, and continueous glucose monitoring (CGM) devices assess glucose levels in this compartment, which are becoming more common.

24.2 Pathophysiology of Hypoglycemia

Under typical circumstances, when plasma glucose levels drop, the body may do one of two things: (1) boost its glucose synthesis via glycogenolysis and gluconeogenesis, or (2) alter its behavior to make you feel hungry and want to eat more.

A decrease in glucose concentration in nondiabetic individuals is accompanied by a decrease in insulin production. It happens when the blood glucose level is still below the critical threshold for human health. When glucose levels drop even further, the secretion of glucagon and epinephrine (along with the less important hormones cortisol and growth hormone) increases, setting off an intense sympathoadrenal reaction that manifests as relevant symptoms. Continued decrease in glucose levels can lead to cognitive decline and serious neurological consequences. Complicated hormonal and metabolic interactions cause hypoglycemia in patients with diabetes. In patients with diabetes and significant beta cell failure, there is a lack of that initial response to hypoglycemia of a drop in insulin. Healthy pancreatic alpha cells generate glucagon when blood glucose levels drop, encouraging the liver to burn glycogen to raise blood glucose. Adrenaline promotes hepatic glucose release and decreases insulin synthesis. Advanced diabetes compromises the sympathoadrenal compensatory responses, notably in chronic type 1 and advanced type 2 diabetics [4].

Insulin, a hormone that helps tissues absorb glucose, has beneficial and harmful consequences. Hypoglycemia can develop from excessive use of insulin or insulin secretagogues despite their therapeutic importance in blood sugar management. Impaired counterregulatory hormones compromise glucose homeostasis in diabetes, increasing hypoglycemia intensity and duration [7].

The brain is more vulnerable during hypoglycemia, as it relies heavily on glucose, and this will lead to cognitive impairment. Hypoglycemia can cause convulsions, unconsciousness, and potentially fatal consequences, such as cardiovascular events, if left untreated. Avoiding these complications requires prompt hypoglycemia diagnosis and treatment. Hypoglycemia occurs when blood glucose falls below normal levels, significantly impacting cognitive function and, in severe cases, precipitating cardiovascular events. In diabetes, compromised counterregulatory hormonal responses exacerbate the severity and duration of hypoglycemic episodes [4].

24.3 Clinical Features

Clinical signs and symptoms of hypoglycemia in adults range from mild to severe and are crucial markers for individuals [8]. Sympatho-adrenal system activation as a counterregulatory response causes autonomic symptoms such as palpitations, tremors, sweat, irritability, anxiety, shaking, and hunger [7]. These indicate the body's physiological response to low blood glucose.

Neuroglycopenic symptoms caused by brain glucose deficiency include confusion, impaired concentration, dizziness, blurred vision, and aberrant behavior [9]. Uncontrolled hypoglycemia can lead to more severe symptoms such as seizures, unconsciousness, and, in difficult situations, coma. Individuals may have different symptoms.

Some people, especially those with long-term diabetes or recurring episodes, may not show the usual warning signs [9], which is described as hypoglycemic unawareness. Healthcare providers should educate individuals with diabetes and their caregivers on effective recognition and management of hypoglycemic episodes. Occasionally, particularly in those under poor glycemic control, symptoms may emerge even when the blood glucose levels are in the reference range, which is related to the brain sensing "relative" hypoglycemia compared with recent ambient levels.

Hypoglycemia is classified into three levels, indicating the severity [10]. Level 1 hypoglycemia is defined as plasma glucose concentration < 70 mg/dL (3.9 mmol/L) but >54 mg/dL (3 mmol/L). When plasma glucose is below 70 mg/dL (3.9 mmol/L), neuroendocrine responses to hypoglycemia usually appear in individuals without diabetes. In patients with diabetes, this level of blood glucose needs immediate intervention due to defective counter-regulatory response, even if they are asymptomatic [11].

Level 2 hypoglycemia is plasma glucose concentration below 54 mg/dL (3 mmol/L) requiring immediate intervention to correct the hypoglycemia. At this level, the neurogenic and neuroglycopenic symptoms are present. Level 3 hypoglycemia is a severe event characterized by a change in the mental status or impairment in the patient's physical ability to function that requires intervention by another person to restore normal glucose levels [11].

The JBDS classifies it into similar categories, mild, moderate, and severe based on the alertness, behavior, and need for assistance.

The Whipple triad is defined by the presence of hypoglycemic symptoms, confirmation of low blood sugar during the occurrence of these symptoms, and the resolution of symptoms upon restoring blood glucose levels to normal. This triad was originally used for patients with hyperinsulinemia secondary to pancreatic insulinoma but has been applicable to diagnose hypoglycemia even in diabetics. However, the sensitivity, specificity, and predictive value of the Whipple triad in diagnosing hypoglycemia in diabetics are questionable [12].

24.4 Impact on Patients

Beyond physiological impacts, hypoglycemia affects cognitive function and increases accident risk, causing psychological issues. The fear of hypoglycemia significantly influences treatment compliance and potentially compromises overall diabetes management [5, 13]. Chronic hypoglycemia can worsen pre-existing illnesses and cause cardiovascular events. Healthcare practitioners must comprehend these consequences to tailor an effective management program and communicate openly with patients [5]. Additionally, UK research highlights the emotional and behavioral elements of hypoglycemia, emphasizing the necessity for a patient-centered approach [14].

24.5 Risk Factors and Recognition

Hypoglycemic episodes may be induced in the hospital setting by a few factors, such as fluctuations in meal ingestion, alterations in the patient's clinical condition, and the administration of specific medications. Moreover, the dynamic nature of the hospital environments, with irregular meal schedules and potential interruptions to regular diabetes care routines, increases the vulnerability to hypoglycemia. In community settings, individuals with diabetes face diverse challenges, including lifestyle variations, medication adherence, and potential social factors that can influence glycemic control.

Commonly, primary antidiabetic medications that induce hypoglycemia include insulin and insulin secretagogues such as sulfonylureas and repaglinide. On the other hand, metformin, pioglitazone, DPP-4 inhibitors, acarbose, SLGT-2 inhibitors, and GLP-1 analogs seldom lead to hypoglycemia.

Individuals, who are elderly, have chronic kidney disease (CKD), or experience pancreatic insufficiency are particularly susceptible to hypoglycemia. Table 24.1 provides a comprehensive list of risk factors associated with hypoglycemia. Healthcare practitioners must recognize these risks to develop targeted preventive strategies, educate patients, and encourage collaborative diabetes treatment in hospital and community settings.

24.6 Management Strategies for Hypoglycemia

A comprehensive approach is required for the management of hypoglycemia in adults to ensure timely resolution and mitigate the risk of potential complications.

Moreover, it encourages further interventions such as adjusting medications, lifestyle modifications, and personalized glycaemic targets. Practical tips on blood sugar monitoring, recognizing trends, and implementing preventive measures are provided. Studies show that implementing patient education programs and leveraging technology for continuous glucose monitoring can significantly reduce the incidence of severe hypoglycemia [15, 16].

Table 24.1 Risk factors for hypoglycemia from LBDS hypo guideline

Medical issues	Reduced carbohydrate intake/absorption
• Previous history of severe hypoglycemia • Long duration of type 1 diabetes • Strict glycaemic control • Duration of insulin therapy in type 2 diabetes • Lipohypertrophy at injection sites • Impaired awareness of hypoglycemia • Severe hepatic dysfunction • Impaired renal function (including those people requiring renal replacement therapy) • Sepsis • Inadequate treatment of previous hypoglycemia • Terminal illness • Cognitive dysfunction/dementia • C-peptide negativity	• Food malabsorption e.g., gastroenteritis, coeliac disease, gastroparesis • Bariatric surgery involving bowel resection
Lifestyle issues	Endocrine disorders
• Increased exercise (relative to usual) • Increasing age • Alcohol • Early pregnancy • Breastfeeding • No or inadequate blood glucose monitoring	• Addison's disease • Growth hormone deficiency • Hypothyroidism • Hypopituitarism

24.7 Emergency Management

In order to restore blood sugar levels, diabetic individuals suffering hypoglycemia need a carbohydrate that acts quickly. After the fast-acting carbohydrate, long-acting carbs are recommended as a snack or meal. Individuals suffering from hypoglycemia must get prompt medical attention. It is important to confirm hypoglycemia by taking a blood glucose reading when it is safe to do so, particularly if there is a suspicion that the individual may also be under the influence of Alcohol. There should be no delay in therapy even if measurement is difficult (as in a patient experiencing a seizure).

After administering acute treatment, it's essential to assess whether hypoglycemia is likely to be prolonged, particularly in cases involving long-acting insulin or sulfonylurea medications. In such instances, individuals may require a continuous glucose infusion to maintain steady blood glucose levels. Consistent monitoring of blood glucose levels may reveal asymptomatic biochemical hypoglycemia (Fig. 24.1).

For a comprehensive assessment, consider the following ABCDE:

(a) Airway.
(b) Breathing.
(c) Circulation.
(d) Disability (using measures such as blood glucose and the Glasgow Coma Scale; GCS).

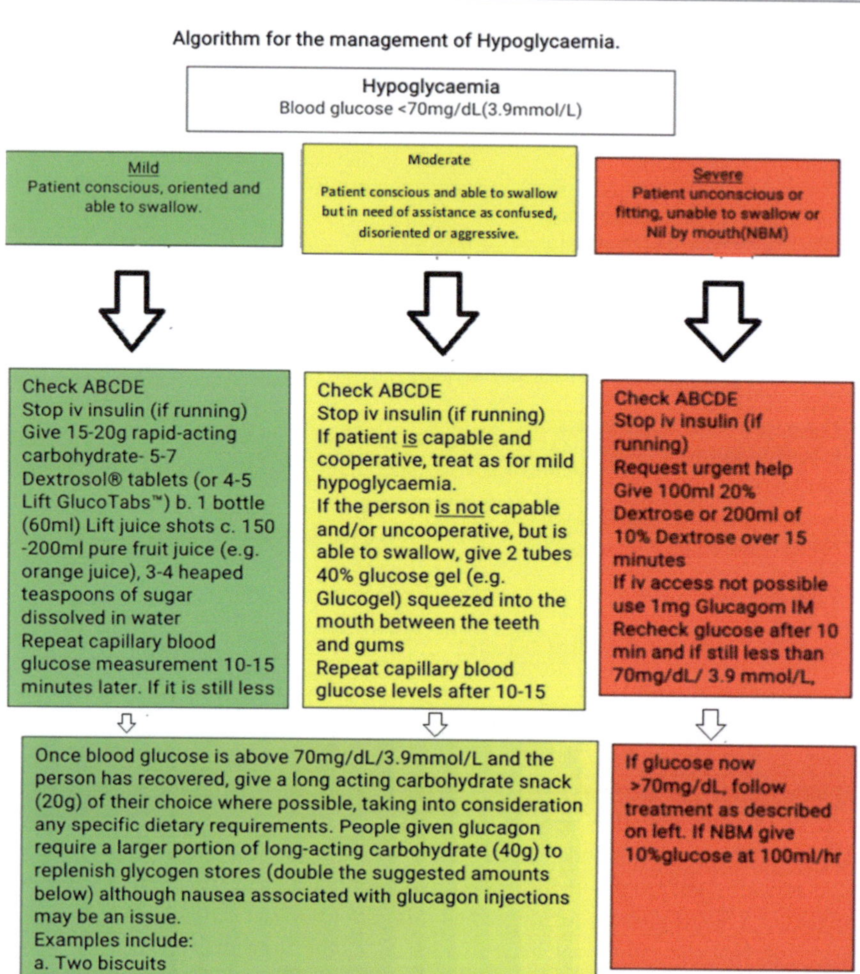

Fig. 24.1 Algorithm for management of hypoglycemia in adults with diabetes in hospital [18]

(e) Exposure (taking into account factors such as direct sunlight and ambient temperature).

Immediate treatment for moderate to mild hypoglycemia, as recommended by the Endocrine Society's clinical practice guideline and the American Diabetes Association (ADA), entails the administration of 15–20 g of rapidly assimilated carbohydrates, including glucose granules or gel. Then, measure blood glucose levels at 15-minute intervals after that and continue consuming carbohydrates until normoglycemia is achieved [17].

- If a patient's blood sugar level is 55–69 mg/dL, the 15–15 rule states that they should consume 15 g of carbohydrates and recheck their sugar level 15 min later.

If it is still below the target range, repeat these steps until it is in the target range. When it reaches the recommended range, a nutritious meal or snack (two biscuits, a piece of bread, two hundred to three hundred milliliters of milk, or the following carbohydrate-containing meal) should be provided.

Examples of items that contain 15 g of carbs:

- ½ cup, or 4 ounces, of either ordinary soda or juice.
- One tablespoon of honey, syrup, sugar, or sugar substitute.
- 3–4 glucose pills
- One bottle of glucose gel, one dosage.

In more severe instances where the patient cannot consume carbohydrates orally, and Intravenous (IV) access is available, IV Dextrose 10% or 20% should be given intravenously. If there is no IV access, it is recommended to administer glucagon intramuscularly or subcutaneously. Healthcare providers and individuals with diabetes should collaborate on developing personalized hypoglycemia management plans, addressing contributing factors such as medication adjustments, meal planning, and physical activity considerations.

24.8 Algorithm for the Management of Hypoglycemia

24.9 Hypoglycemia Prevention

Balancing glycemic targets while preventing hypoglycemia is crucial in diabetes management. In 2015, the American Diabetes Association (ADA) adjusted its preprandial glycemic target from 70–130 mg/dL (3.9–7.2 mmol/L) to 80–130 mg/dL (4.4–7.2 mmol/L), aligning with the findings of the ADAG study. This adjustment was based on empirical data demonstrating that self-monitored blood glucose (SMBG) targets were inconsistent with achieving HbA1C goals [19]. Lower SMBG targets in the empirical data helped avoid overtreatment, providing a safety margin for patients titrating glucose-lowering drugs. Moreover, individuals with type 1 diabetes who develop hypoglycemia as a result of anxiety about hyperglycemia may not always find relief from glycemic target relaxation.

Recognizing precipitating or risk factors (refer to Table 24.1) is crucial for patient, family, and healthcare professional education. Patient education on hypoglycemia awareness, along with nutritional training focusing on a consistent carbohydrate diet to match insulin or insulin secretagogue, proves beneficial.

Regular blood glucose monitoring is vital, with continuous glucose monitoring (CGM) and blood glucose monitoring (BGM) being the most important tools for evaluating treatment efficacy and identifying individuals at risk of hypoglycemia. Electronic prescribing in hospital settings and standardized protocols for managing hyperglycemic complications can also contribute to preventing hypoglycemia episodes.

The Hypoglycemia Assessment Tool (HAT) study underscores the importance of understanding regional variations and predictors of hypoglycemia across diverse populations. Spanning 24 countries, the global HAT study identified factors such as insulin type, age, and diabetes duration as significant predictors of hypoglycemia [20]. Management strategies should be individualized, considering these variables and modifying measures to address each patient's unique needs and characteristics.

24.10 Hypoglycemia and Driving

Ensuring road safety in the context of diabetes management is a crucial priority for healthcare practitioners globally. Individuals with diabetes, particularly those undergoing insulin therapy, face an increased vulnerability to hypoglycemia, posing a specific danger, especially while driving. Hypoglycemia during driving can impair cognitive and motor function, significantly elevating the risk of road traffic accidents [5]. It is imperative to underscore the responsibility of healthcare providers in educating individuals with diabetes on the significance of regular blood glucose monitoring before driving, particularly those undergoing insulin therapy. Acknowledging symptoms and taking preventive precautions before driving are crucial aspects of this educational initiative [6]. Collaboration among healthcare experts, local licensing authorities, and patients is essential for alleviating the impact of hypoglycemia on driving safety. This partnership promotes a balanced state of effective diabetes control and the general welfare of persons navigating highways worldwide [7].

24.11 Team Approach and Community Care

The holistic management of diabetes-related complications requires a collaborative approach. A multi-disciplinary team approach involving healthcare professionals, including nurses and community care providers, is essential. It emphasizes patient, caregiver, and healthcare provider education in preventing, recognizing, and managing hypoglycemia, particularly in high-risk populations.

References

1. ACCORD Study Group, Buse JB, Bigger JT, Byington RP, Cooper LS, Cushman WC, Friedewald WT, Genuth S, Gerstein HC, Ginsberg HN, Goff DC Jr, Grimm RH Jr, Margolis KL, Probstfield JL, Simons-Morton DG, Sullivan MD. Action to control cardiovascular risk in diabetes (ACCORD) trial: design and methods. Am J Cardiol. 2007;99:21i–33i. PubMed Google Scholar

2. ADVANCE Collaborative Group, Patel P, MacMahon S, Chalmers J, Neal B, Billot L, Woodward M, Marre M, Cooper M, Glasziou P, Grobbee D, Hamet P, Harrap S, Heller S, Liu L, Mancia G, Mogensen CE, Pan C, Poulter N, Rodgers A, Williams B, Bompoint S, de Galan BE, Joshi R, Travert F. Intensive blood glucose control and vascular outcomes in patients with type 2 diabetes. N Engl J Med. 2008;358:2560–72. PubMed Google Scholar
3. Duckworth W, Abraira C, Moritz T, Reda D, Emanuele N, Reaven PD, Zieve FJ, Marks J, Davis SN, Hayward R, Warren SR, Goldman S, McCarren M, Vitek ME, Henderson WG, Huang GD, VADT Investigators. Glucose control and vascular complications in veterans with type 2 diabetes. N Engl J Med. 2009;360:129–39. PubMed Google Scholar
4. Cryer PE. Hypoglycemia in diabetes: pathophysiology, prevalence, and prevention. Retrieved from PubMed Central 2013.
5. Seaquist ER, Anderson J, Childs B, Cryer P, Dagogo-Jack S, Fish L, et al. Hypoglycemia and diabetes: a report of a workgroup of the American Diabetes Association and the Endocrine Society. Diabetes Care. 2013;36(5):1384–95. https://doi.org/10.2337/dc12-2480.
6. UK Hypoglycemia Study Group. Risk of hypoglycemia in types 1 and 2 diabetes: treatment modalities' effects and duration. Diabetologia. 2007;50(6):1140–7. https://doi.org/10.1007/s00125-007-0599-y.
7. International Hypoglycemia Study Group. Hypoglycemia, cardiovascular disease, and mortality in diabetes: epidemiology, pathogenesis, and management. Lancet Diabetes Endocrinol. 2019;7(5):385–96. https://doi.org/10.1016/S2213-8587(18)30309-1.
8. Inkster B, Frier BM. The Edinburgh hypoglycemia scale: a tool to assess awareness of hypoglycemia. Diabet Med. 2012;29(1):76–9. https://doi.org/10.1111/j.1464-5491.2011.03403.x.
9. Deary IJ, Hepburn DA, MacLeod KM. Partitioning the symptoms of hypoglycemia using multi-sample confirmatory factor analysis. Diabetologia. 1993;36(8):771–7. https://doi.org/10.1007/BF00400843.
10. Agiostratidou G, Anhalt H, Ball D, Blonde L, Gourgari E, Harriman KN, Kowalski AJ, Madden P, McAuliffe-Fogarty AH, McElwee-Malloy M, Peters A, Raman S, Reifschneider K, Rubin K, Weinzimer SA. Standardizing clinically meaningful outcome measures beyond HbA1c for type 1 diabetes: a consensus report of the American Association of Clinical Endocrinologists, the American Association of Diabetes Educators, the American Diabetes Association, the Endocrine Society, JDRF International, The Leona M. and Harry B. Helmsley Charitable Trust, the Pediatric Endocrine Society, and the T1D Exchange. Diabetes Care. 2017;40:1622–30. PMC free article PubMed Google Scholar
11. Nakhleh A, Shehadeh N. Hypoglycemia in diabetes: an update on pathophysiology, treatment, and prevention. World J Diabetes. 2021;12(12):2036–49. https://doi.org/10.4239/wjd.v12.i12.2036. PMID: 35047118; PMCID: PMC8696639
12. Ademolu AB. Whipple triad: its limitations in diagnosis and management of hypoglycemia as a co-morbidity in Covid-19 diabetics and diabetes mellitus in general—a review. Int J Diabet Endocrinol. 2020;5(2):23–6.
13. Association of Diabetes Care & Education Specialists. Position statement: diabetes management in the school setting. Diabetes Educ. 2018;44(1_suppl):35S–40S.
14. Heller SR, Frier BM, Hersløv ML, et al. Severe hypoglycemia in adults with insulin-treated diabetes: impact on healthcare resources. Diabet Med. 2016;33(4):471–7. https://doi.org/10.1111/dme.12925.
15. Mattishent K, Loke YK. Meta-analysis: association between hypoglycemia and serious adverse events in older patients treated with antihyperglycemic agents. Front Endocrinol (Lausanne). 2021;12:683953. https://doi.org/10.3389/fendo.2021.683953.
16. Cryer PE. Hypoglycemia: the limiting factor in the glycaemic management of type I and type II diabetes. Diabetologia. 2002;4(7):937–48. https://doi.org/10.1007/s00125-002-0822-9.
17. American Diabetes Association. Defining and reporting hypoglycemia in diabetes: a report from the American Diabetes Association Workgroup on Hypoglycemia. Diabetes Care. 2017;40(1):136–44. https://doi.org/10.2337/dc16-1820.
18. Joint British Diabetes Societies for Inpatient Care. The hospital management of hypoglycemia in adults with diabetes mellitus, January 2023.

19. Wei N, Zheng H, Nathan DM. Empirically establishing blood glucose targets to achieve HbA1c goals. Diabetes Care. 2014;37:1048–51.
20. Khunti K, Alsifri S, Aronson R, Cigrovski Berković M, Enters-Weijnen C, Forsén T, et al. Rates and predictors of hypoglycemia in 27,585 people from 24 countries with insulin-treated type 1 and type 2 diabetes: the global HAT study. Diabetes Obes Metab. 2018;20(11):2395–402. https://doi.org/10.1111/dom.13343.

Diagnosis and Management of Infections in Diabetes Mellitus

25

Subramanian Swaminathan and Sudha Teresa

Diabetic patients are vulnerable to infections for a variety of reasons. Not only is the incidence of certain infections more common in such patients, but also the risk of complications and mortality is often higher in this group of patients [1]. Understanding the profile of infections and the specific risks is key to designing preventive interventions that are effective.

Why are infections more common in diabetic patients?

(a) Elevated blood sugars impair neutrophil functioning and also impair chemotaxis. This makes the neutrophil less effective in responding to challenges.
(b) Elevated blood sugar results in glycosuria, which in turn increases the risk of bacterial and fungal colonisation of the urinary tract. Some of the newer medications for diabetes—the sodium-glucose cotransporter 2 (SGLT 2) inhibitors utilise this mechanism to improve sugar control, but this increases the risk of Candiduria and Candidial balanoposthitis.
(c) Renal dysfunction, as result of nephropathy and chronic renal failure (CRF) often noted in patients with long-standing diabetes also impairs immune function and is an added risk for infection.
(d) Liver failure due to non-alcoholic steatohepatitis (NASH) resulting in end-stage liver disease (ESLD), liver failure, and liver cancer increases the risk of attributable infections.
(e) Peripheral sensory neuropathy can impair sensation in the feet and make them more vulnerable to injury, as well as resulting in poor wound healing. Furthermore, the loss of pain results in patients causing further injury to an injured foot.

S. Swaminathan (✉)
Infectious Diseases and Infection Control, Gleneagles Hospitals, Chennai, India

S. Teresa
Infectious Diseases and Infection Control, Kauvery Hospital, Chennai, India

G. Abraham et al. (eds.), *Management of Diabetic Complications*,
https://doi.org/10.1007/978-981-97-6406-8_25

(f) Autonomic neuropathy can impair bladder functioning resulting in retention of urine, increasing the risk of urinary infections. Involvement of the bowel results in impaired movement and bacterial overgrowth.
(g) Vasculopathy of the peripheries results in gangrene of the extremities and poor wound healing.
(h) Over time there are structural changes that happen in the feet due to neuropathy and vasculopathy—the extreme form of which is a Charcot foot. The abnormal shape and pressure points increase the risk of injury and infection.
(i) Patients with diabetes are more likely to require solid organ transplants (renal-nephropathy related chronic renal failure, liver-non-alcoholic steatohepatitis related liver failure and cancer, heart-diabetic cardiomyopathy), and medications for these exacerbate the immune suppression which the diabetes creates.
(j) Patients with diabetes are more often in healthcare settings and around other patients with communicable diseases, which can result in them contracting such infections at a greater frequency.

The lack of prospective studies assessing the exact risk of incidence of different infections in diabetic patients makes exact estimation of attributable risk difficult. One study from the Netherlands showed increased risk of lower respiratory tract infections, urinary tract infections, and skin and mucous membrane infections [2].

In addition, patients with diabetes seem to have an elevated risk of certain unusual infections (like rhino-orbital Mucormycosis and emphysematous cholecystitis), as well as being vulnerable to certain complications as compared to non-diabetic patients (like renal abscess) (Case 25.1).

25.1 Infections in Specific Organ Systems

25.1.1 Urinary Tract Infections

The burden of urinary tract infections is significantly higher in diabetics, and they are more prone to development of complications like renal abscesses. They are also host to more unusual infections like renal limited Mucormycosis.

Diabetic patients have a higher risk of having sterile pyuria and asymptomatic bacteruria. Whilst the risk of pyelonephritis is higher in such patients, treatment of the pyuria or bacteruria does not reduce the risk of urinary infections in the future; in fact, it only increases the probability of a drug-resistant infection, which is more difficult to treat. This challenge is especially an issue in patients undergoing surgery for various reasons. Data now indicates that although diabetics with bacteruria have a higher risk of wound infection, treatment of the same does not reduce the risk of such infections. In fact, it is possible that the bacteruria is a risk marker rather than the risk itself. There are some situations where asymptomatic bacteruria needs to be treated like in pregnant women, immediately after a renal transplant and prior to urological interventions like stenting.

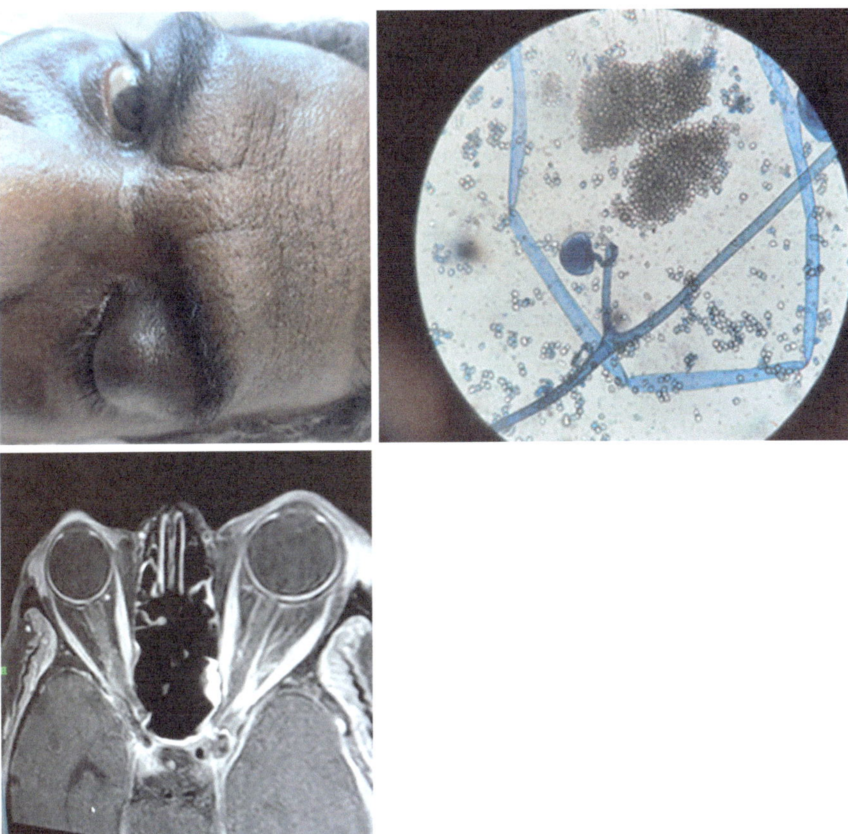

Case 25.1 57/M with uncontrolled DM-2 (HbA1C 11). Recently treated for severe covid with steroid and Remdesvir. Presented with pain and swelling of right eye. CT showed Left eye proptosis with thickening of ipsilateral optic nerve, superior rectus, and superior oblique and medial rectus. Mucosal thickening involving left frontal, bilateral ethmoid, bilateral sphenoid and left maxillary sinuses. Patient underwent FESS and orbital decompression. Histopath showed broad filamentous fungus with angioinvasion. Culture grew mucormycosis. Patient was started on IV Liposomal Amphotericin 5 mg/kg and stepped down to oral posaconazole after 2 weeks

The microbiology of urinary infections mirrors that seen in the general population, with *Escherichia coli* being the most common causative organism. As noted above, there is a higher risk of isolating drug-resistant strains in this group. However, it is important to educate the patient on the proper way to collect the urinary sample—clean the external genetalia; discard the first few ml of voided urine; and collect the midstream sample as a clean catch. Always analyse the Gram stain of the unspun urine with the culture to ensure concordance. Finally, and most importantly, urinary tract infection is a clinical diagnosis, not a microbiological diagnosis. The colony count does not make it significant without appropriate clinical picture. In fact, recent studies have indicated that the cut offs for number of white blood cells (WBCs) per high power field (HPF) should be much higher in diabetics to validate the possibility of a urinary infection. Guidelines do not recommend the routine use of urine cultures for simple urinary tract infections like cystitis but should be part of treatment of complicated or upper tract infections like pyelonephritis.

Treatment of cystitis can be done with nitrofurantoin or cotrimoxazole; upper tract infection often requires parenteral antibiotics, and the choice should be based on the probability of identifying resistant pathogens- in most countries with high rates of extended spectrum beta lactamase (ESBL) producing organisms, a class 2 carbapenem (imipenem or meropenem) would be considered appropriate initial therapy, with step down to simpler agents once culture and susceptibility is available. For most infections, a five-day course is considered adequate. Longer therapy is indicated in those with undrained abscesses, persistent obstruction, or other such complications. Oral step-down therapy should be considered as soon as susceptibility is confirmed; the patient can tolerate oral medications; there is no inoculum issue like obstruction or abscess; and the patient is clinically stable (Case 25.2).

Complications of pyelonephritis include development of renal abscess, which should be suspected in patients who continue to remain septic in spite of appropriate therapy. This may require per drainage for improvement. Another rare complication includes xanthogranulomatous pyelonephritis. Patients with diabetes are also significantly more at risk of development of emphysematous cystitis and pyelonephritis, which requires combination medical and surgical therapy.

In patients with drug-resistant infections like nosocomial infections, the hospital antibiogram could be a valuable resource in deciding choice of initial therapy. Given the risk of carbapenemase-producing organisms (CROs), the options are often limited to a newer beta-lactam/beta-lactamase inhibitor (BI/BLI) based therapy like ceftazidime-avibactam with aztreonam. Colistin-based therapy is a less preferred option. Aminoglycosides like amikacin could also be acceptable alternatives in this situation.

The presence of Candida in the urinary system is not unusual, as it is a common resident. Patients with uncontrolled diabetes and those on SGLT2 inhibitors have a higher risk of Candida in the urine and external genetalia (like balanoposthitis).

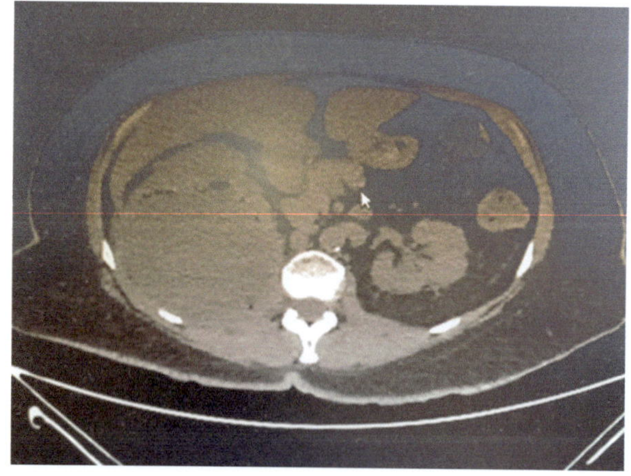

Case 25.2 68 F DM-2/HTN with fever and right sided abdominal pain. CT abdomen showed large right renal abscess, patient underwent USG guided abscess drainage, BL DJ stent was placed, pus grew NON-ESBL Klebsiela pneumonia initially treated with Meropenem and then discharged on oral Ciprofloxacin

Candida overgrowth can also be a consequence of antibiotic use. The presence of Candida does not require specific treatment but should encourage the physican to consider better diabetes control, if relevant. Candida can extremely rarely cause pyelonephritis and sepsis, should be considered in those with obstruction due to stones, and should be confirmed on culture of urine proximal to the obstruction after placement of a stent or a percutaneous nephrostomy. Treatment can be with an echinocandin if the patient is septic, as these agents are superior to azoles in sick patients. However, it is worth remembering that although these agents have high concentrations in the renal parenchyma, they do not enter the urine. The only azole that penetrates the urine is fluconazole, which makes treatment of azole-resistant Candida a challenge, with flucytosine being an option.

In addition, genitourinary tuberculosis is also noted in diabetics and is often missed. Tuberculosis should be suspected in patients with continued local and systemic symptoms who present with persistent pyuria (either with negative cultures or with different organisms being isolated), and not responding to beta-lactam antibiotics, but improving transiently with the use of quinolones. Diagnosis requires a high degree of suspicion and repeated testing. PCR tests on the GeneXpert platform have not been validated for testing of urine but have been often used successfully to confirm the diagnosis. The preferred means of confirmation of diagnosis is by repeated cultures of 24-h urine samples.

Treatment with standard anti-tubercular therapy is indicated, but the concern of drug-resistant infection continues to rise, and without cultures can be difficult to diagnose. Tubercular infection of the ureter or urethra can result in the formation of strictures which can then predispose to the risk of development of urinary tract infections in the future.

Mold infections of the kidney in the form of mucormycosis are being increasingly reported in India. Since there is no other organ system involved, it is unclear exactly how the agent reaches the kidney. This represents an emergency, and in the past always involved a total nephrectomy. However, with the earlier diagnosis, and availability of better medical options, kidney-preserving surgical options are more commonly used today. The gold standard for treatment involves the use of liposomal formulation of amphotericin B, which is less nephrotoxic than conventional amphotericin desoxycholate, but is significantly more expensive. There is now evolving experience with early switch to the newer azole (posaconazole and isavuconazole) in the treatment of this condition, as these are better tolerated and do not have an issue with renal toxicity.

Patients can sometimes present with prostatitis, and whilst these can mimic a urinary tract infection, there are often other symptoms like pelvic pain and strangury. The aetiology of this includes sexually transmitted diseases like gonococcus and Chlamydia, as well as the routine uropathogens. Urinary cultures can be helpful in identifying the pathogen concerned, the use of agents with good prostatic penetration (like quinolones) is advisable. Some patients can develop a chronic bacterial or abacterial prostatitis, which can be notoriously difficult to treat. Diagnosis can be confirmed with urological evaluation of the prostate coupled with quantitative urine cultures pre and post-prostatic massage. Rarely, prostatic abscess has been noted in diabetic patients, and two pathogens of utmost importance include *Staphylococcus aureus* and *Pseudomonas pseudomallei* (melioidosis).

25.1.2 Respiratory Infections

Infections in the respiratory tract are among the commonest problems encountered in this group. The risk of upper respiratory infections is not significantly increased in this group of patients, with the major exception of rhino-orbital Mucormycosis and malignant otitis externa, which will be dealt with later.

Lower respiratory infections are encountered in a higher frequency in this group and result in a higher chance of requiring hospitalisation, ICU care, and mortality. Diabetes increases the risk of hospitalisation in those with influenza, as well as increased risk of death [3]. This association with higher risk of poor outcomes after disease also extends to infections with COVID-19. Furthermore, they can trigger a secondary bacterial pneumonia, which can be more severe is diabetics. Studies have identified diabetes as an independent risk factor for poor outcomes and death in those with pneumonia. In fact, this risk is not just for in-hospital mortality, but this additional 10% excess mortality lasts beyond day 90 of infection and is closely related to uncontrolled blood sugar level at the time of presentation [4].

Most lower respiratory tract infections tend to be viral, similar to those in non-diabetics. The causative organisms of community-acquired pneumonia (CAP) are similar to non-diabetics, with *S. pneumoniae*, *H. influenza*e, and atypical pathogens being important causes [5]. However, certain pathogens are more commonly encountered in this population—uberculosis, *S.aureus*, Gram-negative bacteria (including melioidosis), and fungi like molds [6]. Of note, diabetic patients are more prone to have multi-lobar infiltrates, more likely to have bacteremia, and are more prone to development of complications like pleural effusion [7].

Patients with diabetes have a higher risk of developing active tuberculosis; in addition, there is also a higher risk of drug-resistant tuberculosis. Patients with diabetes have a higher risk of treatment failure and death [8]. Treatment of tuberculosis is complicated by the interaction between rifampicin and oral hypoglycemic drugs which makes glycemic control more difficult.

Fungal infections of the lung are also more common in this population. This includes infections by dimorphic fungi (like Histoplasmosis) and mold infections (like Aspergillosis and Mucormycosis). Histoplasmosis can often be missed as a mimic of tuberculosis and can be often diagnosed by appropriate examination of respiratory secretions or biopsy samples. Treatment is with amphotericin in patients who are very sick and can be stepped down to itraconazole. Aspergillosis is often noted in the presence of additional risk factors like influenza, COPD, steroid use, and old mycobacterial cavity. Voriconazole is the gold standard in treatment, but surgery plays a role in some patients. The rise of pulmonary Mucormycosis in diabetic patients in India is concerning as this is often under diagnosed due to its rapid fatality, poor availability of diagnostics and importantly, a lack of clinical suspicion [9]. Treatment involves aggressive sugar control, early surgical resection, and appropriate antifungals (amphotericin or a newer azole like posaconazole or isavuconazole).

The management of LRTI in diabetics is similar to normal hosts—it relies primarily on a detailed examination of a well-expectorated respiratory sample. The availability of rapid multiplex PCR can complement conventional Gram stain and culture testing in establishing the diagnosis. Treatment guidelines are similar to non-diabetic hosts, and fluoroquinolones are best avoided until the possibility of tuberculosis is excluded in this population.

25.1.3 Skin and Soft Tissue Infections (SSTI)

Abscesses and cellulitis are the commonest SSTI noted in all patients. However, in the ambulatory setting, diabetic patients had a fivefold higher complication rate and a fourfold higher risk of chance of hospitalisation as compared to nondiabetics. In the in-patient setting, diabetic patients with SSTI were more likely to be diagnosed to have bacteremia, endocarditis, septicaemia, or sepsis as compared to non-diabetic patients [10].

Microbiologically, *S. aureus* and Streptococci are the most common causes of infection. Diabetic patients have higher rates of colonisation with MRSA, and empiric therapy should cover this possibility as well. These infections tend to be monomicrobial, as against foot ulcers, which are often polymicrobial. Gram-negative infections are less common and are usually seen in diabetic foot ulcers. Carbuncle is a complex infection involving deeper skin structures with multiple pus points, which can turn gangrenous.

Treatment should be informed by local epidemiology, and simple infections are often best treated with topical agents like mupirocin. Larger infections require antibiotics, and options like clindamycin, cotrimoxazole, and linezolid could be considered. Carbuncle requires rapid surgical drainage along with parenteral antibiotics and aggressive sugar control.

Diabetic foot ulcer is a complex problem, with poor outcomes unless properly managed. It often starts with long-term damage to the foot as complications due to uncontrolled long-term diabetes continue to mount. There is a combination of vasculopathy due to vascular disease and sensory and autonomic neuropathy, which results in chronic trophic changes to the foot. This results in abnormal pressure points and development of callosities and ulcers that do not heal. Infections of these often result, exacerbated by the poor immune function.

Evaluation of a patient with foot ulcer should pay attention to all the above-noted points, in addition to the ulcer itself. Assessment of the size, location, depth, and possibility of bone involvement should be done. In general, if the bone can be reached by a probe in the depth of the wound, infection of the same osteomyelitis is inevitably present. The presence of a remote site non-foot infection is concerning for bacteremia and endocarditis should be excluded [11]. Patients sometimes can present with systemic manifestations, including sepsis and septic shock. This is often noted in patients with other complications like renal injury.

Management starts with debridement of the wound with offloading pressure from the foot. Wound management is done by selecting among various different dressing materials available, and wounds with necrosis or slough can benefit from enzymatic debridement and dressings with hydrocolloids or hydrogels. Close medical follow-up is vital to ensure early intervention and preservation of the foot. It is important to distinguish an infected from an uninfected foot, as 'routine' or 'prophylactic' antibiotics to reduce the burden of bacteria do not facilitate wound healing but do serve to increase colonisation—and subsequent infection—by drug-resistant bacteria. Measures that help include revascularisation and improved sugar control.

Classifying the wound as per International Working Group on Diabetic Foot/IDSA guideline can help decide the disposition of the patient, the choice, and route of antibiotic therapy. Curettage of tissue or bone samples should be sent for conventional microbiological cultures before starting therapy. Superficial swab cultures can be unreliable in identifying the causative pathogen. Initial therapy should cover *S. aureus* and streptococci, in addition to *P. aeruginosa*, which is often seen in tropical countries. Previous cultures should also be considered when choosing the most appropriate initial combination. This should then be adjusted based on culture reports, and a 1–2 weeks duration is considered adequate in absence of bone infection [12].

Charcot foot can often be confused as infection, as it can present with swelling and warmth. MRI imaging can sometimes help clarify, and a non-response to antibiotics should increase suspicion of this condition.

Another infrequent skin manifestation is Fournier's gangrene. This condition usually affects men and involves the skin and soft tissues of the lower abdomen and groin. The use of SGLT2 inhibitors sometimes seems to trigger this condition as well. The initial focus of infection could be cutaneous, gastrointestinal, genitourinary, or traumatic and is unknown in about a third of patients. This is a polymicrobial infection that results in obliterative endarteritis and microthrombosis along facial planes. The extension can be very rapid, making this an emergent situation. Patients usually present with scrotal pain, fever, and skin changes that progress rapidly. The diagnosis is primarily clinical, and radiology is to exclude other conditions like epididymo orchitis. Patient should receive fluids and broad-spectrum antibiotics—Gram positive, Gram negative, and anaerobes, with coverage based on the possibility of drug-resistant bacteria in that setting. Aggressive blood sugar control is vital for control of disease. Early extensive surgical debridement improves survival, limits extent of disease, reduces need for redebridement, and shortens hospital stay. Hyperbaric oxygen therapy has been shown to reduce mortality as well [13].

25.1.4 Gastrointestinal Infections

Patients with diabetes have an elevated risk of oral and oesophageal Candidiasis. Oral Candidiasis can present in many forms—median rhomboid glossitis or central papillary atrophy, atrophic glossitis, denture stomatitis, pseudomembranous candidiasis, and angular cheilitis. When the patient reports odynophagia, oesophageal Candidiasis should be considered.

Patients with diabetes are at an elevated risk of developing emphysematous cholecystitis, especially in men. Patients often present with symptoms similar to those with uncomplicated cholecystitis. Finding crackles on palpation indicates a worse prognosis. The usual causative agents are *Campylobacter* and *Salmonella spp* [14]. Gas can be demonstrated in the wall of the gall bladder on radiology. Surgery (or percutaneous drainage in critically ill) along with antibiotics is the standard of care.

There appears to be an association between hepatitis C and diabetes, up to a third of HCV-infected patients are diabetic. Type 2 diabetes is sometimes considered an extrahepatic manifestation of hepatitis C [15]. Unfortunately, diabetes worsens the outcomes of hepatitis C. There is more severe liver disease and increased fibrosis in the setting of diabetes. Therefore, all patients with hepatitis C infection should be screened for diabetes.

Splenic and liver abscesses, especially in the setting of disseminated abscesses, should raise the concern of melioidosis. Endocarditis and *S. aureus* sepsis are very important differentials, but infection with *Burkholderia pseudomallei* in its septicaemic form should be identified and managed appropriately. For patients with severe disease, drainage as appropriate, good sugar control, and high dose meropenem is appropriate. They will need weeks of therapy, followed up by step-down therapy to cotrimoxazole for a few months.

25.1.5 Head and Neck Infections

Two important infections occur in the head and neck region in diabetic patients—malignant otitis externa and rhino-cerebral Mucormycosis.

Malignant otitis externa is usually seen in elderly diabetics. It affects the external auditory canal and the temporal bone. However, this can spread to the base of the skull and other contiguous areas. Patients usually present with severe ear pain and discharge in the setting of uncontrolled blood sugars. In patients with extension of the disease, facial nerve or other cranial nerve injuries may be noted. Cultures should be taken from the ear drainage, and *P. aeruginosa* is most commonly isolated. *S. aureus* and fungi are sometimes seen as the causative organism. Quinolones are preferred therapy given their penetration, but rising resistance to these agents is a concern. Treatment requires weeks of antimicrobial use. Surgical intervention is reserved for local debridement, drainage of abscess or removal of a sequestrum [16]. Sugar control is also imperative. Unfortunately, recurrence rates of up to 25% have been reported.

Rhinocerebral Mucormycosis is usually noted in patients with poor sugar control, especially those with ketoacidosis. Even in the setting of COVID-19-associated Mucormycosis, diabetes, and uncontrolled blood sugars were an important risk factor. Infection is caused by a group of ubiquitous fungi found in the environment; the commonest being *Rhizopus* spp. The fungus is capable of tissue and angio invasion and extends very rapidly with no concern of anatomical barriers. Patients often present severe orbital pain and nasal discharge which may be bloody or black. Extension into the orbital cavity can result in swelling, diplopia, and proptosis. Further progression through the cribriform plate can result in intra-cranial extension, with risk of cerebral abscess formation, cavernous sinus thrombosis, and internal carotid artery thrombosis. Nasal examination usually shows black necrotic tissue. Examination of scrapings can confirm the diagnosis. Imaging with CT scan and MRI is often needed to understand the extent of the disease. Immediate surgical debridement with aggressive sugar control is key. Medical therapy is based on liposomal formulation of amphotericin B, with the newer azoles—posaconazole and isavuconazole—as alternatives or step-down options [17]. In spite of optimal treatment, mortality remains high.

25.2 Prevention of Infections

This involves multiple interventions, starting with effective glycemic control. Studies have clearly indicated that the degree of hyperglycemia influences the risk of poor outcomes, including mortality. Therefore, it is key to ensure that blood sugar control should be done to achieve metabolic targets appropriate to the host. Other interventions like foot care, screening for neuropathy, vasculopathy, and vision loss periodically are key to preventing occurrence and progression of foot ulcers. Finally, the importance of vaccination in this group is often forgotten. The American Diabetes Association (ADA) and the Advisory Committee on Immunization Practice (ACIP) of the Center for Disease Control (CDC) recommend the use of the seasonal influenza vaccine and the pneumococcal vaccine in this population. Influenza vaccine has been shown to reduce the risk of hospitalisation for pneumonia and is associated with a lower mortality rate. In addition, the use of the vaccine has been demonstrated to reduce the risk of cardiovascular deaths [18]. In addition, those above 50 should also be encouraged to receive the shingles vaccine.

Therefore, it is important to do a detailed assessment in every diabetic patient and ensure that it is repeated at least yearly to document new complications developing which could change the risk status and the need for additional protective measures. Patients need education on the risks so that problems can be avoided and they present to care early in the event of a problem. Preventive measures should be emphasised, and most importantly, glycemic control should be tightened to the best extent possible.

References

1. Seshasai SR, Kaptoge S, Thompson A, Di Angelantonio E, Gao P, Sarwar N, Whincup PH, Mukamal KJ, Gillum RF, Holme I, Njolstad I, Fletcher A, Nilsson P, Lewington S, Collins R, Gudnason V, Thompson SG, Sattar N, Selvin E, Hu FB, Danesh J. Diabetes mellitus, fasting glucose, and risk of cause-specific death. N Engl J Med. 2011;364:829–41.

2. Muller LM, Gorter KJ, Hak E, Goudzwaard WL, Schellevis FG, Hoepelman AI, Rutten GE. Increased risk of common infections inpatients with type 1 and type 2 diabetes mellitus. Clin Infect Dis. 2005;41:281–8.
3. Xi X, Xu Y, Jiang L, Li A, Duan J, Du B, et al. Hospitalized adult patients with 2009 influenza A(H1N1) in Beijing, China: risk factors for hospital mortality. BMC Infect Dis. 2010;10:256.
4. Kornum JB, Thomsen RW, Riis A, Lervang HH, Schønheyder HC, Sørensen HT. Type 2 diabetes and pneumonia outcomes: a population-based cohort study. Diabetes Care. 2007;30(9):2251–7.
5. Ahmed MS, Reid E, Khardori N. Respiratory infections in diabetes. Reviewing the risks and challenges. J Respir Dis. 2008;29(7):285–93.
6. Klekotka RB, Mizgała E, Król W. The etiology of lower respiratory tract infections in people with diabetes. Pneumonol Alergol Pol. 2015;83(5):401–8.
7. Falguera M, Pifarre R, Martin A, Sheikh A, Moreno A. Etiology and outcome of community-acquired pneumonia in patients with diabetes mellitus. Chest. 2005;128(5):3233–9.
8. Dooley KE, Chaisson RE. Tuberculosis and diabetes mellitus: convergence of two epidemics. Lancet Infect Dis. 2009;9:737–46.
9. Chakrabarti A, Das A, Jharna Mandal MR, Shivaprakash VK, George BT, Rao P, Panda N, Verma SC, Sakhuja V. The rising trend of invasive zygomycosis in patients with uncontrolled diabetes mellitus. Med Mycol. 2006;44(4):335–42.
10. Suaya JA, Eisenberg DF, Fang C, Miller LG. Skin and soft tissue infections and associated complications among commercially insured patients aged 0-64 years with and without diabetes in the U.S. PLoS One. 2013;8(4):e60057.
11. Chen SY, Giurini JM, Karchmer AW. Invasive systemic infection after hospital treatment for diabetic foot ulcer: risk of occurrence and effect on survival. Clin Infect Dis. 2017;64(3):326–34.
12. Senneville É, Albalawi Z, van Asten SA, Abbas ZG, Allison G, Aragón-Sánchez J, Embil JM, Lavery LA, Alhasan M, Oz O, Uçkay I, Urbančič-Rovan V, Zhang-Rong X, Peters EJG. IWGDF/IDSA guidelines on the diagnosis and treatment of diabetes-related foot infections (IWGDF/IDSA 2023). Clin Infect Dis. 2023:ciad527.
13. Huayllani MT, Cheema AS, McGuire MJ, Janis JE. Practical review of the current Management of Fournier's gangrene. Plast Reconstr Surg Glob Open. 2022;10(3):e4191.
14. Calvet HM, Yoshikawa TT. Infections in diabetes. Infect Dis Clin N Am. 2001;15:407–20.
15. Elhawary EI, Mahmoud GF, El-Daly MA, Mekky FA, Esmat GG, Abdel-Hamid M. Association of UVV with diabetes mellitus: an Egyptian case-control study. Virol J. 2011;8:367.
16. Tsilivigkos C, Avramidis K, Ferekidis E, Doupis J. Malignant external otitis: what the diabetes specialist should know-a narrative review. Diabetes Ther. 2023;14(4):629–38.
17. Manesh A, Devasagayam E, Bhanuprasad K, Varghese L, Kurien R, Cherian LM, Dayanand D, George MM, Kumar SS, Karthik R, Vanjare H, Peter J, Michael JS, Thomas M, Mathew BS, Samuel P, Peerawaranun P, Mukaka M, Rupa V, Varghese GM. Short intravenous amphotericin B followed by oral posaconazole using a simple, stratified treatment approach for diabetes or COVID-19-associated rhino-orbito-cerebral mucormycosis: a prospective cohort study. Clin Microbiol Infect. 2023;29(10):1298–305.
18. Modin D, Claggett B, Køber L, Schou M, Jensen JUS, Solomon SD, et al. Influenza vaccination is associated with reduced cardiovascular mortality in adults with diabetes: a Nationwide cohort study. Diabetes Care. 2020;43:2226–33.

Musculoskeletal Complications of Diabetes Mellitus

26

Shruti Govindaraj and Anukampattu B. Govindaraj

26.1 Introduction

The musculoskeletal complications of diabetes manifest across a spectrum, involving bones, joints, muscles, and connective tissues [1]. Diabetic arthropathy, characterised by bone metabolism and structure alterations, is emerging as a significant concern, with an increased risk of fractures and delayed fracture healing. Joint manifestations, including diabetic cheiroarthropathy and adhesive capsulitis, contribute to functional impairment and reduced quality of life in affected individuals [2].

Moreover, diabetes-related myopathies and alterations in muscle structure and function contribute to the overall burden of musculoskeletal complications [3].

The pathophysiological mechanisms underlying these complications are multifaceted, involving chronic inflammation, oxidative stress, and microvascular abnormalities [4]. Additionally, the impact of diabetic neuropathy on proprioception and joint integrity further exacerbates musculoskeletal issues. Lifestyle factors, glycemic control, and the duration of diabetes play crucial roles in modulating the risk and severity of these complications [5].

Understanding the musculoskeletal complications of diabetes is paramount for clinicians, as it influences therapeutic strategies and rehabilitation approaches. This review synthesises current research findings, highlighting the need for integrated and multi-disciplinary collaborative care to address individuals' musculoskeletal challenges with diabetes. Furthermore, potential preventive measures, early detection strategies, and therapeutic interventions are discussed to mitigate the impact of

S. Govindaraj
Heartland Hospital, Birmingham, UK

A. B. Govindaraj (✉)
Orthopaedics, MGM HealthCare, Chennai, India
e-mail: govindaraj.ab@mgmhealthcare.in

G. Abraham et al. (eds.), *Management of Diabetic Complications*,
https://doi.org/10.1007/978-981-97-6406-8_26

musculoskeletal complications and improve the overall well-being of individuals living with diabetes.

Some of the common musculoskeletal complications of diabetes are discussed.

Diabetic Cheiroarthropathy, characterised by limited joint mobility, skin changes, and contractures in the hands, poses a significant challenge in individuals with diabetes [1]. Diagnosis of diabetic cheiroarthropathy is primarily clinical, and there is no specific laboratory test that confirms the condition. Hands and fingers show signs of limited joint mobility, thickened skin, and decreased range of motion. One manifestation of this neuropathy is the 'prayer sign' (Fig. 26.1), which involves difficulty or an inability to place the palms of the hands together in a praying position due to stiffness or weakness in the muscles and joints. Early detection and management of diabetes, along with appropriate lifestyle modifications, can help prevent or slow the progression of complications. Individuals with diabetes should have regular check-ups and screenings to monitor their overall health and identify any potential complications. A comprehensive management approach emphasising glycemic control, physical therapy, topical therapies, orthotic devices, pharmacological interventions, patient education, regular monitoring, and lifestyle modifications can help control the condition [6].

Optimal blood glucose levels are crucial in preventing and managing diabetic complications. Striving for target HbA1c levels is foundational to managing diabetic cheiroarthropathy. Joint mobility exercises and stretching techniques are integral to physical therapy to enhance range of motion and prevent joint contractures. Regular use of moisturisers helps manage skin changes associated with cheiroarthropathy, addressing dryness and preventing complications [7]. Customised splints are pivotal in maintaining optimal hand positioning, preventing contractures, and improving functional outcomes. Analgesics and anti-inflammatory medications are considered for pain management, while topical agents such as corticosteroid creams may address inflammation and skin manifestations.

Empowering individuals with self-care practices, including proper hand hygiene, moisturising, and targeted exercises, fosters active participation in managing diabetic cheiroarthropathy.

Regular monitoring through scheduled follow-up with endocrinologists and rheumatologists facilitates ongoing assessment and adjustment of management strategies based on disease progression. Smoking cessation is encouraged, as smoking exacerbates diabetic complications [8]. A healthy lifestyle, including regular exercise, a balanced diet, and weight management, contributes to overall well-being. Early intervention and a multidisciplinary approach involving endocrinologists, rheumatologists, physical therapists, and other healthcare professionals are critical to successful management.

Flexor Tenosynovitis (Trigger Finger) is a condition characterised by inflammation of the flexor tendon sheath, leading to pain, swelling, and restricted joint mobility. Pathologic changes begin with a thickening or nodule within the tendon; when located at the site of the tight first annular pulley, the thickening or nodule blocks smooth extension or flexion of the finger. The finger may lock in flexion, or 'trigger', suddenly extending with a snap. Symptoms start with early morning locking of

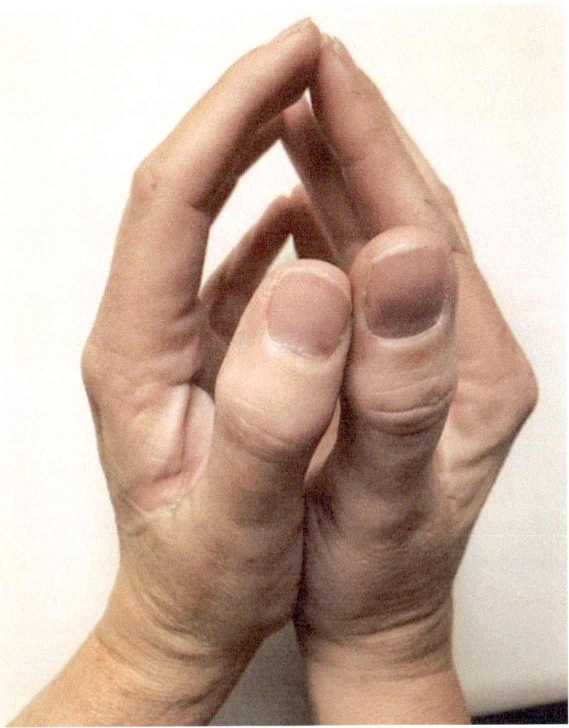

Fig. 26.1 Prayer sign

one or more fingers, relieved with some effort or exercises. Diagnosis is by eliciting the history and clinical examination—a painful nodule at the distal palmar crease of the corresponding finger confirms the diagnosis. A 'triggering test' asking the patient to flex and extend the affected finger confirms the diagnosis of stenosing tenosynovitis. If there is a catching or locking sensation, it may indicate flexor tenosynovitis. Kanavel Signs**:** These are a set of four clinical signs that may be indicative of flexor tenosynovitis in the fingers. The signs include a finger held in slight flexion, uniform swelling along the tendon sheath, tenderness along the course of the tendon, and pain with passive extension of the affected finger. Imaging studies, such as ultrasound or magnetic resonance imaging (MRI), may be used to visualise the structures within the affected finger and assess the extent of inflammation and any potential damage. In some instances, fluid may be aspirated from the affected area to analyse it for signs of infection or inflammation as gripping a cylindrical can or exercise ball, and rehabilitation programs aim to restore range of motion, strength, and functionality.

Nonsteroidal antiinflammatory drugs (NSAIDs) provide analgesia and anti-inflammatory effects, contributing to pain relief and reduction of swelling. Local corticosteroid injections into the tendon sheath can reduce inflammation and improve symptoms. This procedure can occasionally be combined with the percutaneous release of the A1 pulley, which is the causative factor for the triggering action

In recurrent cases the A1 pulley can be released through a pinhole incision using a 16G hypodermic needle under local anaesthesia (Fig. 26.2).

Tenosynovectomy involves surgical removal of the inflamed synovial tissue, which may be considered in cases refractory to conservative measures and after failed injection therapy.

This comprehensive approach to flexor tenosynovitis management combines conservative and interventional strategies tailored to the severity and underlying cause of the condition. Early diagnosis and prompt initiation of appropriate treatments are Simple measures such as adequate rest of the affected hand, ice or warm bath and gentle gripping exercises help reduce strain on the inflamed flexor tendon sheath. Physical Therapy includes specialised exercises such essential for optimal outcomes.

Dupuytren's Contracture This condition affects the palmar fascia, a layer of connective tissue under the skin of the palm. It causes thickening and shortening of the fascia, resulting in nodules and cords that pull the fingers into a permanently flexed, deformed position. It is more common in men than women and may have a genetic pre-disposition. It is also associated with diabetes, especially type 1 diabetes and long duration of diabetes. The cause of this condition is not fully understood, but it may involve fibroblast proliferation, collagen deposition, and cytokine production.

Gentle stretching exercises and hand therapy aim to maintain or improve range of motion and functionality. Night splinting may be employed to prevent the progression of contractures and maintain finger extension.

Minimally invasive interventions such as Intralesional injection of collagenase clostridium histolyticum (CCH), which is an FDA-approved treatment that enzymatically disrupts the collagen cords, allowing for manipulation and straightening of affected fingers, can be effective in the early stages [9]. Percutaneous release of contractures using a hypodermic needle (Needle Aponeurotomy) is a less invasive option that may be suitable for select cases. Open fasciectomy involves surgically removing the affected tissue and is effective for moderate to severe cases.

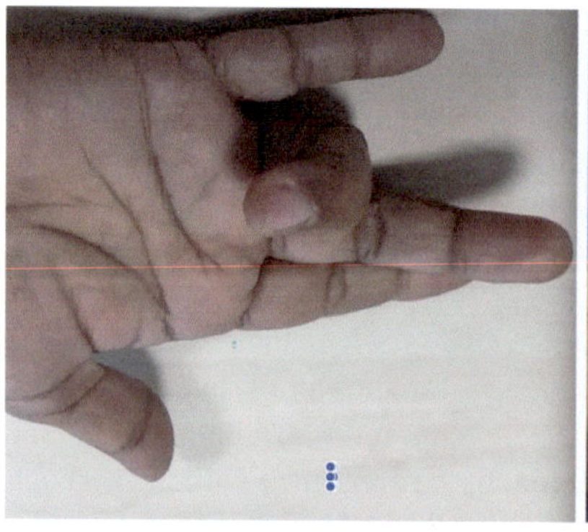
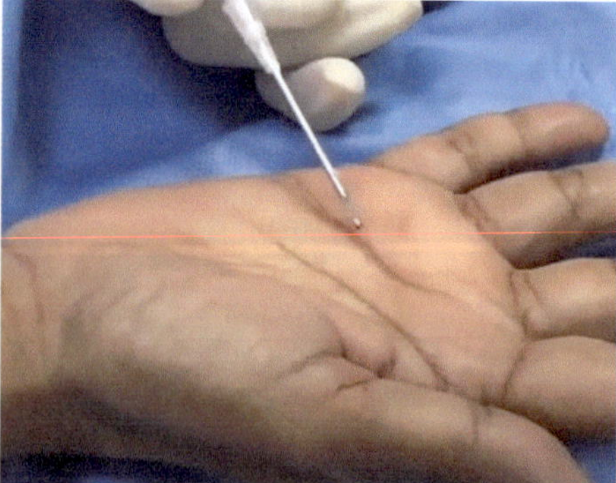

Fig. 26.2 Trigger finger release through pin hole

Removal of only the diseased portion of the fascia (Partial Fasciectomy) leaves healthy tissue intact. Targeted removal of specific cord segments (Segmental Aponeurectomy) may be considered in some instances—limited incisions to release contractures (Fasciotomy) in specific palm areas.

Rehabilitation after surgical intervention focuses on preventing contracture recurrence, restoring function, and optimising hand strength [10]. Providing patients with information about the natural history of Dupuytren' s contracture and realistic expectations for treatment outcomes. Close follow-up with healthcare providers, including hand specialists and physiotherapists, is essential to monitor disease progression and adjust treatment plans accordingly.

Dupuytren's contracture management requires a comprehensive approach that integrates conservative measures, minimally invasive interventions, and surgical options to address the diverse spectrum of disease severity. Tailoring treatment plans to individual patient characteristics and preferences is crucial for optimising outcomes.

Adhesive Capsulitis (Frozen Shoulder) It is a condition that affects the shoulder joint, causing pain, stiffness, and reduced range of motion. It is more common in women than men and may affect both shoulders. It is also associated with diabetes, especially type 1 diabetes and poor glycemic control. This condition's cause is unclear, but it may involve inflammation, fibrosis, and capsular contraction of the shoulder joint. A detailed medical history is essential, including the onset and duration of symptoms, any history of trauma or injury to the shoulder, and any underlying medical conditions (e.g. diabetes, thyroid disorders, dyslipidemia) associated with an increased risk of frozen shoulder. Limited external rotation and abduction are characteristic findings in adhesive capsulitis. X-rays may be ordered to rule out other conditions, such as arthritis or fractures and assess the shoulder's joint space. In some cases, an MRI may be used to visualise soft tissues, including the joint capsule and surrounding structures, helping to confirm the diagnosis and rule out other causes of shoulder pain and stiffness (Fig. 26.3). While there are no specific blood tests for adhesive capsulitis, blood tests may be ordered to rule out conditions such as rheumatoid arthritis or other inflammatory disorders. It's important to note that adhesive capsulitis is a clinical diagnosis, and imaging studies are often used to rule out other potential causes of shoulder pain and stiffness rather than to confirm the diagnosis.

The treatment of this condition includes Nonsteroidal anti-inflammatory drugs (NSAIDs), corticosteroid injections, physical therapy, and surgery [11]. NSAIDs and analgesics may alleviate pain associated with a frozen shoulder. Limiting activities that exacerbate symptoms and avoiding overuse of the affected shoulder can aid in symptom management. Physical therapy is central to maintaining and improving shoulder mobility through a targeted range of motion exercises. Gradual stretching and strengthening exercises enhance flexibility and muscle strength around the shoulder joint [12].

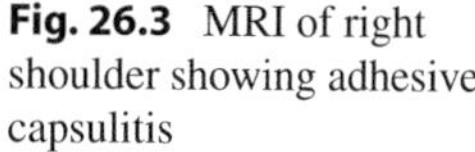

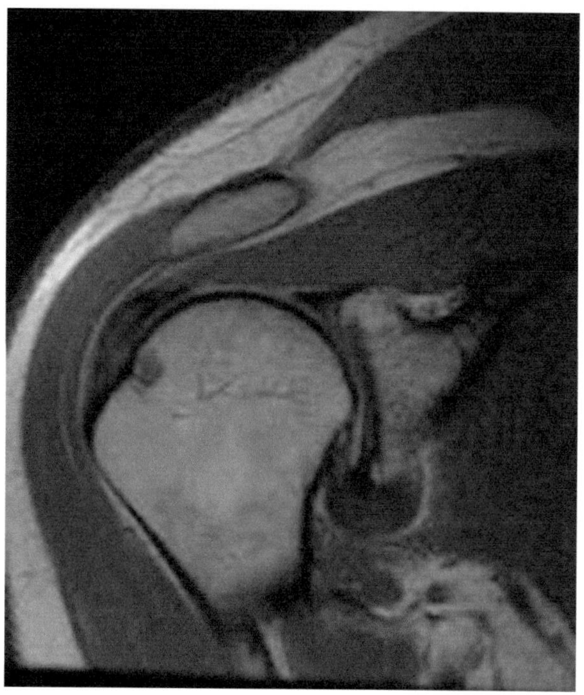

Fig. 26.3 MRI of right shoulder showing adhesive capsulitis

Corticosteroid injections or distension (Hydrodilatation) with saline solution can alleviate inflammation and improve joint mobility. Intra-articular corticosteroid injections may temporarily relieve pain and inflammation [13]. Viscosupplementation with sodium hyaluronate may improve joint lubrication. Manipulation under anaesthesia (MUA) and arthroscopic release may be performed for cases resistant to conservative measures to break adhesions and improve range of motion. Surgical intervention involves releasing tight ligaments and removing adhesions to restore shoulder mobility.

Patients are often prescribed home exercises to reinforce gains made in physical therapy and maintain shoulder mobility. Educating patients about the natural course of the condition, setting realistic expectations, and promoting adherence to prescribed exercises. Continuous follow-up with orthopaedic specialists to monitor progress and adjust treatment plans is essential. This comprehensive approach to managing frozen shoulder integrates various modalities to address pain, inflammation, and impaired range of motion. Individualised treatment plans, considering the stage and severity of the condition, contribute to improved outcomes.

Rotator Cuff Tendinopathy This condition affects the rotator cuff tendon around the shoulder joint. It causes pain, weakness, and reduced range of motion in the shoulder. It is more common in older people and may be related to overuse or injury. It is also associated with diabetes, especially type 2 diabetes and obesity. The cause of this condition is not well understood, but it may involve degeneration, inflammation, and microtears of the tendons. A detailed medical history is crucial. The nature of pain or discomfort, any specific activities that aggravate or alleviate symptoms, and any history of trauma or overuse. Cervical nerve root compression and other causes of shoulder pain radiating down the arm must be excluded. Occasionally, a myocardial infarction can mimic tendinopathy. Ultrasonography may be used to visualise the rotator cuff tendons, assess for signs of inflammation or tears, and guide interventions such as injections. MRI may be recommended to provide detailed images of the soft tissues in the shoulder, including the rotator cuff tendons. It can help identify tears, inflammation, or other structural abnormalities. X-rays may be ordered to evaluate the bones and joint space, ruling out other conditions such as arthritis or bony abnormalities. Reduced subacromial space is diagnostic of cuff tendinoparhy (Fig. 26.4).

Treatment options may include rest, physical therapy, anti-inflammatory medications, corticosteroid injections, and, in some cases, surgical intervention for more severe cases or in the presence of a significant tear. Initial management involves avoiding activities exacerbating symptoms and providing adequate rest to the affected shoulder. Applying ice or heat may help alleviate pain and reduce inflammation. Specific exercises targeting the rotator cuff muscles aim to improve strength, flexibility, and shoulder stability [14]. Techniques such as massage, joint mobilisation, and stretching may be incorporated to enhance the range of motion and reduce pain [15]. Nonsteroidal anti-inflammatory drugs (NSAIDs) are commonly used for pain relief and anti-inflammatory effects.

Intra-articular or subacromial corticosteroid injections can provide short-term relief from pain and inflammation. Platelet-rich plasma (PRP) injections may promote healing and reduce symptoms.

Surgical procedures like acromioplasty may be indicated in cases of subacromial impingement to relieve pressure on the rotator cuff tendons. Surgical

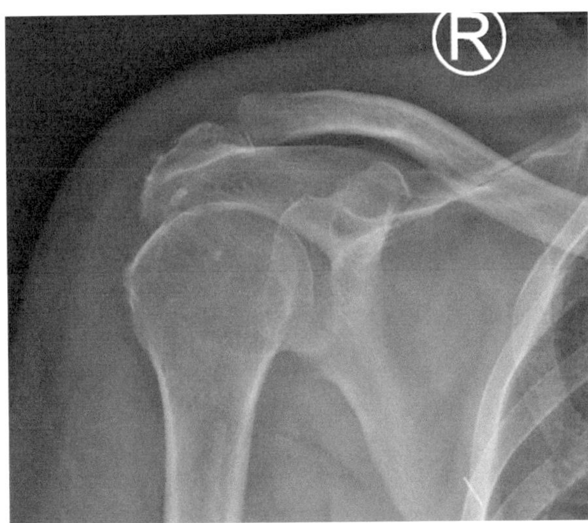

Fig. 26.4 Xray of right shoulder in cuff tendinopathy

decompression of the subacromial space can be performed to address impingement and improve tendon function [16].

Patients are often prescribed specific exercises to continue at home, promoting ongoing shoulder health and preventing recurrence. Educating patients about modifying activities to avoid overuse and prevent exacerbation of symptoms. Providing information about the natural course of rotator cuff tendinopathy, realistic expectations for recovery, and the importance of adherence to treatment plans. Continuous follow-up with healthcare providers, including orthopaedic specialists, to monitor progress, adjust treatment plans, and address emerging issues.

This comprehensive rotator cuff tendinopathy management approach integrates various modalities to address pain, inflammation, and functional impairment. Individualised treatment plans, considering the specific needs and characteristics of the patient, contribute to optimal outcomes.

Carpal Tunnel Syndrome This condition is caused by median nerve compression that runs through the carpal tunnel. It causes numbness, tingling, pain, and weakness in the thumb and first three fingers. It is more common in women than men and may be related to repetitive motions or wrist injuries. It is also associated with diabetes, especially type 2 diabetes and obesity. The cause of this condition is compression or entrapment of the median nerve by swelling or thickening of the surrounding tissues. Symptoms should be elicited, including the nature and location of pain, numbness, tingling, or weakness in the hand and fingers. The presence of a 'Tinel sign' (tapping over the median nerve to elicit tingling or pain) or a 'Phalen manoeuvre' (flexing the wrist to see if symptoms worsen) can support the diagnosis of carpal tunnel syndrome. Nerve conduction studies may be conducted to measure the electrical conduction of the median nerve. These tests can help determine the severity of nerve compression and rule out other conditions with similar symptoms. MRI or ultrasound may be used to visualise the structures within the carpal tunnel and rule out other potential causes of symptoms. Blood tests may be ordered to check for underlying conditions that could contribute to nerve compression, such as rheumatoid arthritis or thyroid disorders.

The treatment of this condition includes splinting, NSAIDs, corticosteroid injections, and surgery. This review provides an overview of evidence-based management strategies for CTS, including conservative measures, splinting, pharmacological interventions, and surgical options [17]. Identifying and modifying activities that exacerbate symptoms, such as repetitive hand movements, can be beneficial [18]. Night-time wrist splinting to maintain a neutral wrist position can alleviate symptoms and improve nerve function. A physical therapy regimen can include specific exercises to stretch and strengthen the wrist and hand muscles. Ergonomic adjustments to workstations, tools, and equipment can reduce strain on the wrists and help prevent exacerbation of CTS symptoms. Physical therapy programs can incorporate techniques to mobilise and promote median nerve sliding.

Local corticosteroid injections into the carpal tunnel can be considered for short-term symptom relief. Surgical intervention involves releasing the transverse carpal ligament to relieve pressure on the median nerve. Minimally invasive endoscopic techniques for carpal tunnel release may be considered in selected cases. Patients can benefit from ongoing exercises to maintain wrist flexibility and strength postoperatively or as part of conservative management. Educating on preventive measures and lifestyle modifications to reduce the risk of symptom recurrence can be beneficial. Individualised treatment plans, considering the specific needs and characteristics of the patient, contribute to optimal outcomes.

Neuropathic Arthropathy This is also known as Charcot joint or diabetic osteoarthropathy. It is a condition that affects the bones and joints of diabetic patients with peripheral neuropathy (nerve damage). It causes progressive destruction and deformity of the affected joints due to loss of sensation and proprioception (awareness of joint position). It can affect any joint but is more common in the feet and ankles. It is more prevalent in patients with type 1 diabetes and long duration of diabetes. The cause of this condition is not fully understood, but it may involve increased blood flow, osteoclastic activity, and inflammatory mediators.

A detailed medical history is essential—a history of neuropathy, diabetes, or other conditions that may contribute to nerve damage, about the onset and progression of joint symptoms, pain, swelling, and changes in joint appearance is crucial. Clinical signs may include joint deformity, swelling, erythema, and temperature changes. Sensory perception, reflexes, and motor function assessment are essential to identify peripheral neuropathy signs. X-rays are commonly used to assess changes in bone structure, joint alignment, and the presence of fractures or dislocations (Fig. 26.5a). An MRI may provide more detailed images of soft tissues, bones, and joints. Blood tests may be ordered to check for underlying conditions associated with neuropathy, such as diabetes or autoimmune disorders.

The treatment of this condition includes immobilisation, off-loading, infection control, and surgery. This review outlines evidence-based management strategies for neuropathic arthropathy, encompassing diagnostic approaches, conservative measures, surgical interventions, and preventive strategies [19]. Non-weight-bearing devices, such as braces or casts, can help offload affected joints and prevent further damage. A range of motion exercises for unaffected joints and gait training may be beneficial to maintaining function and preventing complications [20]. Neuropathic pain may require pharmacological interventions such as gabapentin or pregabalin. Nonsteroidal anti-inflammatory drugs (NSAIDs) may be considered for symptomatic relief.

Surgical procedures, including joint stabilisation and fixation, may be necessary to address severe instability and prevent further deformity (Fig. 26.5b). Surgical debridement can help remove necrotic tissue and reduce the risk of infection.

The involvement of a multidisciplinary team (collaborative care), including orthopaedic surgeons, podiatrists, endocrinologists, and plastic surgeons, is crucial for comprehensive management [21]. Regular wound care is essential to prevent and manage complications such as ulcers and infections. Aggressive management of underlying neuropathy, including glycemic control in diabetic patients, is critical

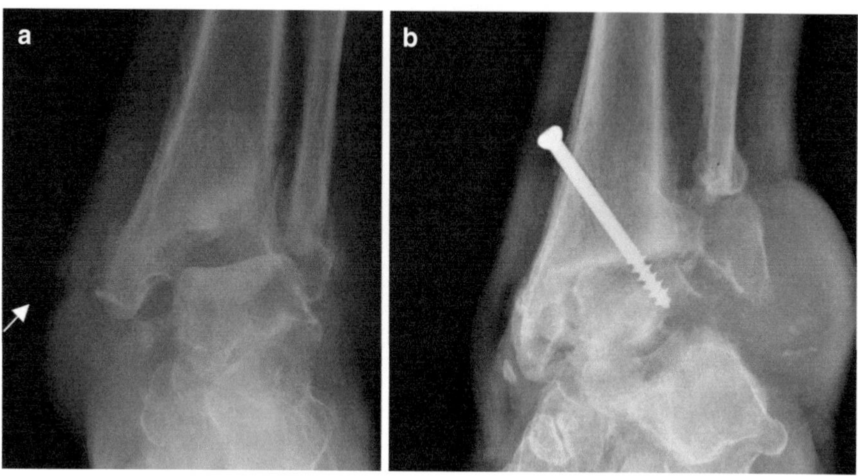

Fig. 26.5 (**a**) Charcot's arthropathy of the right ankle with trophic ulcer; (**b**) Charcot's ankle arthrodesis with a screw with healed ulcer

to prevent the development of neuropathic arthropathy. Patient education on foot care practices, stretching, proper footwear, and regular check- ups can help prevent complications. Continuous follow-up with healthcare providers to monitor disease progression, evaluate treatment effectiveness, and address emerging issues. Individualised treatment plans, considering the specific needs and characteristics of the patient, contribute to optimal outcomes.

Diabetes and Joint Replacement Surgery Prosthetic joint infections occur more often in diabetic patients with poor long-term control of hypoglycaemia. The prevalence of infection after primary total joint arthroplasty was higher in diabetes patients (1.9%) than in non-diabetic patients (1.2%) [22]. Long-term hyperglycaemia has a deleterious effect on the immune system due to reduced leukocyte activity, which can raise the risk of prosthetic joint infection. Diabetic patients experienced longer postoperative stays in the hospital and had stiffer knees [23]. This review examines evidence-based strategies for managing diabetes in the context of joint replacement surgery, encompassing preoperative optimisation, intra-operative considerations, and postoperative care.

Achieving optimal glycemic control before surgery is crucial to minimise the risk of peri-operative complications. Targeting HbA1c levels within recommended ranges is associated with improved outcomes [24]. Comprehensive cardiovascular ris k assessment and management are essential, considering the increased cardiovascular risk associated with diabetes and joint replacement surgery [25]. Strict intra-operative blood glucose monitoring is recommended to maintain euglycemia and prevent peri-operative complications [26] antibiotic prophylaxis is crucial to prevent surgical site infections, considering the increased risk of infection in individuals with diabetes [27]. Close and intensive monitoring of blood glucose levels postoperatively and prompt intervention to maintain glycemic control are essential for preventing cardiovascular complications [28]. Tailored thromboprophylaxis is crucial for individuals with diabetes to reduce the risk of venous thromboembolism after joint replacement surgery. Early mobilisation and structured physical therapy are essential for postoperative care, promoting optimal joint function and preventing complications. Long-term follow-up and monitoring, including regular orthopaedic and endocrinology consultations, are critical for identifying and managing potential complications associated with diabetes and joint replacement. This approach to managing diabetes in the context of joint replacement surgery emphasises the importance of preoperative optimisation, intra- operative vigilance, and postoperative care tailored to the unique needs of individuals with diabetes.

These are some of the musculoskeletal complications that can occur in diabetic patients. They can cause significant pain, disability, and reduced quality of life. Therefore, diabetic patients must maintain reasonable glycemic control, monitor their blood pressure and cholesterol levels, exercise regularly, and have regular check-ups with their healthcare providers. Early diagnosis and treatment of these complications can prevent further damage and improve the outcomes for diabetic patients.

References

1. American Diabetes Association. Standards of medical care in diabetes—2022. Diabetes Care. 2022;45(Supplement_1):S1–S243.
2. Napoli N, Strollo R, Paladini A. The role of inflammation in musculoskeletal pain. In: Handbook of experimental pharmacology, vol. 244. Springer; 2017. p. 105–21.
3. Rhee C, Lee J. Prevention and management of osteoporosis complicating diabetes. Endocrinol Metab. 2018;33(2):149–56.
4. Singh VP, Bali A, Singh N, Jaggi AS. Advanced glycation end products and diabetic complications. Korean J Physiol Pharmacol. 2014;18(1):1–14.
5. Vinik AI, Nevoret ML, Casellini C. The new age of assessment of cardiovascular autonomic function: application of novel indices in the age of COVID-19. Diabetes Technol Ther. 2013;15(12):982–94.
6. Lopes JM, Dourado D, Lopes MB. Diabetic cheiroarthropathy: a concise review. J Rheumatol. 2018;45(1):44–6.
7. Mueck K, Welsch C. Diabetic hand syndrome (cheiroarthropathy). Diabetes Care. 2015;38(6):e88–9.
8. Viswanathan V. Hand disorders in diabetes mellitus. In: Rheumatology in questions. Springer; 2014. p. 127–31.
9. Hurst LC, Badalamente MA, Hentz VR, Hotchkiss RN, Kaplan FT, Meals RA, et al. Injectable collagenase clostridium histolyticum for Dupuytren's contracture. N Engl J Med. 2009;361(10):968–79.
10. McFarlane RM, McGrouther DA, Flint MH. Dupuytren's disease: biology and treatment. Churchill Livingstone; 1990.
11. Neviaser AS, Hannafin JA. Adhesive capsulitis: a review of current treatment. Am J Sports Med. 2010;38(11):2346–56.

12. Page MJ, Green S, Kramer S, Johnston RV, McBain B, Chau M, Buchbinder R. Manual therapy and exercise for adhesive capsulitis (frozen shoulder). Cochrane Database Syst Rev. 2016;2016(6):CD011275.
13. Buchbinder R, Green S, Youd JM, Johnston RV. Oral steroids for adhesive capsulitis. Cochrane Database Syst Rev. 2006;2006(4):CD006189.
14. Littlewood C, Bateman M, Brown K. A self-managed single exercise programme versus usual physiotherapy treatment for rotator cuff tendinopathy: a randomised controlled trial. J Sci Med Sport. 2015;18(2):e74.
15. Page MJ, Green S, McBain B, Surace SJ, Deitch J. Manual therapy and exercise for rotator cuff disease. Cochrane Database Syst Rev. 2016;2016(6):CD012224.
16. Ketola S, Lehtinen J, Arnala I, Nissinen M, Westenius H. Does arthroscopy help in the diagnosis of rotator cuff tears: a systematic review of the literature. Acta Orthop. 2013;84(3):184–9.
17. Page MJ, O'Connor D, Pitt V, Massy-Westropp N. Exercise and mobilisation interventions for carpal tunnel syndrome. Cochrane Database Syst Rev. 2012;2012(6):CD009899.
18. Gerritsen AA, de Krom MC, Struijs MA, Scholten RJ, de Vet HC, Bouter LM. Conservative treatment options for carpal tunnel syndrome: a systematic review of randomised controlled trials. J Neurol Neurosurg Psychiatry. 2002;72(4):373–82.
19. Sanders LJ, Frykberg RG. Charcot Neuroarthropathy. Med Clin. 2019;103(2):273–88.
20. Rogers LC, Frykberg RG, Armstrong DG. The Charcot foot in diabetes. Diabetes Care. 2009;32(7):1875–9.
21. Dalla Paola L, Carone A, Ricci S, Cardillo S, Volpe A. Limb salvage in Charcot foot and ankle osteomyelitis: combined use single stage/double stage of arthrodesis and external fixation. Foot Ankle Surg. 2013;19(4):219–26.
22. Bozic KJ, Lau E, Kurtz S, Ong K, Berry DJ. Patient-related risk factors for postoperative mortality and periprosthetic joint infection in medicare patients undergoing TKA. Clin Orthop. 2012;470:130–7. https://doi.org/10.1007/s11999-011-2043-3.
23. Kurtz SM, Lau E, Schmier J, Ong KL, Zhao K, Parvizi J. Infection burden for hip and knee arthroplasty in the United States. J Arthroplast. 2008;23:984–91. https://doi.org/10.1016/j.arth.2007.10.017.
24. Ruben Diaz and Jenny DeJesus. Managing Patients Undergoing Orthopedic Surgery to Improve Glycemic Outcomes. Curr Diab Rep. 2021;21(12):68.
25. Majd Tarabichi et al. Determining the Threshold for HbA1c as a Predictor for Adverse Outcomes Following Total Joint Arthroplasty: A Multicenter, Retrospective Study; J Arthroplast. 2017;32(9).
26. Peel TN, Cheng AC, Buising KL, Choong PFM. Microbiological aetiology, epidemiology, and clinical profile of prosthetic joint infections: are current antibiotic prophylaxis guidelines effective? Multicenter Study Antimicrob Agents Chemother. 2012;56(5).
27. Bellon F, Solà I, Gimenez-Perez G, Hernández M, Metzendorf M-I, Rubinat E, Mauricio D. Perioperative glycaemic control for people with diabetes undergoing surgery. Cochrane Database of Systematic Reviews 2023, Issue 8. Art. No.: CD007315.
28. Stefano R. Muscatelli, MD Michael A. Charters, MD Brian R. Hallstrom, MD. Time for an Update? A Look at Current Guidelines for Venous Thromboembolism Prophylaxis After Hip and Knee Arthroplasty and Hip Fracture; Arthroplasty Today, 10, P105–107. August 2021.

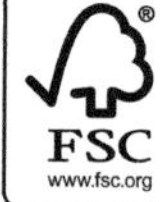

MIX
Papier aus verantwortungsvollen Quellen
Paper from responsible sources
FSC® C105338

If you have any concerns about our products,
you can contact us on
ProductSafety@springernature.com

In case Publisher is established outside the EU,
the EU authorized representative is:
Springer Nature Customer Service Center GmbH
Europaplatz 3, 69115 Heidelberg, Germany

Printed by Libri Plureos GmbH
in Hamburg, Germany